CHOLESTEROL *Explained*

DR WARRICK BISHOP
MBBS FRACP FCSANZ
Preventive Cardiologist

DR KARAM KOSTNER
MD PhD FRACP FCSANZ
Associate Professor of Medicine
Cardiologist, Lipidologist

with

Penelope Edman

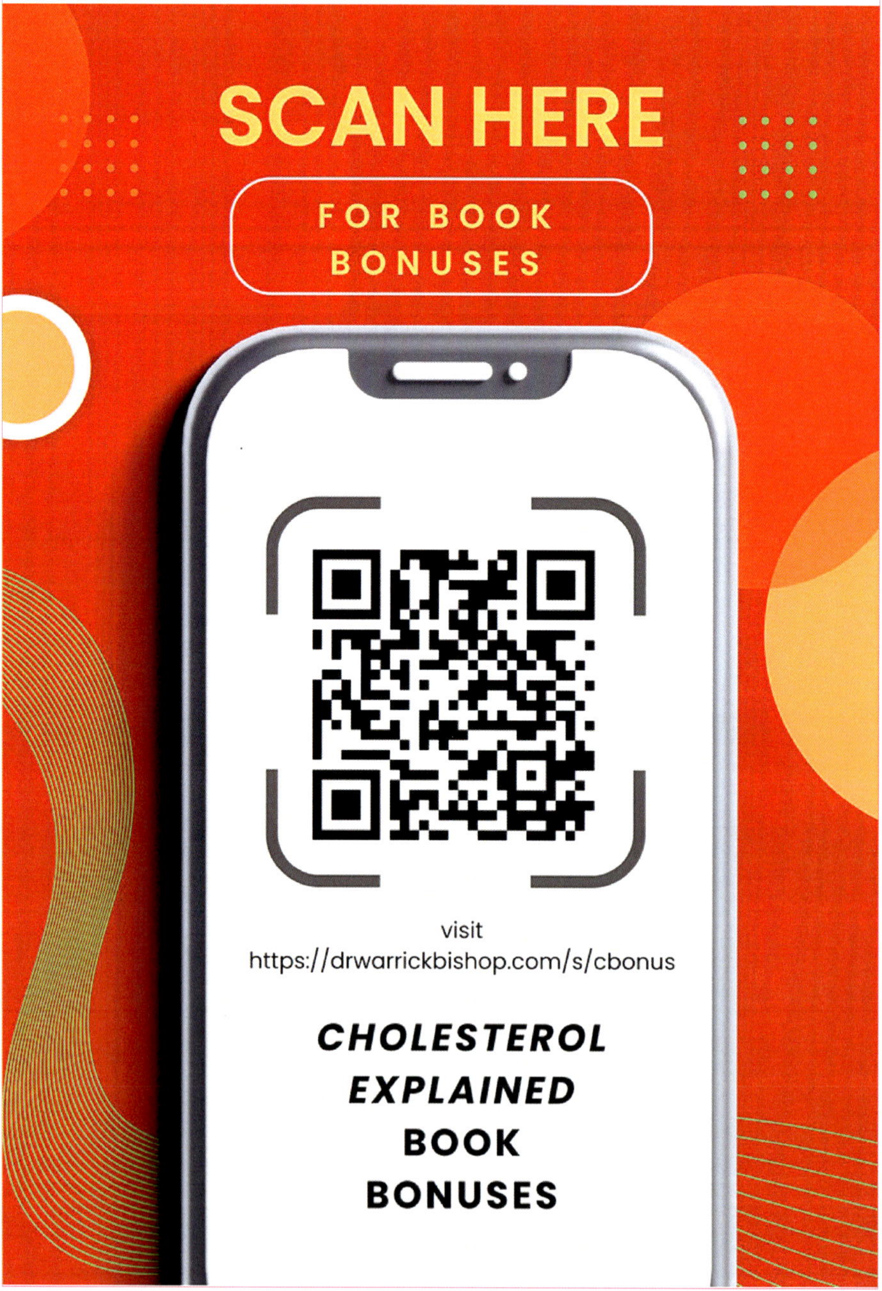
SCAN HERE
FOR BOOK BONUSES
visit
https://drwarrickbishop.com/s/cbonus
CHOLESTEROL EXPLAINED BOOK BONUSES

CHOLESTEROL *Explained*

understanding the science, significance, tests, management options, and controversies

This book is for you, if you

- want to learn more about one of the most important risk factors of heart health
- have elevated cholesterol levels
- want to manage and improve your cholesterol levels effectively
- believe that prevention is better than cure
- have a family history of high cholesterol or cardiovascular disease
- would enjoy an informative read about the controversies and science surrounding cholesterol and its therapies
- are a medical, nursing or other health professional student seeking a 'taster' that puts you 'ahead of the game' in your learning
- are a proactive doctor wanting the latest information on cholesterol risk management and treatment advances
- are a collaborative healthcare professional who recommends informative books to your patients to foster their pursuit of healthy living.

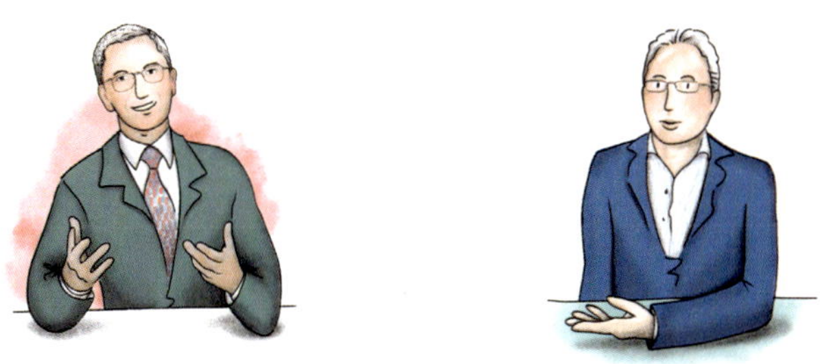

This book is for you if you have a heart.

PUBLISHER'S NOTE

The authors and editors of this publication have made every effort to provide information that is accurate and complete as of the date of publication. Readers are advised not to rely on the information provided without consulting their own medical advisers. It is the responsibility of the reader's treating physician or specialist, who relies on experience and knowledge about the patient, to determine the condition of, and the best treatment for, the reader. The information contained in this publication is provided without warranty of any kind. The authors and editors disclaim responsibility for any errors, mis-statements, typographical errors or omissions in this publication.

AI use disclaimer. In preparing this book, the authors made limited use of artificial intelligence tools, including ChatGPT, to assist with spelling, grammar, clarity and some artwork. All scientific and clinical content, interpretations, recommendations and conclusions are solely those of the authors.

National Library of Australia Cataloguing-in-Publication entry

Authors:	Dr Warrick Bishop MBBS FRACP FCSANZ Dr Karam Kostner MD PhD FRACP FCSANZ
Writer:	Penelope Edman, *PAGE 56*
Title:	Cholesterol Explained
ISBN:	Ebook: 978-0-9756310-8-9
	Paperback (IngramSpark): 978-0-9756310-9-6
	Paperback (Amazon KDP): 978-1-7645264-0-1
	Hardcover (IngramSpark): 978-1-7645264-1-8
	Hardcover (Amazon KDP): 978-1-7645264-2-5
Subject:	Cardiac healthcare
Publisher:	Dr Warrick Bishop MBBS FRACP
Designer:	Cathy McAuliffe, *Cathy McAuliffe Design*
Illustrator:	Cathy McAuliffe, *Cathy McAuliffe Design*

dedicated to
Max and Ella Bishop and Sean Dwyer
and
Max, Kathleen and Alex Kostner,
our fine children
who we love and cherish
and want to live as well as possible
for as long as possible

Superior doctors prevent the disease.
Mediocre doctors treat the disease before the event.
Inferior doctors treat the full-blown disease.

an ancient Chinese proverb

CONTENTS

TAKING CHARGE OF CHOLESTEROL LEVELS

medications, treatments

CHOLESTEROL IS NOT THE ENEMY

controversies, myths, mysteries

MEET THE AUTHORS

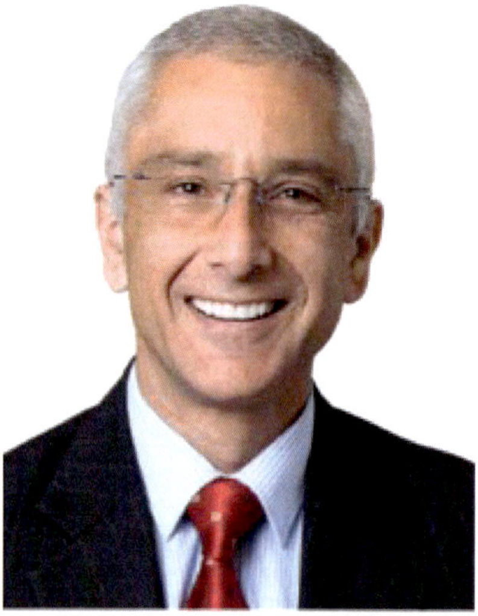

WARRICK BISHOP

is a practising cardiologist passionate about helping people live as well as possible for as long as possible. He is particularly interested in preventing heart attacks by using cardiac CT imaging, managing cholesterol, and giving attention to diet. He is devoted to educating patients, believing that well-informed individuals make the best healthcare decisions.

Warrick graduated from the University of Tasmania School of Medicine, Hobart, Tasmania, Australia, in 1988. He worked in the Northern Territory before undertaking specialist training in Adelaide, South Australia. He completed his advanced training in cardiology in Hobart, becoming a Fellow of the Royal Australian College of Physicians in 1997. He has worked predominantly in private practice.

In 2009, Warrick undertook training in CT coronary angiography, becoming the first cardiologist in Tasmania to receive this specialist accreditation. This area of imaging aligns well with his interest in preventive cardiology, which was the focus of his first book, *Have You Planned Your Heart Attack?* (2016). He is a member of the Society of Cardiovascular Computed Tomography (SCCT).

Warrick is also a member of the Australian Atherosclerosis Society and a participant on the panel of 'interested parties' developing a model of care and a national registry for familial hypercholesterolaemia. He has also developed a particular interest in diabetes-related risk of coronary artery disease, specifically linked to dietary guidelines and lipid profiles.

While a member of the Clinical Issues Committee of the National Heart Foundation of Australia, which provides input on significant issues related to managing heart patients, Warrick contributed to the committee's 2021 position paper on coronary artery calcium scoring for the primary prevention of cardiovascular disease in Australia.

Warrick enjoys a strong social media profile, having founded the Healthy Heart Network in 2018. (In 2026, this will become the Healthy Life Network.) Warrick has presented on heart health issues on a TEDx stage, once in Australia and once in the United States of America.

In 2023, he and his wife, Chelle, became franchise owners of OsteoStrong Hobart. In 2025, Warrick further strengthened his commitment to education and disease prevention, opening Longevity Labs Hobart in partnership with others.

He has authored numerous articles and the books *Have You Planned Your Heart Attack?*, *Know Your Real Risk of Heart Attack*, *Atrial Fibrillation Explained*, *Cardiac Failure Explained*, *Cardiac Rehabilitation Explained* (in collaboration with Dr Alistair Begg, of Adelaide, South Australia), *10 Commandments of Heart Health Explained* (in collaboration with Dr Karam Kostner, of Brisbane, Queensland), and now, *Cholesterol Explained* (in collaboration with Dr Kostner).

Warrick focuses all his public endeavours on helping people stay healthier for longer through education and support.

He is a keen intermittent faster who values family and friends, music, travel, and keeping himself as well as possible for as long as possible.

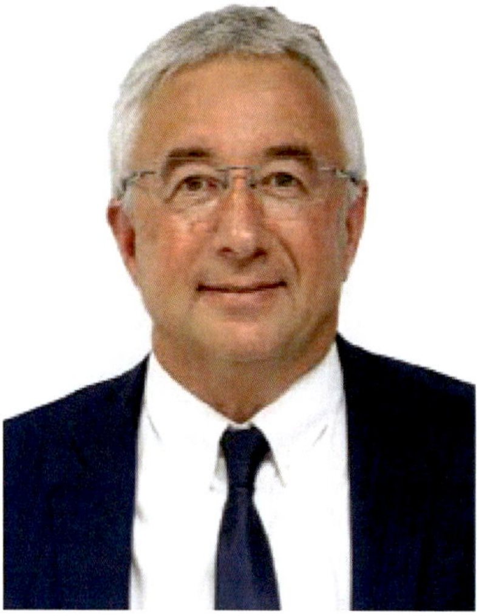

KARAM KOSTNER

is Associate Professor of Medicine at the University of Queensland (UQ) and Director of Cardiology at both the Mater Public and Mater Private Hospitals in Brisbane, Queensland, Australia. As a cardiologist and one of the most experienced lipidologists in the country, he manages a large public and private lipid clinic. He is also a director of Cholesterol Care Australia, a specialist cholesterol clinic and research facility in Brisbane and he is a senior cardiologist with Heart of Australia, which delivers specialist healthcare services and testing to rural, remote, and First Nations communities across Queensland.

Karam's clinical interests are preventive cardiology and lipid disorders. His passion combines helping people with high cholesterol, and researching new and emerging therapies for patients with elevated cholesterol.

Karam has been at the forefront of cardiovascular research for the past 20 years, and, as a principal investigator, he has conducted more than 65 clinical trials, including many trials on lipid-lowering therapies. His team developed an extracorporeal lipid removal technique termed lipid apheresis, and the first patients worldwide were trialled by his team in Brisbane. Furthermore, together with his father, Professor Gerhard Kostner, he is developing a medication to reduce lipoprotein(a). This is currently in the experimental stage.

Karam completed his education and most of his medical studies in Austria. He undertook two years of post-doctoral work at the Royal Brisbane Hospital in affiliation with the University of Queensland, Brisbane (1991-93). On his return to Austria, he undertook special training in internal medicine (1994-98), graduating as an Internal Medicine specialist. Karam then undertook cardiology training between 1998 and 2000, to become a specialist in cardiology in March 2001. Also in 2001, when aged 33, he was awarded an associate professorship in medicine in Austria.

He returned to Australia, also in 2001, settling in Brisbane and continuing his cardiology and research career at the Mater Hospitals and UQ.

Government and medical bodies regularly consult Karam about approval of and funding for new and established lipid-lowering therapies.

Having published more than 150 peer-reviewed papers, four book chapters, and several review articles and editorials, Karam has also delivered numerous invitational lectures at cardiovascular meetings, and is past president of the Cardiac Society of Australia and New Zealand (CSAN), Queensland branch.

Currently, he is an associate editor of *Atherosclerosis* and *The Journal of Preventive Cardiology* and an associate editor and cardiovascular section editor of the *European Journal of Clinical Investigation* (a peer-reviewed medical journal that covers a wide range of clinical research and investigations in various fields of medicine). Karam is a founding member of the editorial board of *Advances in Lipoprotein(a) Research.*

He is a regular reviewer for many journals, as well as being a National Health and Medical Research Council grant reviewer. (The NHMRC is the leading body for health and medical research in Australia, responsible for providing funding, setting guidelines, and promoting research excellence in health and medicine.)

Throughout his career, Karam has also organised, or sat on the committee of many national and international conferences and has been the chair and organiser of the World Congress of Clinical Lipidology on four occasions (the most recent being in June 2025, in Vienna, Austria).

This is his second collaboration with long-time friend and colleague Dr Warrick Bishop. Their first book was *10 Commandments of Heart Health Explained* (2024).

Outside of work, Karam loves outdoor activities such as skiing and hiking with his family, and friends. He is a very keen fisherman.

a very special connection - next page

a very special connection

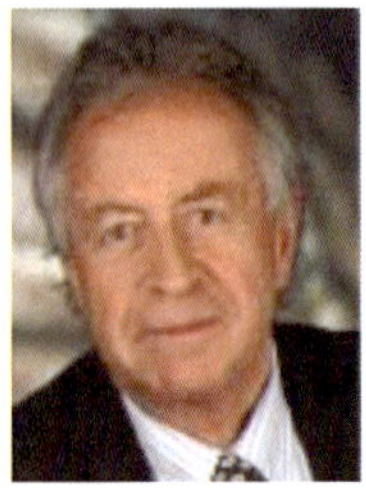

Karam's father, Emeritus Professor Gerhard Kostner of the Medical University of Graz, Austria, has dedicated his life to lipoprotein and lipid research. He was one of the first researchers to put lipoprotein(a) on the map and has published hundreds of studies identifying it as a risk factor, defining the threshold at which it becomes clinically significant, and investigating its metabolism. He also discovered a unique therapy to lower lipoprotein(a). Prof. Kostner was one of the first to utilise Mendelian randomisation (MR) studies[1] and explore antisense oligonucleotide (ASO) therapy for lipoprotein(a)[2], leading to significant advances in the field. Momentously, at one of the many conferences he has organised, American researchers Michael Brown and Joseph Goldstein presented their work (for the first time) that later earned them the 1985 Nobel Prize in Physiology or Medicine for discoveries that revolutionised the understanding of cholesterol metabolism. Their discovery of the low-density lipoprotein receptor led to the development of statins and other transformative therapies. Prof. Kostner is the founding editor-in-chief of the journal, Advances in Lipoprotein(a) Research.

1 *Mendelian randomisation (MR) is a genetic research method that helps determine whether an observed association between a biomarker, like lipoprotein(a) [Lp(a)], and a disease, such as cardiovascular disease (CVD), is causal or a correlation. It uses naturally occurring genetic variations that influence levels as a type of 'natural experiment', avoiding confounding factors that affect traditional observational studies. In relation to cholesterol and cardiovascular risk, MR studies have shown:*

Lp(a) is causally linked to CVD, independent of low-density lipoprotein cholesterol (LDL-C) and other cholesterol fractions.

A high Lp(a) level is genetically determined, meaning medications and lifestyle changes don't significantly lower it, unlike LDL-C.

Lowering Lp(a) could reduce cardiovascular risk, supporting the need for targeted therapies.

2 *Antisense oligonucleotide (ASO) therapy is a cutting-edge approach to lowering Lp(a). It works by targeting the LPA gene, which encodes apolipoprotein(a), the protein component of Lp(a). ASO binds to the messenger RNA (mRNA) of the LPA gene, blocking production of Lp(a) before it is formed. Key points about ASO therapy for Lp(a):*

Pelacarsen (formerly IONIS-APO(a)-LRx) is the most advanced ASO in clinical trials. It has shown up to 80 per cent reductions in Lp(a) levels in trials. The Lp(a) HORIZON trial assessed its impact on cardiovascular outcomes.

Since high Lp(a) increases cardiovascular risk independently of LDL-C, antisense therapy offers a promising treatment option for people with genetically elevated Lp(a), especially those already optimally treated for LDL-C but still at high risk.

FOREWORD

"The only books that influence us are those for which we are ready and which have gone a little further down our particular path than we have yet got ourselves."

E. M. Forster, *Two Cheers for Democracy* (1951)

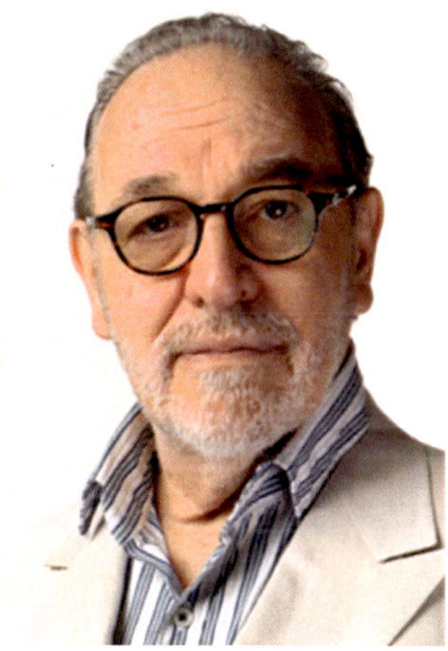

You are perusing this book because you are ready to know more about cholesterol and reading further will influence you in many beneficial ways.

Almost everyone has heard about cholesterol. Some may already know their cholesterol number, others may be receiving treatment for high cholesterol, and a few may be managing patients with high cholesterol with or without coronary disease. Yet the majority, including healthcare professionals, will not have a deep understanding of the nature of this major risk factor that causes atherosclerosis and leads to coronary disease and heart attacks.

The academic literature on this subject is extensive and highly complex. This has led to much misunderstanding and many myths about the importance and value of treating cholesterol. Knowledge continues to grow exponentially as advances are made in precision and personalised medicine, with the development of many new treatments and the publication of several clinical outcome trials.

Quality healthcare also requires participatory medicine, shared decision-making processes, and patient-centric practice. This is the ideal time for cholesterol to be explained to the public to optimise quality health care in preventing cardiovascular disease.

Doctor Warrick Bishop and Associate Professor Karam Kostner are two highly experienced preventive cardiologists with particular expertise in imaging and lipidology. They are well placed to write a book on cholesterol that addresses these modern needs in clinical practice.

With consummate clarity and brevity, they separate the wheat from the chaff in both scientific and popular literature, and beautifully demystify cholesterol not only for the public but also for multidisciplinary healthcare professionals and undergraduate students of medicine and allied health specialties.

I strongly commend the authors on a wonderful exposition on cholesterol that will have a major impact in implementing better care of patients and is well aligned with the recommendations of all major international guidelines on the prevention of cardiovascular disease.

GERALD F. WATTS
DSc MD PhD FRACP FRCP FCSANZ FESC

Winthrop Professor of Cardiometabolic and Internal Medicine
Senior Physician
Departments of Cardiology and Internal Medicine, Royal Perth Hospital
Medical School, University of Western Australia, Perth

Chair, Familial Hypercholesterolaemia Network and Registry, Australian Atherosclerosis Society

PREFACE

Thank you for taking the time to read this book.

Cholesterol is at the heart of one of medicine's biggest and on-going debates. The mixed messages and confusion surrounding its treatment are the stimuli for this work. If you want more information about your medical journey or feel overwhelmed by the many opinions online about cholesterol and statins, we wrote this book for you.

Cholesterol is a vital biochemical compound found naturally in our bodies and certain foods. It is produced by most animal cells and plays a crucial role in the structure of animal cell membranes. Because of this, we – humans – can't live without it. And, it also supports several essential processes in the body.

Although cholesterol is a critical element of our biological makeup, it is the most important treatable risk factor for cardiovascular disease, as it can build up in our arteries and cause serious damage. Here, it becomes a component of plaque or, more formally, atherosclerotic plaque[1], and is implicated in coronary artery disease. Reducing cholesterol levels can slow, minimise or even reverse this process. We look forward to sharing more information about this with you as the book unfolds.

We also know there are many questions. These need consideration, discussion, and where possible, answers. Some of the most common questions asked of us are:

- What does cholesterol do in our body?
- Why is cholesterol such an important risk factor for heart disease?
- What are the different cholesterols?
- Is elevated cholesterol always bad; does it always need treatment?
- Can cholesterol be too low?

---

1 *Plaques within the body vary by type. For example,* ***atherosclerotic*** *plaques in arteries contribute to cardiovascular disease,* ***dental*** *plaque leads to tooth decay and* ***amyloid*** *plaques in the brain are linked to Alzheimer's disease.*

- Does high cholesterol run in families?
- Does exercise and/or diet lower cholesterol?
- What are the side effects of cholesterol-lowering medications?
- When can I stop taking my cholesterol-lowering medication?
- Is cholesterol linked to inflammation?

We will answer these questions and more.

We will also address:

- concerns about memory in association with lowering cholesterol,
- treating cholesterol in individuals who are not ill,
- the role of the pharmaceutical industry in the cholesterol debate,
- whether cholesterol-lowering medications can reduce plaque and calcium in our arteries, or even unblock them, and
- confusion, controversies, and unanswered questions.

We appreciate your interest in *Cholesterol Explained: understanding the science, significance, tests, management options, and controversies.* We believe this book is needed.

It is structured to first explain the science of cholesterol, then explore how to manage it, and finally address common controversies and myths. Given the complexity of the subject, we encourage you to read it in its entirety first to gain a solid overview, then even read it again before returning to sections of particular interest.

Please enjoy what follows and benefit from our efforts to share what we do know, what we know we don't know, and, of course, respect that we don't know what we don't know.

Wishing you good health!

Warrick Bishop, Hobart, Tasmania, Australia

Karam Kostner, Brisbane, Queensland, Australia

CHOLESTEROL BASICS

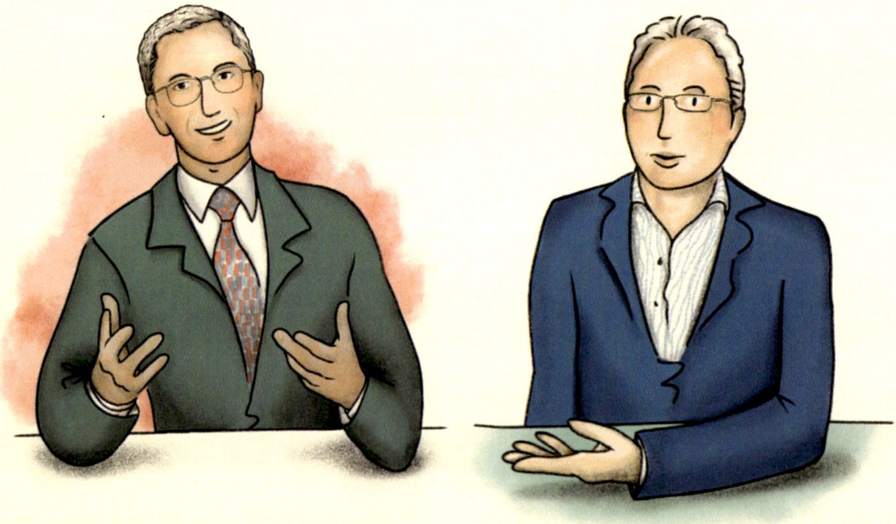

10 ESSENTIALS TO GET YOU STARTED

1. **Cholesterol – friend AND foe, in the cells and blood:** Your body requires cholesterol. It is essential for life. Every cell in the human body needs cholesterol ***and*** most also make their own for vital functions such as building cell membranes, producing hormones, synthesising vitamin D, and aiding digestion. ***However***, high levels of low-density lipoprotein cholesterol (LDL-C), often called 'bad' cholesterol, increase the risk of clogged arteries and the possible development of heart disease and stroke, while high-density lipoprotein cholesterol (HDL-C), or 'good' cholesterol, generally helps remove excess cholesterol from the tissues. Knowing and managing these levels are significant steps towards protecting your heart's health.
2. **Your body makes most of it:** A large majority of your cholesterol (about 80 per cent) is produced within the body, so only a small amount comes from dietary sources. For most people, dietary cholesterol has little effect on overall cholesterol levels.
3. **The danger of plaque build-up:** LDL-C can lead to atherosclerotic plaque build-up in arteries. This increases the risk of heart attacks, strokes, and other cardiovascular issues. (In Australia, cardiovascular disease [CVD] accounts for 24 per cent of all deaths – 118 deaths a day or one CVD death every 12 minutes.[1])
4. **Medications save lives:** The use of medication is essential for those who have had an event (heart attack, stroke, stent, surgery) and may prevent an event for those who have not had one. Statins, ezetimibe, and other medications effectively lower LDL-C and reduce cardiovascular risk. They are safe and effective and work well alongside lifestyle changes and nutraceuticals.

1 *(Australian) Heart Foundation - Key statistics - cardiovascular disease: https://www.heartfoundation.org.au/your-heart/evidence-and-statistics/key-stats-cardiovascular-disease?*

5. **Lifestyle matters:** Diet and exercise can help manage cholesterol, but they work best in conjunction with medications. Specific nutraceuticals can complement medical treatments.
6. **Not all risks are the same:** Understanding your lipid profile numbers and knowing your cardiovascular risk are essential. High LDL-C does not always indicate the presence of plaque in the arteries, nor does low LDL-C guarantee healthy arteries. A cardiac scan can provide a more accurate picture.
7. **Genetic risks you can't ignore:** Familial hypercholesterolaemia (FH) and elevated lipoprotein(a) [Lp(a)] are inherited conditions that can significantly increase CVD over a lifetime. They may require treatment from an early age.
8. **No symptoms - silent risk:** High cholesterol does not cause any symptoms, so regular monitoring is essential.
9. **Prevention is power:** Early detection (atherosclerosis is a many-years-long process) offers the best outcome. Regular cholesterol checks, cardiac scanning, healthy habits, and appropriate treatment can stop problems before they start. Heart disease can be preventable.
10. **It is not just about cholesterol:** Cholesterol is just one piece of the healthy heart puzzle. Other factors such as blood pressure, smoking, diabetes, and genetics also affect heart disease risk. A comprehensive approach to heart health is best.

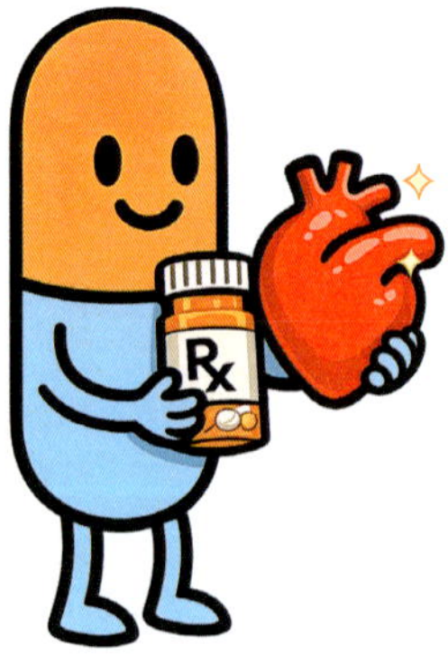

Medications are essential for effectively lowering LDL-C in high-risk patients. This significantly reduces the risk of cardiovascular events such as heart attacks and strokes. While lifestyle changes and nutraceuticals can complement treatment, medications remain the cornerstone of managing cholesterol and plaque build-up.

KEY CHOLESTEROL TERMS

These essential cholesterol-related terms and brief definitions can be a heavy read, but they will help, as familiarity will clarify and enhance your understanding of the complex concepts discussed throughout the book.

Lipids – A broad group of naturally occurring molecules that include fats, oils, waxes, sterols (such as **cholesterol**), fat-soluble vitamins (A, D, E, K), and other related compounds that are insoluble in water. Lipids are essential for various biological functions. While all fats are lipids, not all lipids are fats.

Dyslipidaemia – The umbrella term for any abnormality in blood lipids, whether that be high LDL cholesterol, high triglycerides, or low HDL cholesterol. **Hyperlipidaemia** is a subset of dyslipidaemia, referring specifically to an excess of lipids in the blood. Within this group, **hypercholesterolaemia** describes elevated LDL cholesterol levels, while **hypertriglyceridaemia** refers to raised triglycerides.

Cholesterol – A sterol alcohol in the lipid family. This waxy substance, found in all body cells, is crucial for cell membrane structure and hormone production. Low-density lipoprotein cholesterol (LDL-C), 'bad' cholesterol, contributes to plaque build-up in arteries, increasing the risk of heart disease, while high-density lipoprotein cholesterol (HDL-C), 'good' cholesterol, **generally** helps remove excess cholesterol from tissues and transport it back to the liver, in a process called reverse cholesterol transport.

Four key categories related to cholesterol and cardiovascular risk exist:

- *hypercholesterolaemia* – persistently high cholesterol levels, increasing cardiovascular risk;
- *primary prevention* – managing cholesterol before a cardiovascular event (e.g., heart attack or stroke) to reduce future risk;
- *secondary prevention* – managing cholesterol after a cardiovascular event, as these individuals are at high risk for further events, and

- *familial hypercholesterolaemia* – a genetic disorder causing dangerously high LDL-C from a young age, significantly increasing the risk of early heart disease. (see *FH*)

Lipoproteins – Complexes of lipids and proteins (see *apolipoproteins*) that transport cholesterol and other lipids around the body via the bloodstream. Lipids are not water-soluble and need these protein-coated particles to move them through the aqueous environment of the blood. Think of them as vehicles that transport cholesterol through the bloodstream. There are several types of lipoproteins, and each has a distinct role to play. Of particular (negative) note is lipoprotein(a) [Lp(a)], an inherited lipoprotein that closely resembles LDL-C but has another specialised protein, called apolipoprotein(a), attached to it. This unique structure causes Lp(a) to be more of a problem than LDL-C. [see *Lipoprotein(a)*]

Apolipoproteins – Specialised proteins that join with lipids to form lipoproteins (transporters of cholesterol). *Apo* indicates proteins that can associate with lipoproteins or exist separately. There are several main classes of apolipoproteins in the body. Each contributes uniquely to the regulation of lipid and cholesterol levels. The ones that concern us are:

- ApoA, associated with HDL-C
- ApoB, associated with LDL-C and Lp(a), and
- apo(a), associated uniquely with Lp(a).

Chylomicrons – Lipoproteins that transport dietary lipids (triglycerides [TG] and cholesterol) from the intestines via the lymphatic system to various locations in the body after food has been ingested and digested.

Very-low-density lipoproteins (VLDL) – Produced in the liver, these lipoproteins transport mainly triglycerides (TG) and some cholesterol to body tissues. As they offload TG, they transition into intermediate-density lipoprotein (IDL) particles and eventually become LDL particles, primarily carrying LDL-C.

Intermediate-density lipoproteins (IDL) – Transitional lipoproteins formed during the metabolism of VLDL. IDL are an intermediary step in TG and cholesterol transport and are further metabolised into LDL particles.

Low-density lipoproteins (LDL) – Lipoproteins that are remnants or end products of VLDL metabolism: *the carriers of the cholesterol.*

LDL cholesterol (LDL-C) - The measured cholesterol carried by LDL particles: *the cargo*. Increased LDL-C is linked to the build-up of atherosclerotic plaques in the arteries, increasing the risk of heart disease.

Lipoprotein(a) [Lp(a)] - A unique lipoprotein closely related to LDL. High levels of Lp(a) are genetically determined and strongly associated with an increased risk of CVD. Lp(a) levels are not significantly influenced by diet and are challenging to lower with conventional lipid-lowering treatments. Clinical trials on potential treatments are currently underway (late 2025).

High-density lipoproteins (HDL) - Lipoproteins that transport cholesterol away from tissues and back to the liver, where it can be re-processed as VLDL or excreted from the body: *the carriers*.

HDL cholesterol (HDL-C) - The measured cholesterol carried by HDL particles: *the cargo*. High levels of HDL-C can be associated with lower cardiovascular risk.

Triglycerides (TG) – A type of fat (lipid) that circulates in lipoprotein particles in the blood, primarily after eating. They are the most common form of fat in the body and are stored in fat cells for energy. Elevated TG levels are associated with an increased risk of heart disease, especially when combined with other risk factors such as high LDL-C, low HDL-C, and insulin resistance.

Lipid profile (standard) - A blood test that measures total cholesterol (TC), LDL-C, HDL-C, TG, TC to HDL-C ratio, and non-HDL-C levels (cholesterol in particles).

Atherosclerotic plaque (often referred to as plaque) - The sticky build-up of cholesterol, cellular waste products, calcium and fibrin in the inner lining of an artery that hardens, narrows, or blocks the artery, reducing blood supply. This can lead to a lack of blood to the heart muscle (heart attack), to the brain (stroke), or to the legs (peripheral artery disease [PAD]).

Statins - A class of drugs used to lower LDL-C levels in the blood, primarily to prevent CVD and cardiovascular events. Statins work by inhibiting an enzyme in the liver, HMG-CoA reductase, (see next page), which is involved in cholesterol production. This leads the liver to increase the number of low-density lipoprotein receptors (LDLR) on its surface, enhancing the removal of LDL-C from the bloodstream.

Beta-hydroxy-beta-methylglutaryl coenzyme A reductase (HMG-CoA reductase) - An enzyme (a biological catalyst) that has a central role in cholesterol synthesis in the liver and is targeted by statin drugs.

Proprotein convertase subtilisin/kexin type 9 (PCSK9) **inhibitors** - Newer cholesterol-lowering medications that increase the liver's ability to remove LDL-C from the blood.

Cholesterol absorption inhibitors - Medications, such as ezetimibe, that prevent cholesterol absorption in the intestines.

Family risk or family history of heart disease – Refers to a first-degree relative (parent, sibling, child) who, if a male, has had a coronary artery event (such as a heart attack) before the age of 55 years, and if a female, before the age of 60 years. This generally does not relate to heart rhythm or heart valve problems, nor does it relate to a 90-year-old uncle.

Familial hypercholesterolaemia (FH) – A genetic disorder characterised by very high cholesterol levels, specifically high LDL-C from birth, leading to premature coronary artery disease (CAD) (below).

Cardiovascular disease (CVD) - A group of disorders that affects the heart and blood vessels, including CAD (below), stroke, cardiac failure (CF), and peripheral artery disease (PAD), often caused by atherosclerosis or other heart health factors.

Coronary artery disease (CAD) - Atherosclerotic plaque build-up causes hardening, narrowing or blocking of the coronary arteries that supply blood to the heart muscle. This can lead to angina (chest pain), heart attack (complete blockage of an artery), cardiac failure (when the heart does not pump as well as it should), arrhythmias (electrical malfunctions within the heart), and sudden cardiac death (generally from an arrhythmia).

DOCTORS' COMMENT: Think of CVD as the forest, and CAD as one especially critical tree. Throughout this book, we'll use both terms. Whenever CVD is used, CAD is always implied. When CAD is used, it refers specifically to the heart. Both CVD and CAD are serious health concerns, and both are worth preventing.

CLARIFYING SOME CHOLESTEROL LANGUAGE

Cholesterol is complex and fascinating. In the coming pages, we will clearly explain its intricate and vital role in the body. There is much to learn – and even admire. Before we go further, a few key concepts need to be understood, as they will shape everything that follows, especially your appreciation of cholesterol.

understanding the term 'cholesterol'

When the word 'cholesterol' is used, it can refer to one of two things:

- cholesterol as an **organic molecule** that is in every body cell, or
- cholesterol **in the blood**, which is transported **within lipoprotein particles** and measured as 'cholesterol' in blood tests. This is the form that is crucial in assessing cardiovascular risk.

Although both refer to the **same** lipid molecules, their descriptions are **not interchangeable**. 'Cholesterol' has **two entities** serving **two very distinct functions** within the body.

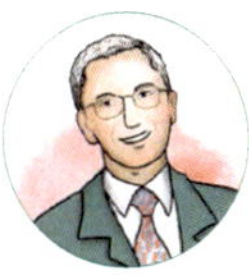

Using 'cholesterol' interchangeably brings confusion to the cholesterol conversation.

cholesterol, the molecule

Cholesterol is **needed** by **all** cells and **produced** by **most** of the body's cells (all except non-nucleated cells such as red blood cells). Although we also receive a **small** amount of cholesterol from certain foods, the impact of **dietary cholesterol** on blood cholesterol levels is **small** for most people. While human life cannot be sustained without it, cholesterol remains the **most significant treatable risk factor** for cardiovascular disease (CVD).

The difference arises because cholesterol (the molecule) – which comes from some food, or is naturally manufactured in the intestines, the liver, and most body cells – cannot be transported alone through the bloodstream to where it is needed in the body.

Cholesterol (the molecule) is **hydrophobic,** meaning it does not mix well with water. Blood is about 55 per cent plasma, and plasma is about 90 per cent water. With our blood's high water content, cholesterol needs help travelling around the body. Enter apolipoproteins and lipoproteins!

cholesterol, within the lipoprotein particle

Apolipoproteins are **specialised proteins** that join with lipids (one of which is cholesterol) to form the **lipoproteins** that **transport** the cholesterol through the blood.

apolipoproteins (proteins) + **lipids** (including cholesterol and triglycerides)

= **lipoproteins**

(the transporters of cholesterol, triglycerides, and other lipids throughout the body)

There are several lipoproteins. The most well-known are low-density lipoproteins (LDL) and high-density lipoproteins (HDL). Lipoproteins vary in nature and size depending on where they originate: the intestines or the liver. Because we are familiar with it, let's focus briefly on LDL and LDL-C.

LDL is the **transport particle**.

LDL cholesterol (LDL-C) is the **cholesterol being transported** around the body in the blood. This LDL-C, **measured in a lipid profile**, can become a **primary component of plaque formation.** So, cholesterol in the bloodstream is really cholesterol in the transport lipoproteins (the particle) - and each has its very particular function.

Yet, **all cholesterol molecules are the same,** regardless of which lipoprotein carries them. The **difference** lies in the **apolipoprotein** (the specialised protein - let's call it 'protein' for now) that helps form the particle. These proteins act like 'docking stations' for the cell interaction and **define how the particle behaves**.

These apolipoproteins - the protein **company** that the cholesterol keeps as it circulates - are where our 'cholesterol concern' and heart health intersect. (Please note, there is a lot more detail to come soon.)

is CAD really a disease?

Now that we have clarified the language, let's challenge a deeper assumption: what do we mean by 'disease'? A strong scientific link exists between cholesterol, cardiovascular disease (CVD) – affecting the heart, brain, or legs – and coronary artery disease (CAD), which affects the heart alone. We believe the term 'disease' can misrepresent the pre-clinical or pre-event stages of CVD, including CAD.

A **disease**, by definition, alters function or causes symptoms, and we typically think of it developing over a **recent** and relatively **short** time. In contrast, CVD and CAD result from atherosclerosis, a **process** that develops **slowly** over many years and can start at an early age[1].

In matters of the heart, many people do not experience symptoms before a major event, such as a heart attack. The underlying process – atherosclerosis, the plaque build-up in the coronary arteries – has been occurring **silently**, unnoticed over **years** rather than days or weeks. The process may have started as early as the person's teens and taken decades to reach the point when the atherosclerotic plaque leads to a symptom or loss of function.

where is the boundary between risk factors and disease?

DR KOSTNER:

> *Twenty-first century research is challenging how we distinguish between cardiovascular **risk factors** and cardiovascular **disease**. Emerging data from a multiethnic study[2] suggest that patients with risk factors such as diabetes, hypertension (high blood pressure), or hypercholesterolaemia – but without diagnosed heart disease – can still show signs of regional myocardial dysfunction (impaired heart muscle contraction).*

---

1 *Autopsies on young people who have died unexpectedly, e.g., from a violent death, have revealed lipid-rich plaques in the coronary arteries.*

2 *The Multi-Ethnic Study of Atherosclerosis (MESA), an ongoing study investigating subclinical cardiovascular disease and its progression in a diverse cohort of participants, including African American, Caucasian, Chinese, and Hispanic individuals.*

Rosen, B, Saad, M, Shea, S. et al. Hypertension and Smoking Are Associated With Reduced Regional Left Ventricular Function in Asymptomatic Individuals: The Multi-Ethnic Study of Atherosclerosis. JACC. 2006 Mar, 47 (6) 1150–1158. https://doi.org/10.1016/j.jacc.2005.08.078

This raises an important question: ***Is the line between having risk factors and having actual disease as clear-cut as we once thought?***

There's no established precedent for these findings, nor a clear mechanism to explain them. However, it is possible that ***cardiovascular risk factors themselves have a direct effect on heart muscle function, even before traditional signs of 'disease' appear****. If this is true, it reinforces the idea that CAD is a* ***continuum****, starting with risk factors that affect the heart and progressing to clinically evident disease.*

'high cholesterol'

We'd also like to address the concept of 'high cholesterol'. 'High cholesterol' (hypercholesterolaemia) can refer to total cholesterol (TC) – a broad measure including all lipoproteins – or, more specifically, to elevated LDL-C. Clinically, when cardiologists talk about 'high cholesterol', they typically mean high LDL-C.

The current distinctions are very high, high, borderline high, near optimal/above optimal and optimal. Each level has a measurement range. For example, when it comes to LDL-C which is the cholesterol within the particle we are most concerned about, very high is 4.9 mmol/L or above (Australia) or 190 mg/dL or above (USA), while high is 4.1-4.8 mmol/L (160-189 mg/dL) (Please see the following page for further details).

What is very important here is that the levels are on a **continuum** and that **'high cholesterol' encompasses borderline high, high and very high, with each presenting a different clinical picture.** There is no question that those in **the high and very high groups will need modification of risk** (medication) over their lifetime. It is not so clear-cut for the patients who are borderline high or below. As the term 'high cholesterol' is used very broadly in cholesterol conversations, it can often refer to levels that are borderline high and below. This can cause confusion for those in the genuinely high, very high, or even the very, very high ranges.

A CLOSER LOOK

understanding cholesterol levels

	TOTAL CHOLESTEROL		LOW-DENSITY LIPOPROTEIN CHOLESTEROL	
very high	300 mg/dL* or above	**7.8 mmol/L** or above**	190 mg/dL* or above	**4.9 mmol/L** or above**
high	240 - 299	**6.2 - 7.7**	160-189	**4.1 - 4.8**
borderline high	200 - 239	**5.2 - 6.1**	130-159	**3.4 - 4.0**
desirable	less than 200	**less than 5.2**	less than 130	**less than 3.4**

Note: these targets are **general recommendations** *for the* **broader population.**
Much **lower levels** *would be the targets for individuals who have had a heart attack, stroke or peripheral artery disease. These will be discussed later.*

* **USA measurement**: milligrams of cholesterol per deciliter of blood – mg/dL
** **Australian measurement:** millimoles of cholesterol per litre of blood – mmol/L

high-risk factors for CVD

established disease

- previous cardiovascular event: heart attack, stroke, stent placement, or bypass surgery (secondary prevention – always high risk)
- documented atherosclerotic disease in arteries (coronary, carotid, peripheral)

major modifiable risk factors

- high low-density lipoprotein cholesterol (dyslipidaemia)
- high blood pressure (hypertension)
- diabetes mellitus (especially type 2)
- smoking
- overweight and obesity
- unhealthy diet (excess saturated/trans fats, refined carbohydrates, salt)
- physical inactivity
- excess alcohol intake

non-modifiable risk factors

- age (risk increases with age)
- sex (men are at higher risk earlier; women's risk rises after menopause)
- family history of premature CVD (early heart attack, stroke, or sudden death in a first-degree relative)
- genetic conditions (e.g. familial hypercholesterolaemia, high Lp(a))

emerging risk factors

- chronic kidney disease, inflammatory conditions (e.g. rheumatoid arthritis, lupus), gut microbiome imbalance, poor sleep, psychosocial factors (such as isolation, depression, chronic stress), polycystic ovarian syndrome, early menopause, and even exposure to various pollutants.

WHY CHOLESTEROL IS IMPORTANT

We now know that cholesterol is essential for life. Found in every animal cell, it plays a vital role in maintaining our health. Cholesterol - absent in plant cells but ubiquitous in animal cell membranes - plays five key roles in maintaining the human body's overall health by:

1. providing structural integrity to cell membranes;
2. serving as the basis for steroid hormone production;
3. enabling vitamin D synthesis;
4. forming bile acids and salts, and
5. facilitating the movement and metabolism of fat-soluble vitamins.

cell membranes

The cell membrane, a **phospholipid bilayer**[1], is stabilised by the presence of cholesterol. Think of the membrane as a brick wall around the cell. Cholesterol is like the mortar. Without it, the wall would either collapse or become too rigid to function properly. Cholesterol prevents the membrane from becoming too stiff while still holding important proteins in place, ensuring they stay where they are needed. This balance helps the cell maintain its shape and function properly.

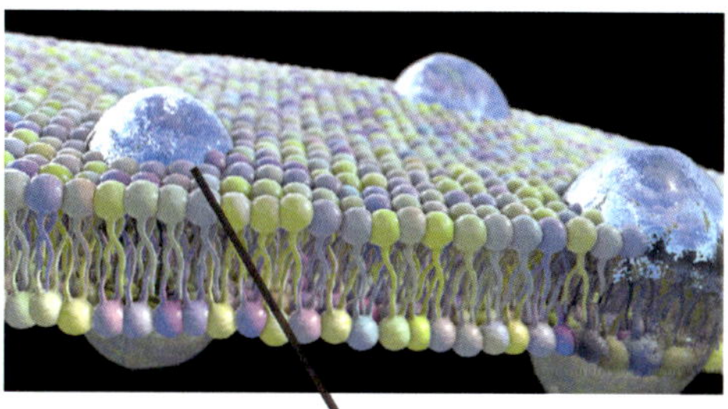

a 3-D representation of a cell membrane

1 *A phospholipid bilayer is a fundamental structure that forms the basis of all cell membranes. It consists of two layers of phospholipids – molecules that have a hydrophilic (water-attracting) head and two hydrophobic (water-repelling) tails. These phospholipids are arranged into two parallel layers, with the hydrophobic tails facing inward and the hydrophilic heads, outward, allowing the bilayer to form a barrier permeable to specific molecules but not others. This structure is crucial for the functionality of cells, helping to maintain the cell's internal environment and facilitate the transport of substances in and out.*

While much endogenous production[2] of cholesterol occurs within the liver (cholesterol the molecule and cholesterol within the particles), **all nucleated cells**[3] within the body are capable of synthesising cholesterol (cholesterol in the molecular form).

Cholesterol is also involved in **cell signalling[4] pathways**, primarily as a precursor in the synthesis of steroid hormones. Steroid hormones are important signalling molecules that regulate a wide range of physiological processes.

Cholesterol is essential for the formation of **lipid rafts** in the cell membrane (see the diagram on the previous page). These special regions within the cell's outer layer act like tiny, floating islands on the cell's surface. These 'islands' are important because they organise and manage proteins, which are essential for the cell's operation. They help move these proteins to where they're needed and initiate processes that allow the cell to communicate and respond to what's happening around it. So, cholesterol keeps cells functioning well and helps them 'talk' to each other.

steroid hormone production

Steroid hormones regulate essential functions: **testosterone** and **oestrogen** influence reproduction, **cortisol** manages stress, and **aldosterone** controls blood pressure. Cholesterol is their starting material, produced in the adrenal cortex, testes and ovaries, placenta, brain, and adipose tissue. Its widespread production highlights cholesterol's vital role in hormonal balance, stress response, reproduction, and overall regulation.

---

2 *Cholesterol produced by the body (not from food).*

3 *Nucleated cells contain a membrane-bound nucleus with DNA inside. Most cells in the body are nucleated. The most notable exception is red blood cells which lose their nucleus to carry more oxygen. Non-nucleated cells obtain their cholesterol from blood lipoproteins, particularly LDL and HDL.*

4 *Cell signalling is a complex system of communication that governs basic cellular activities and coordinates cell actions. It's essential for cells to process information from their environment and other cells. This process involves various signalling molecules, such as hormones and neurotransmitters, which can influence or trigger a response inside the cell. The signalling mechanisms can be simple, involving just a few molecules, or incredibly complex, involving networks of reactions. These processes are crucial for numerous biological functions, including growth, division, death, and specialisation of cells.*

vitamin D

Cholesterol is also a precursor to the formation of vitamin D3. A precursor is an initial substance that can undergo transformation or conversion into another substance. In vitamin D synthesis, cholesterol acts as a precursor because it can be converted into vitamin D3 through a series of chemical reactions triggered by sunlight (ultraviolet B energy). Vitamin D is essential for calcium absorption, bone health and immune function.

bile acids and bile salts

Cholesterol in the liver can be converted into bile acids, which join with amino acids to form bile salts. More water-soluble and detergent-like, bile salts are highly effective at breaking down dietary fats into smaller units for digestion in the small intestine. They also aid the absorption of fat-soluble vitamins. After use, bile salts are reabsorbed and recycled to the liver, while bile acids are stored in the gallbladder.

fat-soluble vitamins

Cholesterol is closely connected to the movement and processing of the fat-soluble vitamins, A, D, E, and K (which are stored in the body's fatty tissues for later use). From their site of absorption in the intestine, each of these vitamins needs to be transported into the bloodstream and then to their respective destinations for use. Because vitamins A, D, E, and K don't dissolve in water, they hitch a ride with cholesterol and triglyceride-carrying lipoproteins to reach the cells that need them.

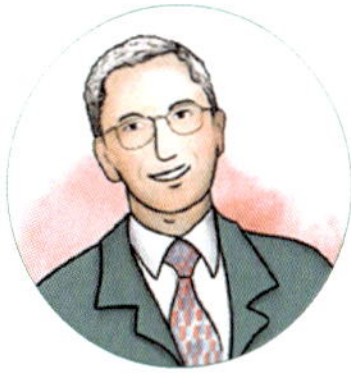

The body can produce as much cholesterol as it needs in its cells. Lowering cholesterol in the blood, even to very low levels, does not negatively influence any of the above functions.

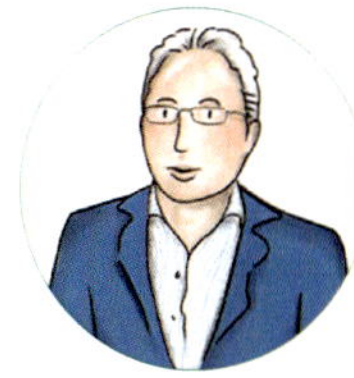

This book draws from clinical experiences of world-leading specialists, case studies, research data, and current best recommendations.
These details will help separate 'the fats' from fiction, answer your questions, and enhance your understanding.
You can then participate in informed discussions with your medical advisers to meet your specific needs or be well-versed during the next dinner conversation.

As expressed in the Preface
we encourage you to read the book as a whole,
at least once, to gain an overview
of this very complex topic.
Along the way, you'll notice that some themes reappear.
This is deliberate, to reinforce key concepts from different angles.
Our aim is not only to inform but to help you,
together with your medical advisers,
to stay curious while feeling confident and equipped
to make sense of cholesterol and its role
in your best health journey.

UNDERSTANDING CHOLESTEROL

an essential human molecule yet a significant cardiovascular risk factor

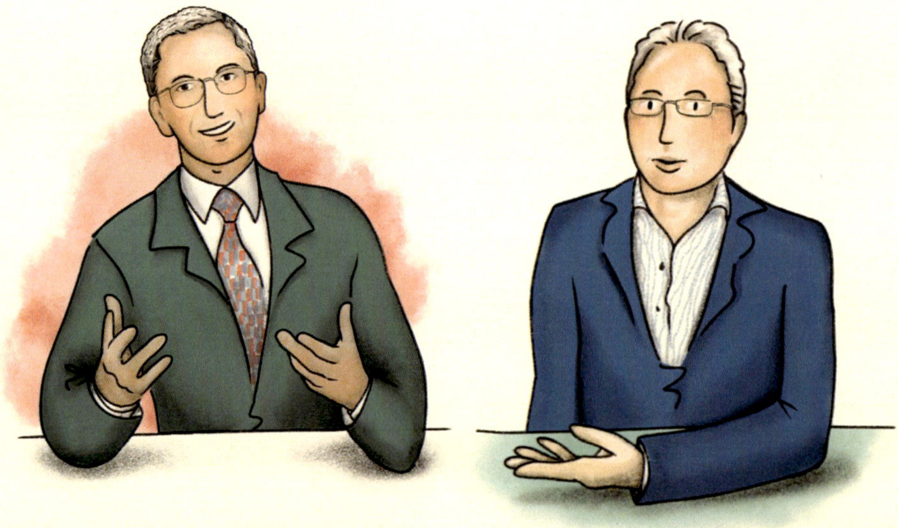

chapter 1

CHOLESTEROL: THE SCIENCE AND SIGNIFICANCE UNPACKED

High cholesterol is more common than most realise. More than 40 per cent of Australian adults live with it[1]. Globally, the figure is 39 per cent. According to the World Heart Federation[2], high cholesterol causes 4.4 million deaths a year, while elevated low-density lipoprotein cholesterol (LDL-C) alone accounts for nearly a quarter of all heart-related deaths.

what is cholesterol?

Cholesterol is a pale yellow/whitish waxy solid with the chemical formula $C_{27}H_{46}O$ and a melting point close to 150°C.

Perhaps not too dissimilar to a pale, crumbly cheese, but with a much higher melting point – although this possibly is not the most helpful description of cholesterol when your doctor tells you that yours is 'high' and you need to do something about it!

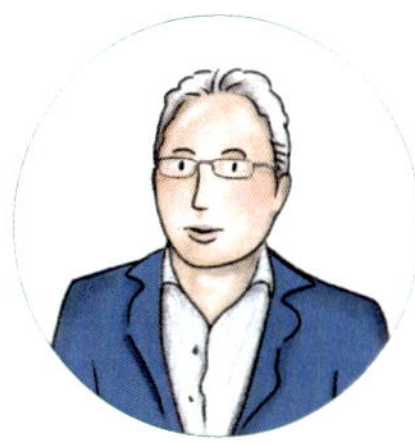

The word cholesterol is derived from two Greek roots, *chole*, meaning bile, and *stereos*, solid, combined with the chemical suffix, *-ol*, applied in organic chemistry to compounds that have a reactive OH tail also known as an 'alcohol'.

cholesterol

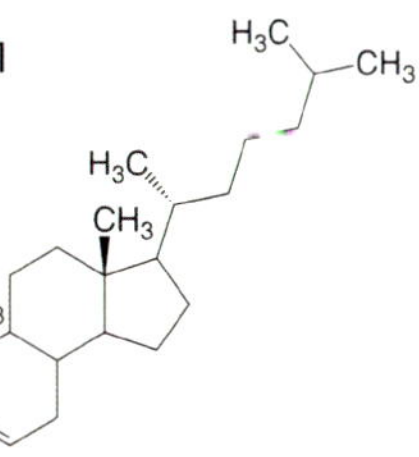

Chemically, cholesterol is a **steroid alcohol**, which means it is a chain of hydrocarbons (steroid) with an OH (alcohol) tail attached and it belongs to a

1 *The Heart Foundation (Australia) website - https://www.heartfoundation.org.au/bundles/for-professionals/key-statistics-risk-factors-for-heart-disease*

2 *World Heart Federation website - https://world-heart-federation.org/ and search 'cholesterol' or use http://bit.ly/3IE5oI6*

group called **lipids**. Lipids are a family of compounds that includes fats and other important molecules including, **cholesterol, triglycerides (TG), phospholipids,** and **fatty acids**. They are essential for cell membranes, energy storage, and hormone production, but because they are not water-soluble, they must be transported in the blood by lipoproteins.

Most of the cholesterol in your body (about 80 per cent) is not in its pure form. Instead, it is bonded with a fatty acid to create what's known as a cholesteryl ester, making it more water-soluble. This means there are two types of cholesterol in the body:

- **unesterified** (or 'free') **cholesterol** – unattached cholesterol that is found on the surface of lipoproteins and in cell membranes and can move between the two, and
- **cholesteryl esters** – cholesterol bonded to fatty acids via a bond between the cholesterol's hydroxyl group (-OH) and the fatty acid's carboxyl group (COOH). The result is a cholesteryl ester (used for transport and storage) and a water molecule (a by-product). Cholesteryl esters are hydrophobic (not water-soluble), and more lipid-soluble than free cholesterol, making them ideal for storage and transport in lipoproteins such as low-density lipoproteins (LDL) and high-density lipoproteins (HDL).

Think of it like this: free cholesterol is like cargo on the deck of a ship, easy to access and move, while cholesteryl esters are securely packed below deck, stored and ready for transport[3]. But ***please*** be aware...

essential, yet ...

All cholesterol in all particles is the same. The heart health impact of cholesterol in the bloodstream depends **entirely** on the lipoproteins carrying them: LDL particles cause problems, HDL particles generally do not. When too many LDL particles circulate in the blood, they can become trapped in artery walls. Over time, the body's immune response tries to 'clean up' these deposits, but instead, it fuels inflammation, thickening the plaque and narrowing the arteries. Plaque can block the coronary arteries

---

3 *For simplicity, we'll now use 'cholesterol' as a single term, but remember that in reality it exists in two forms: free cholesterol (found primarily in cell membranes) and cholesteryl esters (carried in lipoproteins).*

(heart) leading to a heart attack or other coronary artery disease (CAD) complications. It can also affect the carotid arteries (neck), increasing the risk of a stroke or the peripheral arteries (legs), causing pain and cramping while walking (claudication).

This ongoing process, known as **atherosclerosis**, is what turns cholesterol from a vital substance into a potential threat. So, cholesterol, the molecule on its own, **isn't** the problem. Instead, think particles!

LDL particles, with their associated apolipoproteins, are the primary transporters of cholesterol in the blood. LDL particles are **more likely** to penetrate artery walls in association with inflammation, which can lead to atherosclerosis, heart attacks, and strokes. This is why **LDL-C** is the **primary focus** of cholesterol-lowering strategies. Reducing LDL **directly lowers** cardiovascular risk. In contrast, **HDL,** although it contains the same cholesterol molecule, generally plays a **protective** role by helping to remove excess cholesterol from the circulation.

transport

As we have intimated, cholesterol transport is governed by a range of lipoproteins - complex particles that consist of **cholesterol, TG,** and specialised proteins, the **apolipoproteins.** Lipoproteins originate in the intestines and the liver. For example, **chylomicrons** are formed in the intestine, after **dietary cholesterol** is absorbed. Other lipoproteins, such as **HDL**, are secreted from the **liver.** On the other hand, **LDL** is the **waste end-product** of **very-low-density lipoproteins** (VLDL), which are made in the **liver**.

It is crucial to understand that the impact cholesterol (the molecule in the blood) has on heart health is about **the company** it keeps:

- the **type** of lipoprotein carrying the cholesterol and
- the impact of the various **apolipoproteins** also being carried by the lipoprotein.

A lipoprotein's **apolipoproteins** influence how the lipoprotein behaves, affecting cholesterol's ability to contribute to plaque. The main culprit is apolipoprotein B (ApoB), which is contained in lipoproteins such as LDL and Lp(a) – the lipoproteins most linked to plaque build-up and heart disease.

DR BISHOP:

Everyday conversation often confuses cholesterol (the molecule) with the cholesterol carried within the lipoprotein particles in the bloodstream. A clear distinction is needed to prevent confusion.

Understanding that different particles have different proteins is very important. These proteins act like a towbar on a car. As the shape of the towbar determines what trailer it can attach to, so the protein determines what cells the lipoprotein can attach to.

When cholesterol is transported by a certain particle that is associated with a certain protein, for example, HDL (the particle) with ApoA (the protein), it's generally protective. However, problems arise when cholesterol travels with a different particle and protein, for example, LDL with ApoB!

Cholesterol's impact depends on this context – the ***company it keeps*** *(the proteins with which it is associated). This is crucial.*

levels

Although we derive some cholesterol from our food (about 20 per cent), most cholesterol is produced **naturally** within the body (about 80 per cent). It is also **genetically** determined. Some people absorb more cholesterol than others, which is important when it comes to therapy. While cholesterol is essential for building healthy cells, the risk of developing heart disease – heart attack, stroke, blocked blood vessels – rises and falls with the rise and fall of the amount of LDL-C in the blood.

Cholesterol is in a constant, dynamic **interplay** between what the body **produces**, what we **consume** through diet, and how it **circulates** to meet the body's needs.

As high cholesterol levels do not produce any symptoms, regular testing is highly recommended. Even then, it is hard to begin to predict who will have a cardiovascular event.

A CLOSER LOOK

cholesterol's building blocks

To understand cholesterol and its role in the body, it's helpful to break down some key components of fats and lipids.

HYDROCARBONS & FATTY ACIDS: THE FOUNDATION OF FATS

Hydrocarbons are molecules made of carbon and hydrogen atoms, forming either chains or rings. They come in two main types:

- **saturated** hydrocarbons – contain only single bonds between carbon atoms, making them stable;
- **unsaturated** hydrocarbons – contain double or triple bonds, making them more flexible and reactive.

Fatty acids are hydrocarbons with an added carboxyl group (COOH). They form the building blocks of fats and oils and play a key role in energy storage and cell function.

- **Saturated** fatty acids have only single bonds, making them more solid at room temperature.
- **Unsaturated** fatty acids have one or more double bonds, making them more fluid. These include:
  - **monounsaturated** fatty acids (MUFA) – one double bond.
  - **polyunsaturated** fatty acids (PUFA) – multiple double bonds.

Not all fatty acids are good. Some, like **trans fats** (found in processed foods), can raise LDL-C and increase cardiovascular risk.

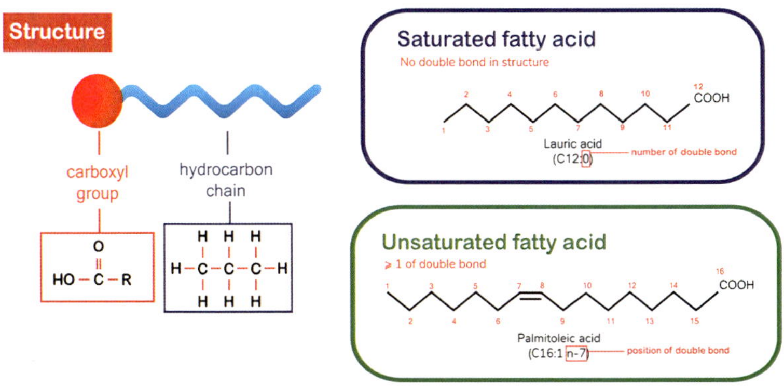

FREE FATTY ACIDS: ENERGY IN MOTION

Free fatty acids (FFA) are unattached fatty acids that the body uses as a major energy source. In the bloodstream, FFA bind to albumin (a transport protein). High levels of FFA can indicate metabolic issues such as obesity, diabetes, and metabolic syndrome. While all FFA are fatty acids, not all fatty acids are FFA. Many fatty acids exist in esterified forms, such as those found in TG and phospholipids.

GLYCEROL, TRIGLYCERIDES & PHOSPHOLIPIDS

Glycerol is a three-carbon alcohol that forms the backbone of key lipid molecules.

Triglycerides (the body's primary form of stored fat and energy reserve) are three fatty acids attached to glycerol.

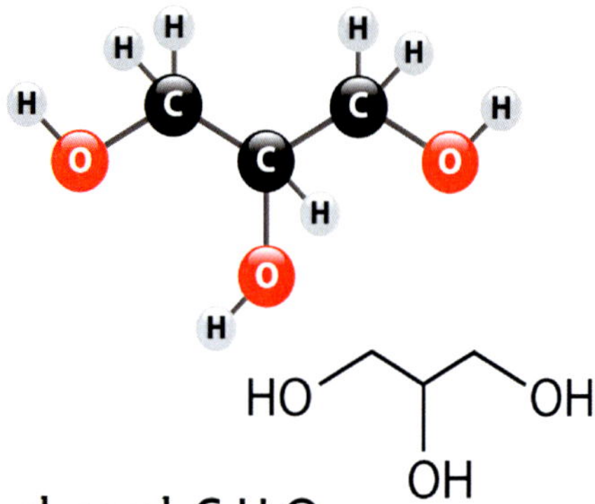

glycerol $C_3H_8O_3$

Phospholipids (essential for cell membranes and lipoproteins) are two fatty acids + a phosphate group attached to glycerol. Phospholipids have a water-soluble phosphate 'head' and a fat-soluble fatty 'tail', allowing them to form cell membranes, and transport cholesterol in lipoproteins.

TRIGLYCERIDEs

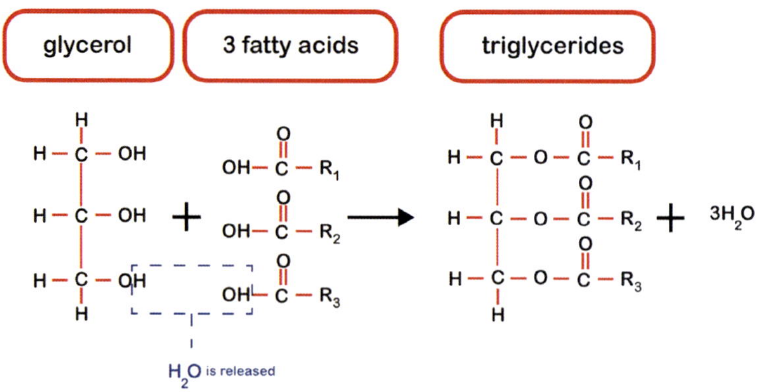

Understanding these basic structures helps explain how fats are stored, transported, and used in the body – critical knowledge for managing cholesterol and overall health.

cholesterol management foundations

Lowering cholesterol involves medications.

Lifestyle changes can have an impact and are important for reasons other than their effect on lipids. Nutraceuticals may be of assistance. Being well educated about cholesterol and its risks is a great advantage.

medications

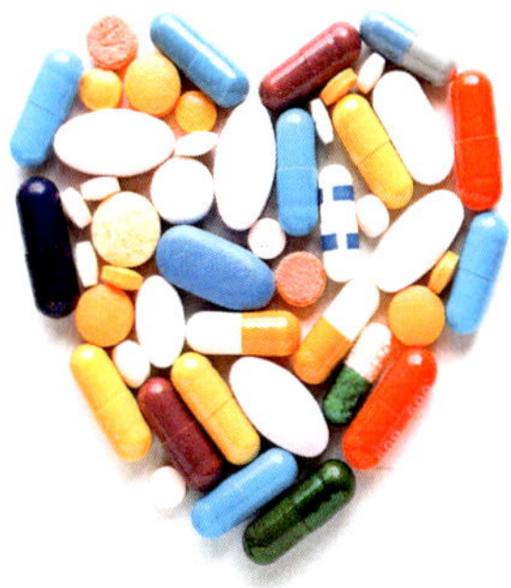

Medications are necessary to lower cholesterol levels, especially in high-risk patients, those who have had an event, and those who have a significant amount of plaque in their coronary arteries.

Cholesterol production, especially within the liver, involves several steps. One key step is carried out by an enzyme called beta-hydroxy-beta-methylglutaryl coenzyme A (HMG-CoA) reductase. Statins (the most commonly used cholesterol-lowering medications) work by blocking this enzyme, thus reducing the body's production of cholesterol. Other drugs, such as ezetimibe and PCSK9 inhibitors, are now available and work on different pathways in cholesterol metabolism.

Follow your doctor's advice and take your medication as directed. Always speak with your doctor if you believe adjustments are needed. **Do not stop taking your medication** because you feel well. Remember, increased cholesterol causes no symptoms. Your medication will continue to work in the background to keep your cholesterol under control.

If you stop, your cholesterol levels will rise, plaque will build up again, and your risk of CVD will increase.

lifestyle changes

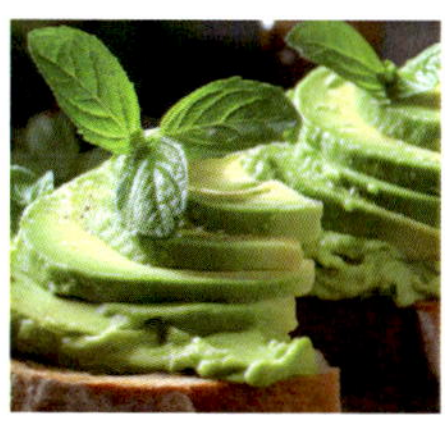

Diet, especially the use of the Portfolio Diet, physical activity, and weight loss **support medications** to lower LDL-C levels and can also affect HDL-C and TG levels.

nutraceuticals

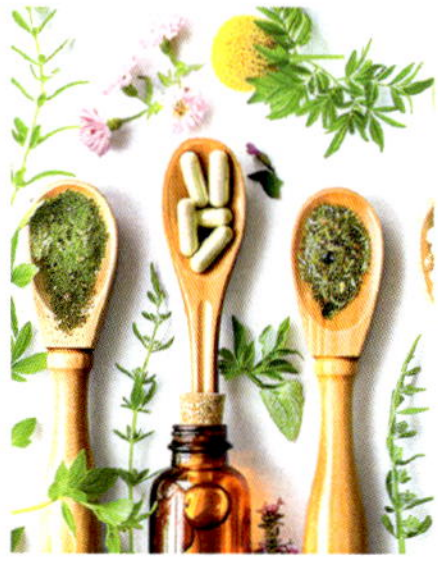

Some people choose to use nutraceuticals (supplements from natural foods) as part of their approach to lowering cholesterol. While nutraceuticals do not replace medications, they **may** offer additional **support**. Options like plant sterols, fibre, and soy can have a small effect on lipids and can contribute to overall cardiovascular health.

education

Understanding cholesterol and its health risks enables informed decisions. Knowing about LDL-C, HDL-C, and TG is key to managing heart health and preventing CVD. Awareness of how diet, weight, and regular exercise affect cholesterol helps you and your doctor manage it proactively, boosting your heart health and overall well-being.

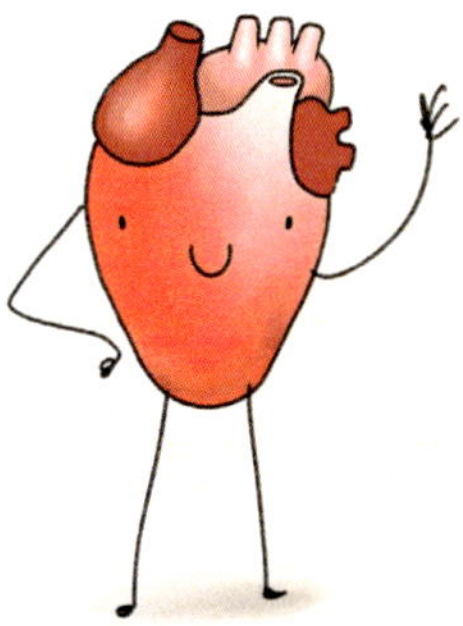

change is possible

- with the help of education
- through seeking medical advice and using medications when needed, supported by lifestyle adjustments and consideration of nutraceuticals
- asking for the support and encouragement of others

We will cover the subject matter of this chapter in much more detail throughout the book.

IMPORTANT POINTS

CHOLESTEROL UNPACKED

- Most cholesterol is produced naturally within the liver, the intestines and most cells in the body and is essential to our body's health. Even so, high LDL-C levels in the blood are associated with the formation of plaque in the arteries and the possibility of serious heart health problems.
- Cholesterol is a pale yellow/whitish waxy solid produced naturally in the body and found in some foods we eat.
- All animals – including humans – need cholesterol as an essential building block for our cells.
- Chemically, cholesterol is a steroid alcohol with the formula $C_{27}H_{46}O$. It is part of the lipid family.
- Cholesterol is insoluble in water, so it is transported around the body (through the bloodstream) by lipoproteins, ball-like particles containing mainly TG, cholesterol and proteins.
- The company that cholesterol keeps in the blood – lipoproteins and apolipoproteins – determines the impact cholesterol has on heart health.
- Medications are needed to lower elevated cholesterol levels. Lifestyle changes, nutraceuticals, and education play important supportive roles.
- As high cholesterol does not have any obvious symptoms, your levels should be checked regularly!

We need cholesterol to sustain life – and yet it can cause havoc, too!

Which organ in the body contains the most cholesterol?

The brain. About a quarter of the body's total cholesterol is found in the brain, where it plays a crucial role in nerve signalling and brain function. The brain makes its own cholesterol locally because cholesterol from your bloodstream can't cross the blood-brain barrier. Brain cholesterol is essentially in its own isolated ecosystem.

How much cholesterol does the body produce a day?

You make about three to four fast-food burgers worth of cholesterol daily, producing roughly 1000 mg (1 g) of cholesterol (the weight of a bank note). Your liver is basically running a cholesterol factory 24/7, and it down-regulates production when you eat more (though not always perfectly).

Were early cholesterol researchers criticised?

Frequently. Many early findings were controversial, and debates about cholesterol's role in heart disease were often heated – a reminder that medical understanding evolves through challenge, not certainty.

Do insects have cholesterol?

Most insects cannot produce cholesterol themselves and must source it from their diet. Despite this, cholesterol remains vital for their growth, development, and cell membranes.

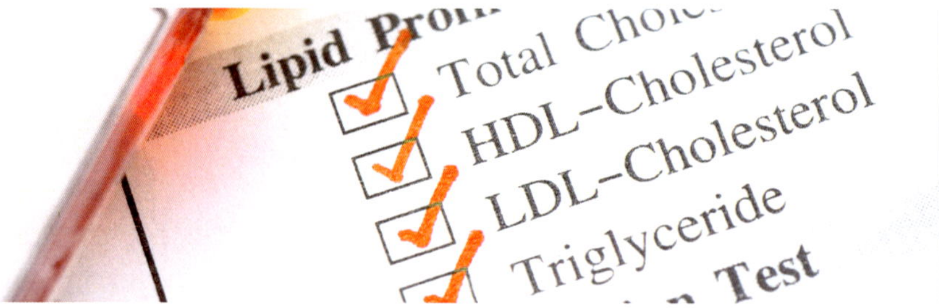

Your lipid profile: A vital blood test measuring total cholesterol (TC), LDL-C, HDL-C, triglycerides (TG), TC/HDL-C ratio, and non-HDL-C levels. These measurements reflect the amount of cholesterol in the various lipoprotein particles. Knowing your lipid profile helps identify cardiovascular risks and guide personalised strategies for managing cholesterol levels.

chapter 2

CHOLESTEROL AND PLAQUE: UNDERSTANDING THE PERIL

The heart-cholesterol-plaque relationship is complex and nuanced. Cholesterol's **movement through the bloodstream** is what determines its **impact** on heart health. When the delicate balance of cholesterol transport is disrupted, plaque can begin forming in arteries, turning cholesterol from indispensable to harmful.This plaque build-up, known as **atherosclerosis,** can lead to **atherosclerotic cardiovascular disease** (ASCVD)[1] and primarily affects the heart, brain (remember, a stroke is significant), and legs. However, in this book our focus is in the coronary arteries, where it drives the development of coronary artery disease (CAD).

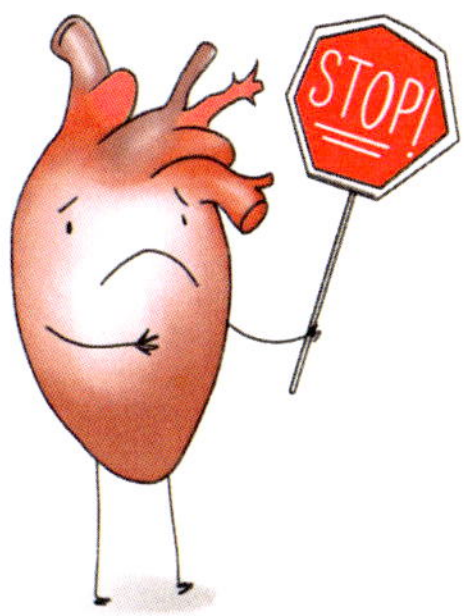

Often silent for years, CAD can reduce blood flow and oxygen supply to the heart muscle, leading to angina, heart attacks, or even sudden cardiac death (SCD).

the heart

No one needs to be convinced about the importance of the heart for a healthy, well-functioning body. The heart is a large muscle that pumps blood to supply our tissues with nutrients and oxygen while removing waste like carbon dioxide. Critical to the heart's operation are the major coronary arteries: the **right** coronary artery, the **left main** coronary artery, which almost immediately divides into the **left anterior descending** artery (LAD), and the **circumflex** artery. These 'fuel lines' carry blood from the heart's major pumping chamber, the left ventricle, to the heart muscle so it can contract rhythmically, pumping blood to the body around 100,000 times a day and more than 35 million times a year!

1 *We will refer to ASCVD as cardiovascular disease or CVD for the remainder of the book.*

These major arteries comprise fewer than 350 mm in total length and are less than five millimetres in diameter at their widest. A single build-up of plaque, even 10 mm long, can cause a critical blockage. This lack of redundancy makes the system highly vulnerable.

We all know people who have suffered heart problems, and it is very likely that someone close to us has experienced a heart attack or died after one. Although 'heart attack' is not a medical term, it is widely used to describe a severe coronary event that can be life-ending, life-threatening, or requiring hospitalisation. Such events usually result from a complete or near-complete blockage of a coronary artery. Symptoms that may point to trouble in the coronary system include:

- angina[2], or chest pain on exertion
- shortness of breath on exertion, and
- acute coronary syndrome (ACS), manifested by chest pain at rest (for example, unstable angina[3]), that could lead to damage or death of part of the heart (heart attack).

These are most commonly caused by the build-up of plaque in the artery, which leads to a narrowing of the vessel through which the blood flows.

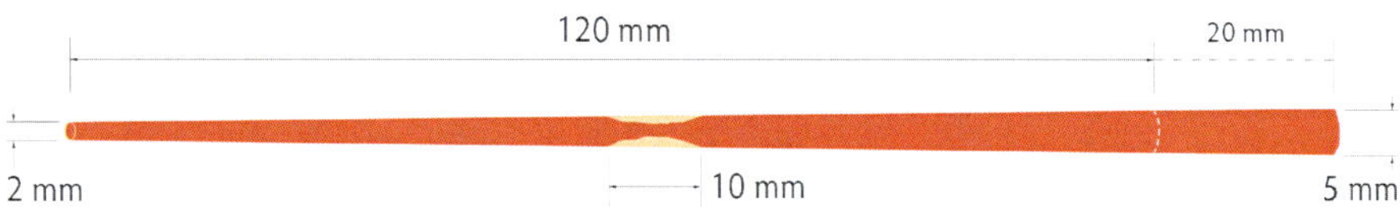

2 *Angina pectoris, commonly called angina or stable angina, has its roots in the Latin words "angere" meaning to strangle and "pectus" meaning chest. Angina is chest pain or discomfort that occurs when the heart muscle does not receive enough blood due to narrowed coronary arteries. The pain – which is the pain of 'cramp' similar to what one may feel in a leg muscle deprived of blood after severe and prolonged exertion – occurs typically during physical exertion or stress and subsides with rest or medication. Stable angina is predictable in onset and eases at rest, but the quality of pain is the same as in unstable angina.*

3 *Unstable angina is more serious than stable angina. It occurs unexpectedly. Unstable angina can happen even at rest and is usually caused by the sudden reduction of blood flow to the heart due to a rupture of plaque in a coronary artery. This pain, although identical in quality to stable angina, is a warning sign of an impending heart attack and requires immediate medical attention.*

plaque

Atherosclerotic plaque (or plaque, for simplicity) is a mixture of cholesterol from the blood, inflammatory cells, scavenger cells, scar tissue, and calcium that accumulates as a lesion or plaque in the artery's wall. Its development can begin early in a person's life. Plaque is localised and often occurs at sites of 'wear and tear' within the artery. A person's circumstances, including age and sex, if the person smokes, has high cholesterol levels, high blood pressure, and/or diabetes, can combine to **influence** the development of CAD.

CAD is a patchy process. Autopsies have shown that generally a focal, localised plaque has led to the life-ending event. Within the same artery, there can be areas that may not be affected to the same extent or even at all.

Conceptually, most people can cope with symptoms like shortness of breath or chest pain on exertion, seeing them as manageable warning signs. Yet CAD is unpredictable; a seemingly tolerable level of disease can still give rise to SCD.

Autopsies after CAD-related SCD show that about **60 per cent** of the culprit plaques have been **flow-limiting**, or tight, before the event that led to death and, were **likely** to have given a clue by way of a **symptom**, such as chest pain or shortness of breath on exertion. This leaves about **40 per cent** that have been **non-flow limiting** before the event. In this case, the person has **no warning** and no chance to seek help.

The heart attack strikes suddenly. One in six will die – often a seemingly fit and healthy person.

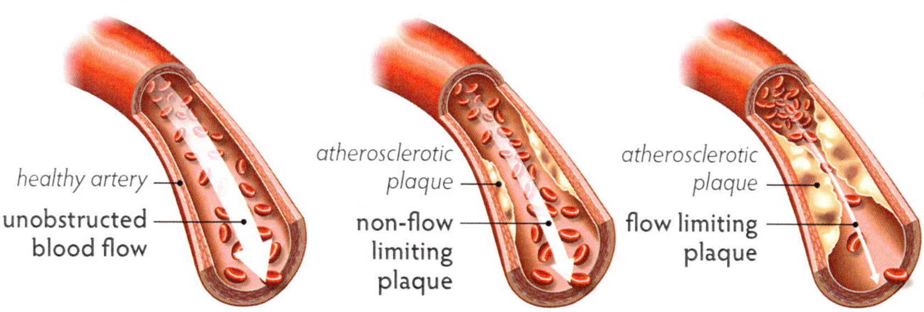

The components of non-flow-limiting (NFL) and flow-limiting (FL) plaque are the same, but are present to different degrees.

what goes wrong?

If we were to cut through the artery in cross section – either flow-limiting or non-flow-limiting – we would see the same structural components:

- the wall of the artery;
- the lumen (or inside space) of the artery;
- the plaque, which has built up under the inner (endothelium) layer of the artery wall and is beginning to intrude into the lumen, and
- a fibrous cap that encases the plaque, separating it from the blood.

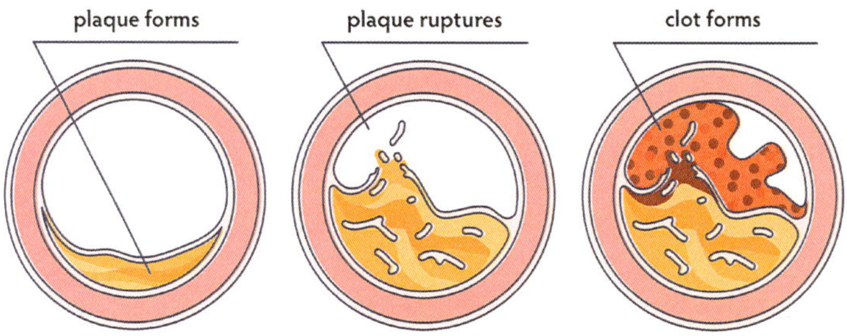

Plaque can cause havoc within the arteries in several ways:-

- **narrowing** (stenosis): Plaque reduces the space inside the artery (lumen), restricting blood flow and reducing oxygen delivery to tissues. This can cause symptoms like chest pain (angina). Good data suggest that if there were a narrowing of greater than 50 per cent, then the particular plaque involved could have event rates of over five per cent per annum. Over 10 years, this would be an event rate of approximately 50 per cent and, this alone, places the person in a high-to-very-high risk category;
- **rupture/thrombosis:** Plaques can rupture, exposing their contents to the bloodstream. This triggers clot formation (thrombosis), which suddenly blocks the artery and leads to acute events such as heart attacks or strokes;
- **destabilisation of the arterial wall:** Even without rupture, plaque erosion can destabilise the arterial wall and trigger clot formation, leading to partial or complete artery blockage;
- **aneurysm formation:** Plaque weakens the arterial wall, increasing the risk of bulging (aneurysm). If an aneurysm ruptures, it can cause life-threatening complications;

- **chronic inflammation:** The body's immune response to plaque creates inflammation in the arterial walls. Chronic inflammation further damages the arteries and promotes plaque instability;
- **reduced elasticity** (arterial stiffness): Plaque build-up reduces the elasticity of arteries, impairing their ability to regulate blood flow. This increases blood pressure, further stressing the heart;
- **embolisation:** Small fragments of plaque or blood clots can break off and travel through the bloodstream, potentially blocking smaller blood vessels and causing tissue damage in downstream organs, and
- **critical blockage in major arteries:** In coronary (heart) arteries, plaque build-up can lead to angina or heart attack. In carotid (neck) arteries, it can cause a stroke. In peripheral (arms and legs) arteries, it can result in peripheral artery disease (PAD).

dangerous

There are two types of plaque. **Calcified** plaque, which contains calcium but little cholesterol, is hardened, older, and generally more stable but, if it narrows the artery, it can cause angina. **Non-calcified** plaque is softer, cholesterol-rich, and more likely to rupture, potentially triggering a heart attack. These characteristics make it the more dangerous of the two. Plaques can be mixed.

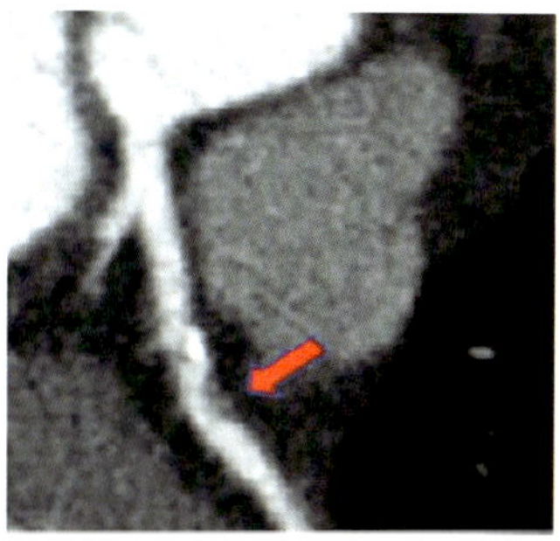

The dark spot on the coronary artery (arrowed) is a non-calcified, 'fatty' or unstable plaque, while the white spot above it is calcified (stable) plaque. Intensive treatment for an unstable plaque may **change** it to a stable plaque! (see from p 127 for more details)

When a **rupture** of the plaque's fibrous cap occurs, blood encounters the plaque contents. Platelets – the small particles responsible for blood clot formation when any abnormality is detected in the inside lining of the artery – rapidly start to cling together to form a clot that may progress to a complete blockage of the artery.

The **biggest concern** is that if it is a non-flow-limiting plaque, it will give no warning. Even a microscopic tear in the plaque's fibrous cap can lead to a clot, which can then rapidly block off that artery and be potentially life-ending.

A CLOSER LOOK

key statistics: cardiovascular disease (CVD)

The term cardiovascular disease covers several medical conditions affecting the heart and blood vessels, most commonly coronary artery disease (CAD), cardiac failure (CF), arrhythmia (electrical malfunction causing an irregular heartbeat), and stroke.

Even in the era of the COVID pandemic, CVD was the most common cause of death in the world and remains one of the most common causes of hospitalisations in the Western world.

Globally[1], it claims an estimated 17.9 million lives a year, about 32 per cent of all deaths.

The World Health Organization says that 85 per cent or about four out of five CVD deaths are due to heart attacks and strokes.

Of the annual 17 million premature deaths (under 70 years of age) due to non-communicable diseases in 2019, 38 per cent were caused by CVD.

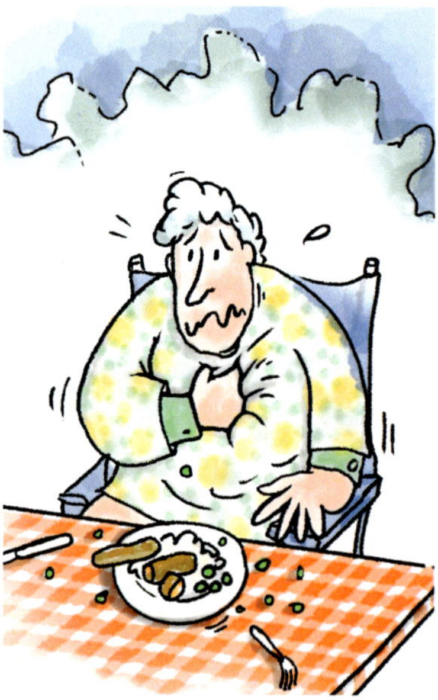

In Australia[2],

- one in four of all deaths is attributed to CVD as the underlying cause, meaning that one Australian dies of CVD every 12 minutes;
- the death rate is 40 per cent higher for men than women;
- 75 per cent of Australians are at risk of developing CVD, and
- CVD affects about one in six Australians and two out of three families.

Most people have a friend or a relative who has CVD. Many premature deaths from CVD are preventable.

---

1 *World Health Organization; https://www.who.int/news-room/fact-sheets/detail/cardiovascular-diseases-(cvds)*

2 *Heart Foundation; https://www.heartfoundation.org.au/bundles/for-professionals/key-stats-cardiovascular-disease*

IMPORTANT POINTS

CHOLESTEROL AND PLAQUE

- The major coronary arteries are critical to the heart's life-giving purpose of pumping blood and nutrients around the body and removing waste. They form a very vulnerable system.
- Atherosclerotic plaque (plaque) is the build-up of LDL particles and Lp(a) (and their cholesterol loads) and other material in an artery wall. That build-up leads to cardiovascular disease (CVD). In the heart, this is coronary artery disease (CAD), making plaque build-up a significant cardiac risk factor.
- Plaque can be flow-limiting (with symptoms including chest pain and shortness of breath on exertion) or non-flow-limiting (no symptoms – no warning before death strikes!).
- The structural components of both types of plaque are the same – the wall of the artery, the space inside the artery, the plaque and a fibrous cap separating the plaque from the blood.
- Even a microscopic tear can cause the fibrous cap of the plaque to rupture. Plaque's contents encounter blood, and the platelets (responsible for forming clots so that we don't bleed to death) go to work. A clot may progress to completely blocking the artery – and, potentially, a heart attack.
- Intensive treatment of the more dangerous non-calcified, cholesterol-rich, unstable plaque can transform it to a stable, calcified plaque and save lives.

Let's get to know more about the complexity of cholesterol as a risk factor.

cholesterol curiosities

Do pets have high cholesterol like humans?

Rarely. Dogs and cats process fats and cholesterol differently from humans. Even with high blood cholesterol, they are far less prone to developing atherosclerotic plaque unless another condition, such as diabetes or hypothyroidism, is present.

Do egg-laying animals use cholesterol differently?

Yes. Cholesterol is essential for embryo development, which is why egg yolks are naturally rich in cholesterol. It plays a key role in the formation of cell membranes and in supporting early growth.

Do wild animals develop atherosclerosis?

Very rarely. In the wild, most animals remain active, lean, and metabolically healthy throughout life. Atherosclerosis is more commonly seen in captive animals with restricted movement or altered diets.

Does cooking change the cholesterol content of food?

No. Cooking does not remove cholesterol, although it can change the structure of fats that accompany it.

Do cholesterol levels increase with age?

Often, yes. Cholesterol levels tend to rise with age, partly due to hormonal changes and metabolic shifts.

Was cholesterol always considered potentially harmful?

No. For much of the 20th century, cholesterol was regarded mainly as an essential biological substance. Its connection to cardiovascular disease gradually became evident through population studies, pathology findings, and clinical trials.

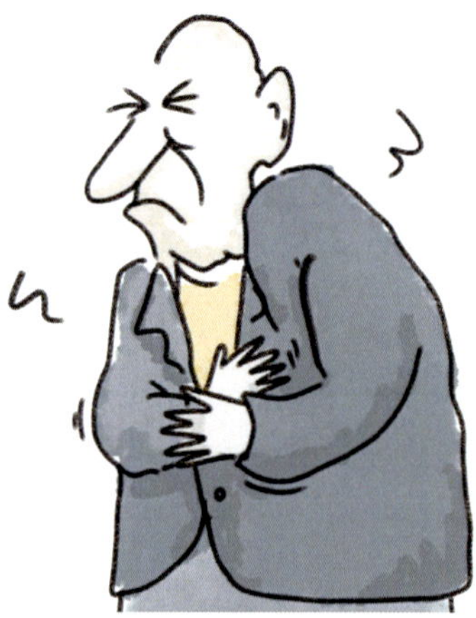

Ten to 15 per cent of people who suffer a heart attack die, and many will have no warning.

chapter 3

CHOLESTEROL TRANSPORT: ON THE MOVE

Building on the foundational concepts of cholesterol, we now delve deeper into the complexities of this life-sustaining and fascinating molecule as we explore cholesterol in the blood. This chapter provides important background for later chapters. You don't need to absorb every detail on first reading; it can be revisited as needed.

lipids

We call cholesterol a 'lipid', but what does that mean? Lipids are naturally occurring molecules – including fats, oils, hormones, and components of cell membranes – that do not mix with water (are hydrophobic). Along with proteins and carbohydrates, they are key building blocks of living cells.

Some examples of lipids are

- ***free fatty acids***, the building blocks of many lipids and include saturated, unsaturated, and polyunsaturated fatty acids;
- ***triglycerides***, the most common type of fat in the body and in food (three fatty acids attached to a glycerol molecule);
- ***phospholipids***, the key components of cell membranes (forming the bilayer) and the outer surface of lipoproteins. Their amphipathic nature (two fatty acid 'tails' and a phosphate-glycerol 'head') helps regulate movement of substances in and out of cells;
- ***sterols***, found in plant and animal cells where they are essential for maintaining cell membrane integrity and fluidity. Common examples include **cholesterol** (animals) and phytosterols (plants);
- ***waxes***, esters of fatty acids and long-chain alcohols, often found in plants and animals as protective coatings, and
- ***others***, including fat-soluble vitamins (such as vitamins A, D, E, and K), monoglycerides, and diglycerides.

Lipids are an essential component of all living cells, necessary for structure, function and energy storage. It is important to remember that while **all fats are lipids, not all lipids are fats**[1].

cells

Let's look more closely at the basic building blocks of life, the cells, where the lipid, cholesterol, plays a crucial role.

A biological cell is the fundamental structural and functional unit of all living organisms. Cells vary in size, shape, and function, but share key features: a cell membrane, cytoplasm, and genetic material (DNA or RNA). Some exist as independent organisms, while others specialise and form complex multicellular organisms, such as humans[2] and other animals. Cells are classified into prokaryotic cells, which lack a nucleus, and eukaryotic cells, which have a nucleus and membrane-bound organelles. These specialised units serve as the **foundation** of tissues and organs, enabling life to function at every level.

For our purposes, it is important to understand that a cell is not a solid sphere - an impression often given in illustrations. Instead, the cell membrane is a **dynamic, fluid**, and **porous** structure, regulating what enters and exits the cell. Cholesterol is a key component, maintaining membrane **fluidity, stability**, and **function**. Without it, membranes would become too rigid or too permeable, disrupting essential cellular processes.

Beyond structure, cholesterol plays a vital role in cellular **metabolism**,

---

1 *While all fats are lipids, not all lipids are fats means all fats belong to the lipid family, but the lipid family is much larger and includes other molecules that are not fats. Remember, FATS are composed of glycerol and three fatty acids and are primarily used for long-term energy storage and insulation). CHOLESTEROL is a lipid but not a fat; it is a sterol and plays key roles in cell membranes and hormone synthesis. PHOSPHOLIPIDS, which form the structural foundation of cell membranes, are lipids but not fats. TRIGLYCERIDES are both lipids and fats.*

2 *The smallest known cells are a group of tiny bacteria called mycoplasmas ... Cells of humans typically have a mass 400,000 times larger than the mass of a single mycoplasma bacterium, but even human cells are only about 20 μm across. It would require a sheet of about 10,000 human cells to cover the head of a pin, and each human organism is composed of more than 30,000,000,000,000 cells. [Britannica, https://www.britannica.com/science/cell-biology]*

signalling, and **transport**. It influences how cells communicate and respond to their environment, supporting hormone production, immune function, and nutrient exchange.

So, cholesterol is far more than simply a molecule linked to heart disease. It is essential for cell function and survival. Understanding its role at this cellular level helps clarify why it is vital for life, even as we work to manage its impact on health.

in the bloodstream

While we now know that cholesterol (the molecule) is critical to all cells, the remainder of the book will focus on **cholesterol that circulates within the bloodstream via lipoprotein particles**.

As we touched on earlier, there are two forms of that cholesterol: free cholesterol and cholesteryl esters. This cholesterol originates from two primary sources.

Firstly, the **liver**, which produces **about 80 per cent** through a pathway involving the enzyme beta-hydroxy-beta-methylglutaryl coenzyme A reductase (HMG-CoA reductase). The liver is important for how cholesterol in the blood is processed, recycled, and balanced in the body.

Secondly, the **diet**, focusing on foods that are high in cholesterol and, interestingly (as we will explain later), foods high in saturated fats.

The amount of cholesterol in the blood is also influenced by:

- the **intestines**, which play a significant role in how cholesterol from food is processed;
- **genetics**, which can determine how the body produces, processes, and clears cholesterol. Some people are very good **producers** of cholesterol in the body (hyper-responders) while others are very good **absorbers** of dietary cholesterol (hyper-absorbers). Genetics can also predispose individuals to familial hypercholesterolaemia (FH) or other lipid disorders, and
- nucleated **cells** which produce their own cholesterol, a minimal amount of which enters the blood.

liver

The liver, the central organ for cholesterol production, acts as the body's 'Grand Central Station' for lipid transport. At some stage of the process, all lipid transport is associated with the liver. Lipids are transported from:

- the **intestines** (where they are absorbed after ingestion/ digestion) to the liver, and
- the **liver** (where they are synthesised/reabsorbed/excreted/ recycled) to all parts of the body, and then back to the liver for processing, recycling or excretion.

transport logistics

As lipids are hydrophobic (water-repelling), they experience significant challenges in the bloodstream, which is just over 50 per cent water. Blood (or plasma) lipids include **TG, phospholipids, cholesterol, cholesteryl esters,** and unesterified long-chain **free fatty acids** (FFA). Of all the plasma lipids, FFA are metabolically the most active. They, too, are packaged into lipoproteins and help transport lipids – although not cholesterol – in the blood plasma.

in the circulation

Think about the fats in the milk you have in your refrigerator. As fats are not water-soluble and lighter than water, they 'float'. If the milk is not

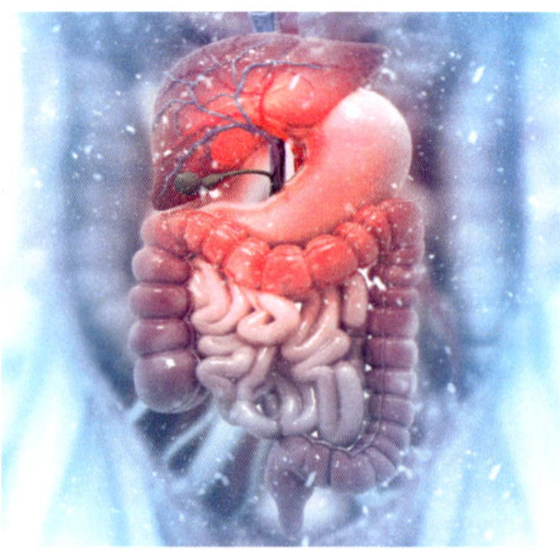

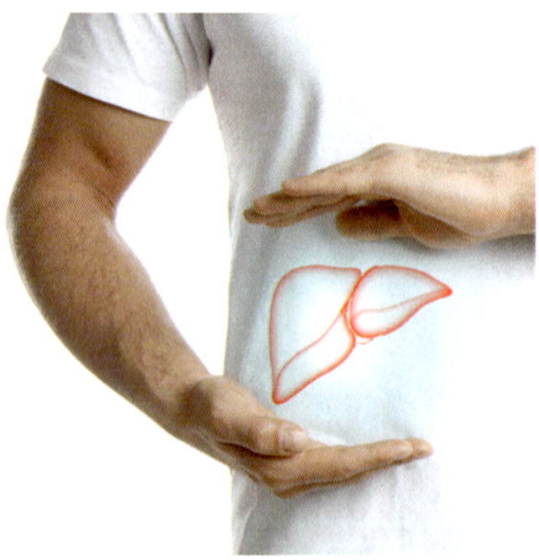

The human digestive system (left), shows the liver in the top left and the intestines in the lower half of the graphic; (right) shows the placement of the liver within the body.

homogenised, the fats will clump and float to the 'surface' like 'cream'. If the milk is homogenised, the fats are pulverised into such small particles that they 'float in suspension' in the milk, giving the illusion of being dissolved, but they are not.

The body doesn't have an inbuilt homogenisation process. Because the bloodstream is predominantly water, as is milk, lipids do not dissolve and so they 'should' clump together and float in the bloodstream. Physics tells us that, under these conditions, if you stood upright for any time, the lipids would float to the highest point – upwards, towards your brain! *Not good*! However, the body prevents this.

imagine ...

Think of it this way: highly specialised transport bubbles or pods (vehicles) move lipids (passengers) around the body (city).

Think ***vehicles***:

- small cars, family cars, mini-buses, and buses.

Think ***passengers***:

- men carrying a bag of shopping, and
- three-armed women carrying three bags of shopping, a bag in each hand.

Each vehicle can

- change size depending on the number of passengers,
- carry both types of passengers at the same time, and
- load and offload passengers as required.

As the vehicle picks up or drops off a passenger, it adjusts its size to fit its load. A small car becomes a family car, then a mini-bus, and then a bus as it takes on more passengers. Similarly, it shrinks as it drops off its passengers. This means the vehicle never travels half empty; **it is always the right size to hold its contents**. *How cool!*

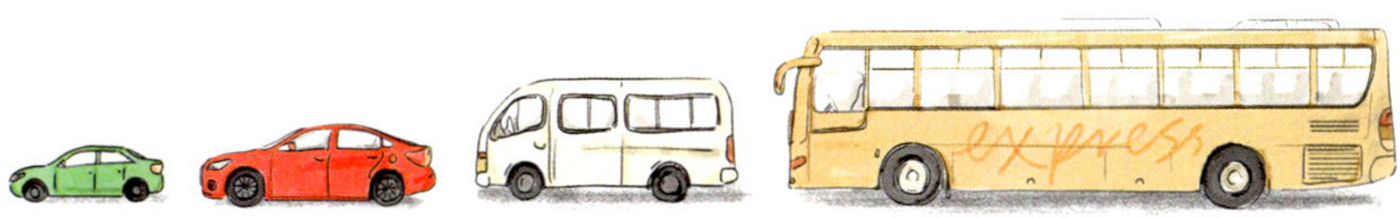

human body

Now, let's move this to our human transport system. The **vehicles become lipoproteins** (the carriers) and the **passengers become cholesteryl esters** and **TG** (the cargo).

Our vehicles (the lipoproteins) have two major structural components:

- **a chassis** (the specialised lipid – **phospholipid**[3]) that helps provide structure and stability to the vehicle (the lipoprotein), and
- **a docking connector** (the specialised protein – **apolipoprotein**) that defines where the vehicle (the lipoprotein) can dock and exchange its cargo (cholesteryl esters and TG).

what is a lipoprotein?

We know that lipoproteins are **complex particles** that **transport lipids** (including cholesterol and TG) through the blood. They consist of:

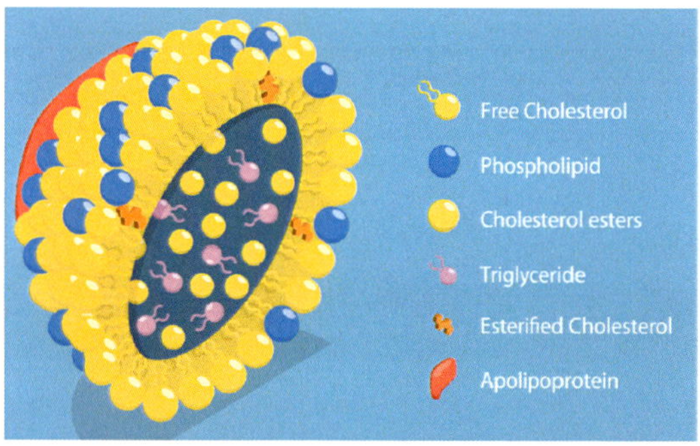

- a **core** of hydrophobic **lipids** (primarily cholesteryl esters and TG), and
- a **shell** of amphipathic[4] molecules, including **phospholipids**, **free cholesterol**, and **apolipoproteins** that stabilise the particle and allow it to interact with enzymes, receptors, and other lipoproteins.

As we will see in the coming pages, they are categorised into several

3 *Remember, phospholipids are both hydrophilic (water-loving) and hydrophobic (water-repelling). This dual property allows phospholipids to form a protective outer layer around the lipoproteins.*

4 *Amphipathic refers to a molecule with both hydrophilic (water-attracting) and hydrophobic (water-repelling) regions. This duality allows amphipathic molecules to interact with both water and lipids, making them essential for the structure and function of biological membranes and lipoproteins. For example, phospholipids in the lipoprotein shell have a hydrophilic head (interacts with water) and a hydrophobic tail (interacts with lipids in the core). This amphipathic nature helps stabilise lipoproteins in the aqueous environment of the bloodstream.*

types based on their **density** and **function** (including LDL and HDL) and to a lesser extent, size. **Each** has a **specific** role in transporting different types of lipids throughout the body.

A lipoprotein *(think of the inside and outside of our vehicles)* has

- an **outer, hydrophilic** (*hydro*, water; *philic,* love) surface (duco or exterior finish) that **loves** to be exposed to water and travels happily through the blood, and
- an **inside, hydrophobic** (*hydro*, water; *phobic*, fear) surface (leather seats) that **hates** water, where the lipids are carried.

Just as our imaginary vehicles can adjust their size to the number of passengers being carried, so can the lipoproteins.

male passengers	**cholesterol**
female passengers	**glycerol**
shopping bags	**fatty acids**
male + 1 shopping bag	**cholesteryl ester** (cholesterol + 1 fatty acid)
female + 3 shopping bags	**triglyceride** (glycerol + 3 fatty acids)

So, as more lipids are put into the lipoprotein, the bigger the lipoprotein becomes (small car ➡ car ➡ mini-bus ➡ bus). As the **lipoprotein grows**, the **density** (the protein:lipid ratio) of the particle **lessens**. Additionally, the woman with three shopping bags (TG) takes up more room than the man with one bag (cholesteryl ester).

So, the **largest lipoprotein particle** packed with the **most TG** (women with three shopping bags) will have the **lowest density** while the **smallest** lipoprotein particle containing the **least** TG will have the **highest** density.

apolipoproteins

As we have mentioned, apolipoproteins are a key component of the lipoprotein shell. These specialised proteins bind to hydrophilic lipids to help form cholesterol-carrying lipoproteins that can function in our watery bloodstream. The name breaks down like this: *apo* – meaning the protein part of, referring to the protein component of the lipoprotein; *lipo* – the fat or lipid; *protein* – the structural component made from amino acids. Apolipoproteins direct lipoproteins to where they are needed, enabling the transport of essential lipids and vitamins to cells.

Remember we said earlier that the company cholesterol keeps is crucial? **These apolipoproteins are that company**. Three are particularly important to us: **apolipoprotein A** (ApoA), **apolipoprotein B** (ApoB), and **apolipoprotein(a)** [apo(a)].

(You will learn more about these in the next chapter when we look at the specific lipoproteins with which they are associated.)

The apolipoproteins in the human body are **numerous and specialised**, each playing a distinctive role in lipid transport and metabolism. These roles range from maintaining lipoprotein structure to enzymatic activation and receptor binding. Despite their diversity, they work in harmony. However, ApoB-100 and apo(a) stand out as the **'bad' company** cholesterol can keep. *More soon!*

cell receptors

Just as apolipoproteins are specialised proteins involved in lipid transport and metabolism, cell receptors are **specialised proteins** that facilitate **communication between cells and their environment.** These receptors, including those that recognise apolipoproteins, play a

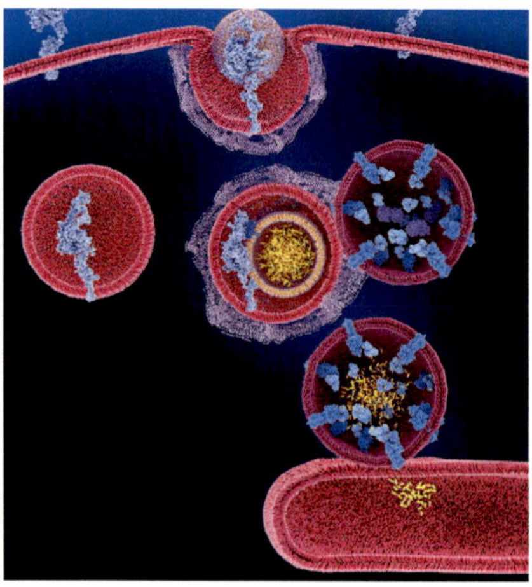

This graphic illustrates the **LDL receptor as a docking station** and the process of **endocytosis**. The docking of LDL particles onto the LDLR allows liver cells to bind and internalise LDL particles, removing them from the blood. Once bound, the cell membrane wraps around the LDL particle-receptor complex, forming a small pocket. This pocket then pinches off, creating a vesicle that transports the LDL inside the cell. Inside the cell, the vesicle will fuse with lysosomes, where LDL is broken down to release cholesterol for cellular use. It is as if the cell 'swallows' the substance – in this case, an LDL particle – in a tightly controlled process.

crucial role in cholesterol regulation, signal transduction, and the cellular uptake of lipoproteins. Cell receptors are found on the cell surface or inside the cell, where they bind to specific molecules - such as hormones, neurotransmitters, or lipoproteins - to trigger a cellular response. Membrane receptors embedded in the cell membrane respond to external signals, while intracellular receptors regulate gene expression in response to hormones.

LDL receptors

The most important cell receptors involved in cholesterol and lipid transport are the **low-density lipoprotein receptors** (LDLR). These membrane proteins are widely expressed, particularly on hepatocytes[5] and other cells where they act as 'docking stations'[6], and play a central role in regulating blood LDL-C levels. LDL particles bind to LDLR through their apolipoprotein B-100 (ApoB-100), in a manner often likened to a key fitting into a lock. (See the illustration on the previous page.)

The main function of the LDLR[7] is to **clear** LDL particles from the circulation by mediating their uptake into liver cells through endocytosis[8]. Within the liver, LDL particles are broken down: some of their cholesterol is converted into bile acids, which facilitate the digestion and absorption of dietary fats, while the remainder is repackaged into new lipoproteins and released back into the bloodstream for delivery to peripheral tissues. There, cholesterol is used for cell membrane synthesis and.

Properly functioning LDLR are essential for maintaining cholesterol homeostasis. Mutations or deficiencies in the LDLR gene impair LDL clearance, leading to elevated circulating LDL-C levels and an increased risk of atherosclerosis.

---

5 *The main functional cells of the liver, they are important in metabolism, detoxification, and protein synthesis.*

6 *This metaphor of a docking station where a ship or vehicle can attach itself for loading or unloading is very apt for LDL receptors and LDL particles as this 'docking' allows the liver cells to take up the LDL particles, removing them from the blood. (see graphic previous page)*

7 *The LDL receptor (LDLR) is present on all nucleated cells, but it is most abundant in the liver, which contains about 70% of the body's total LDLR pool.*

8 *Endocytosis is a process in which a cell takes in substances from outside by engulfing them with its cell membrane. The cell membrane wraps around the substance and forms a small pocket. This pocket then pinches off, bringing the substance inside the cell. It is as if the cells 'swallow' things, in this case LDL particles.*

IMPORTANT POINTS

CHOLESTEROL TRANSPORT

- The term 'lipid' encapsulates several naturally occurring molecules (including cholesterol) that do not mix well with water. Lipids are an essential component of all living cells.
- A cell is the basic unit of life, enclosed by a membrane and housing molecules vital for its function and survival. A cell is not a solid shape as the membrane is fluid and porous. Cholesterol helps regulate its fluidity and stability.
- About 80 per cent of blood cholesterol is produced in the liver. Other contributors are food, the intestines, genetics, and cells.
- Because lipids do not mix with water (are hydrophobic) and the body does not have its own homogenisation process, apolipoproteins (specialised proteins) combine with lipids to form lipoproteins (hydrophilic – water-loving). These lipoproteins transport the lipids, including cholesterol and TG, from the liver and intestines around the body and back again.
- Cell receptors are another specialised protein that have a crucial communication role between cells, lipoproteins, and their environment.
- LDL receptors (LDLR) help keep cholesterol levels in check as they remove LDL particles from the bloodstream.
- Genetic deficiencies in LDLR can reduce LDL uptake, raising LDL-C levels and atherosclerosis risk.

Now, it's time to discover more about the fascinating lipoprotein, that complex particle designed to transport hydrophobic molecules through the watery environment of the bloodstream.

chapter 4

LIPOPROTEINS EXPLAINED: TRANSPORT, TYPES, RISK

In the bloodstream, cholesterol transport does not automatically translate into harm. Risk emerges when certain lipoproteins dominate, persist, or behave differently. How does cholesterol transport become cardiovascular risk?

the good, the bad, the very bad, and the ugly

DR KOSTNER:

> *In the world of lipoproteins (and their content), not all players are equal. Some protect your heart, with cholesterol keeping 'good' apolipoprotein 'company', while others increase your risk of CVD by associating with 'bad' apolipoproteins.*

Dr K. puts the key lipoproteins (carriers) and lipids (cargo) that influence cardiovascular risk into context before we look at them more closely:

high-density lipoproteins (HDL), 'the good': HDL acts as the body's cholesterol cleaner, helping to transport excess cholesterol back to the liver for disposal. HDL is produced mainly in the liver.

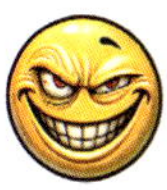

low-density lipoproteins (LDL), 'the bad': LDL is the primary carrier of cholesterol to tissues, but **excess** LDL particles can deposit cholesterol in artery walls, leading to plaque build-up and increasing the risk of CVD. It is formed as a waste product or the remnant of very-low-density lipoprotein (VLDL) metabolism.

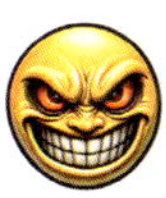

lipoprotein(a) [Lp(a)], 'the very bad': Lp(a) is an LDL-like particle that carries an extra, specialised protein, apolipoprotein(a) [apo(a)], that makes it stickier and more prone to promoting clot formation. An elevated Lp(a) level is a significant and independent risk factor for heart disease and stroke. It is **genetically** determined.

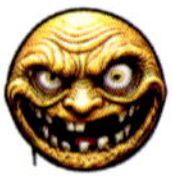

triglycerides (TG) 'the ugly': Triglycerides – a lipid that is a fat and one of the contents of lipoproteins – can contribute to atherosclerosis and, when levels are elevated, can amplify the harmful effects of LDL. They are produced in both the intestines (from dietary fat) and the liver (either 'new' or repackaged).

apolipoproteins and risk

What sets these lipoproteins apart – and determines whether they protect or harm your heart – is the **apolipoprotein** 'company' they carry. These **specialised proteins** guide lipoproteins to their **destinations**, influence their **function**, and ultimately shape their **impact** on cardiovascular health. Each type of apolipoprotein is linked to specific lipoprotein particles, defining their role in lipid metabolism and cardiovascular risk.

Apolipoprotein A **(ApoA)** is the major protein component of high-density lipoproteins **(HDL)** and plays a critical role in **reverse cholesterol transport** – removing excess cholesterol from the tissues and bloodstream. This helps prevent cholesterol build-up in arteries and is why HDL-C is termed 'good'. ApoA has two main types:

- **ApoA-I** is the major protein in HDL. It helps remove cholesterol from tissues, supports HDL formation, and activates lecithin-cholesterol acyltransferase (LCAT), an enzyme that helps process cholesterol. Higher levels of ApoA-I are linked to better heart health;
- **ApoA-II** is the second most common HDL protein. It helps stabilise HDL particles but its role in heart health is still debated.

Apolipoprotein B **(ApoB)** is essential for the transport of lipids in the bloodstream, and its main forms also have distinct roles:

- **ApoB-100** is found in VLDL, IDL (intermediate-density lipoproteins), and LDL and is directly linked to atherosclerosis, as it facilitates LDL-C delivery to tissues, including artery walls;
- **ApoB-48**, in contrast, is unique to chylomicrons and plays a role in transporting dietary lipids from the intestine. Unlike ApoB-100, it does not bind to LDL receptors (LDLR) and is rapidly cleared from circulation as chylomicron remnants are taken up by the liver.

The difference between ApoB-100 and ApoB-48 lies in their length.

ApoB-48 is a shorter form, lacking the LDLR-binding domain. While ApoB-100 is associated with 'bad' cholesterol and cardiovascular risk, ApoB-48 is involved in fat digestion and transport, with lower impact on atherosclerosis.

Apolipoprotein(a) **[apo(a)]** is the unique protein component of lipoprotein(a). Lp(a) resembles LDL but has this additional apo(a) protein attached to the ApoB-100 protein on the LDL particle. This gives Lp(a) its distinctive properties, including a strong tendency to promote atherosclerosis, thrombosis, and inflammation.

lipoprotein classes

remember

apolipoproteins (proteins) + **lipids** (including cholesterol and triglycerides) = **lipoproteins**

(the transporters of cholesterol, triglycerides, and other lipids throughout the body)

While apolipoproteins determine a lipoprotein's fate, it is the **structure and composition** of the lipoproteins themselves that dictate how cholesterol and other lipids **travel** through the body. Understanding these lipoprotein classes helps us see how they interact with cholesterol metabolism and cardiovascular risk.

In addition to FFA[1], the five main lipoprotein classes play a vital role both physiologically and in clinical assessment. We have already introduced two of them - HDL and LDL. The others are chylomicrons, very-low-density lipoproteins and intermediate-density lipoproteins. And not forgetting our 'very bad' and 'the ugly', Lp(a) – a lipoprotein, but different – and TG, which also play significant roles here. Let's get to know them better.

chylomicrons

Chylomicrons, which are central in transporting dietary fats to tissues and the liver, are produced in the enterocyte cells[2] in the lining of the

1 *Remember, free fatty acids also help transport lipids in the blood by binding to albumin, a blood protein that keeps them soluble. This allows FFA to circulate and serve as an energy source.*

2 *Enterocytes line the small intestine and play a key role in digesting and absorbing nutrients, especially fats, sugars, and amino acids. They reassemble monoglycerides and fatty acids into triglycerides (TG) and package these into chylomicrons, while also maintaining the protective barrier between the intestinal contents and the bloodstream.*

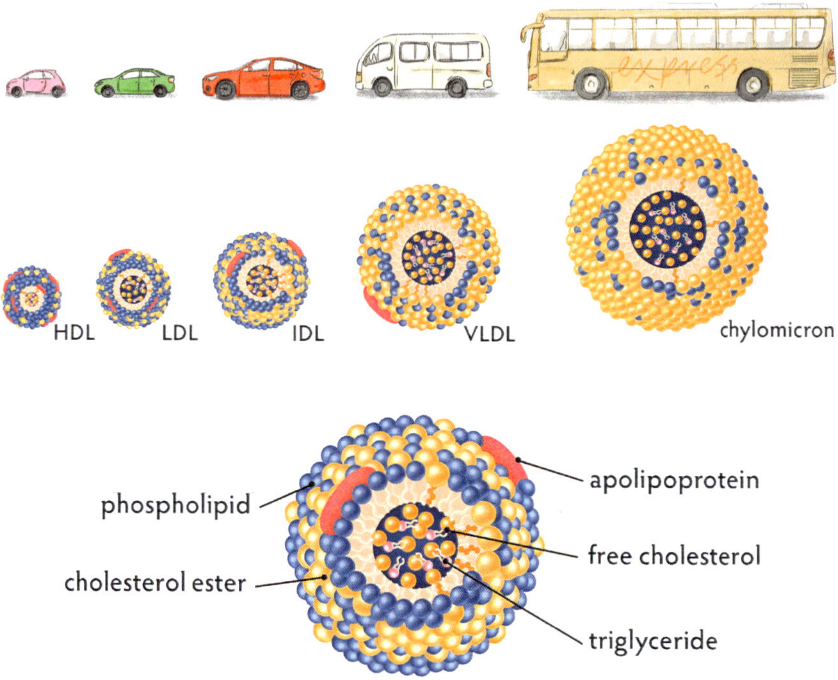

top: the five main vehicles **middle:** each of the five main lipoproteins and its structure
bottom: lipoprotein structure

intestines. This occurs after dietary lipids – including TG, cholesterol, and fat-soluble vitamins – are absorbed from food in the small intestine. They are packaged with apolipoproteins (mainly ApoB-48) to form nascent (immature) chylomicrons, which are released into the lymphatic system and enter the bloodstream through the thoracic duct[3].

In the bloodstream, nascent chylomicrons interact with HDL, which donate apolipoproteins (such as ApoC-II, ApoC-III, and ApoE) to form mature chylomicrons. ApoC-II activate **lipoprotein lipase** (LPL)[4], which

3 *The thoracic duct is the largest lymphatic vessel in the body, transporting lymph (including dietary fats in the form of chylomicrons) from the intestines and other tissues into the bloodstream via the left subclavian vein (a large blood vessel located beneath the clavicle, or collarbone, on the left side of the body. It plays a key role in returning blood from the upper body to the heart).*

4 *Lipase is an enzyme that breaks down TG into free fatty acids (FFA) and glycerol, aiding in fat digestion and lipid metabolism. Lipases are essential in processes such as dietary fat absorption (for example, pancreatic lipase) and lipoprotein metabolism (for example, lipoprotein lipase). LPL handles TG delivery to tissues as it hydrolyses TG in chylomicrons and VLDL to release FFA for energy or storage.*

break down TG in the chylomicrons into FFA and glycerol. ApoC-III, on the other hand, inhibit LPL activity and slow chylomicron clearance. The free fatty acids are either taken up by tissues for energy or stored as fat in adipose tissue. The water-soluble glycerol is released into the bloodstream and transported to the liver, where it can produce glucose or be recycled to form new TG.

After most TG are removed, the chylomicrons become **chylomicron remnants**, which are smaller and more dense, and contain **mostly cholesterol,** and some remaining TG. The liver removes chylomicron remnants from circulation through the use of a special protein, LDLR-related protein 1 (LRP1), which binds to ApoE. The lipids are recycled for other metabolic processes or converted into bile acids for excretion.

This whole process occurs over a few hours after a person has eaten a meal rich in fat.

very-low-density lipoproteins (VLDL)
intermediate-density lipoproteins (IDL)

Once the remnants of chylomicrons are cleared by the liver, the liver has its own way to dispatch lipids – enter VLDL, the liver's lipid delivery vehicle.

VLDL consist of mainly TG and some cholesterol in their core and are associated primarily with ApoB (specifically, ApoB-100). They are synthesised in the liver and secreted into the bloodstream to transport TG and cholesterol to tissues. As VLDL circulate, lipoprotein lipase breaks down the TG releasing FFA, which are taken up by muscle (for energy) or adipose tissue (for storage).

After losing a significant portion of their TG load, VLDL become smaller and more dense, transforming into IDL. Some IDL are taken up directly by the liver via LDLR on liver cells, which recognise ApoB-100 and ApoE on the IDL particle. The rest are further metabolised by hepatic lipase[5]. Losing more TG, they turn into cholesterol-rich LDL.

---

5 *ibid. (lipase) hepatic lipase is located on the surface of liver cells only and primarily hydrolyses TG and phospholipids in IDL and HDL, aiding in their conversion to LDL or smaller HDL particles.*

low-density lipoproteins (LDL)

LDL particles are formed as VLDL lose TG through lipoprotein lipase and hepatic lipase, passing through the intermediate IDL stage.

As IDL particles become more dense and cholesterol-rich, they transition into LDL – the body's main cholesterol transporters. LDL carry ApoB-100, which enables them to bind to LDLR on cells and deliver cholesterol for normal cellular function, helping maintain lipid balance. When LDL levels become too high or clearance is impaired (as in familial hypercholesterolaemia), excess LDL can remain in the bloodstream, where it may increase the risk of oxidation and trigger inflammation, promoting cholesterol deposition in artery walls, driving plaque formation and CVD.

Think of it like a car parked near the ocean. Prolonged exposure to salt air increases the risk of rust.

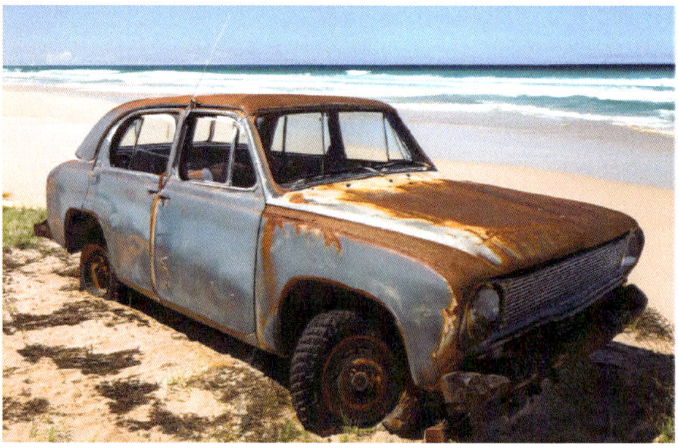

Similarly, prolonged exposure of high concentrations of LDL particles to the bloodstream increases the **likelihood** of plaque build-up.

The liver plays a crucial role in regulating LDL levels by removing particles through LDLR. Cardiovascular risk rises when this process is overwhelmed.

lipoprotein(a)

Lp(a) is often called a cholesterol paradox. Although it is structurally similar to LDL, its impact on heart disease is not only far **greater,** but also **independent** of routine cholesterol levels.

Lp(a) shares many of LDL's properties but is even more atherogenic due to the presence of the additional protein, **apo(a),** which is **unique** to Lp(a). This extra component makes Lp(a) **more prone** to promoting **plaque build-up** and **clot formation**.

A CLOSER LOOK

lipoprotein(a): inherited risk

Lipoprotein(a) [Lp(a)] is an **independent genetic risk factor** for CVD and plays a **major role** in heart attacks and strokes. It is especially dangerous if other risk factors such as high LDL-C are present and is often responsible for **younger patients** having cardiovascular events such as heart attacks and strokes.

GENETICALLY DETERMINED

Lp(a) levels are almost entirely **inherited**.

HIGHLY ATHEROGENIC DESPITE NORMAL CHOLESTEROL

A person can have normal or even low LDL-C levels but still face high cardiovascular risk if Lp(a) is elevated. This creates a paradox where 'normal' cholesterol does not guarantee low risk.

PRO-THROMBOTIC AND PRO-INFLAMMATORY

Lp(a) consists of an LDL particle to which a glycoprotein called apo(a) is attached. Apo(a) promotes **clotting** and **plaque formation, progression,** and **rupture**. This makes it even **more dangerous** than LDL-C alone, increasing the risk of heart attacks and strokes, **even in people without high cholesterol**.

INCREASED VALVULAR CALCIFICATION

Raised Lp(a) levels are also linked with premature development of calcified aortic stenosis.

POOR RESPONSE TO STANDARD LDL-C LOWERING THERAPIES

While most cholesterol-lowering drugs, including statins and ezetimibe, **do not** lower Lp(a), Dr K. recommends **early aggressive** LDL-lowering and **treatment of other risk factors** to **lower the risk** <u>**associated**</u> with significantly elevated Lp(a). Possible new treatments are under development. (See page 172.)

EVOLUTIONARY HYPOTHESIS: WHY DO WE HAVE IT?

Dr W. finds this very intriguing: Some researchers, including the famed, double Noble Prize-winning Linus Pauling, have explored the origins of Lp(a) and its potential evolutionary role. One theory suggests that Lp(a) evolved as a protective mechanism when humans and Old World monkeys lost the ability to produce vitamin C. It may have helped stabilise blood vessels in times of a lack of vitamin C, but in modern humans this adaptation has become a liability, contributing to CVD instead of preventing it.

Unlike LDL, which responds to medications and can be influenced by diet and lifestyle, Lp(a) levels are primarily determined by **genetics** and remain relatively **stable** throughout life. This makes it an independent and significant risk factor for CVD, one that standard cholesterol treatments currently (2026) do not effectively address.

atherogenic lipoproteins

The lipoproteins discussed above all contribute to plaque build-up in the arteries and share a common feature: **they contain ApoB-100**. Collectively known as atherogenic lipoproteins, they include **LDL**, which transports cholesterol to cells but can also deposit it in artery walls; **Lp(a)**, a particularly harmful LDL variant that promotes both plaque formation and clotting; and **TG**-rich particles such as VLDL, IDL, and remnant lipoproteins (RLP). These remnant particles are partially metabolised VLDL and chylomicrons that are cholesterol-rich and readily taken up by artery walls without needing prior oxidation, making them especially atherogenic.

These cholesterol- and TG-carrying particles play a central role in the development of atherosclerosis and CVD. Their regulation is therefore a major focus of both prevention strategies and treatment approaches.

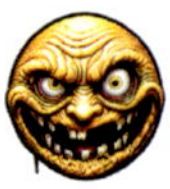

triglycerides (TG)

Beyond atherogenic lipoproteins, another important factor in cardiovascular risk is TG, the primary form of fat transported in the blood.

TG are carried by chylomicrons, which transport dietary-derived fats, and VLDL, which deliver liver-produced TG.

Elevated TG levels often accompany an excess of atherogenic lipoproteins, further contributing to plaque formation.

Managing TG levels, alongside LDL and Lp(a), is crucial for cardiovascular health.

high-density lipoproteins (HDL)

While the lipoproteins we have just discussed promote plaque build-up, HDL generally play the opposite role – removing excess cholesterol (reverse cholesterol transport) and returning it to the liver for disposal. Often called the cholesterol clean-up crew, HDL help protect against atherosclerosis by preventing cholesterol accumulation in artery walls.

HDL is synthesised in the liver and intestines as a disc-shaped, lipid-poor particle, primarily composed of ApoA-I and phospholipids. It gathers free cholesterol from peripheral tissues, including macrophages in arterial walls[6]. The enzyme lecithin-cholesterol acyltransferase (LCAT) esterifies the free cholesterol, allowing it to move into HDL's core and forming mature, spherical HDL particles.

Once mature, HDL particles transport cholesterol back to the liver for disposal or reuse. It interacts with the scavenger receptor class B type I (SR-BI) to deliver cholesterol directly to the liver. Some cholesterol is also transferred to LDL or VLDL via the cholesteryl ester transfer protein (CETP) for indirect removal. The liver eventually clears HDL particles, recycling ApoA-I and other particle components into new HDL particles.

Beyond cholesterol transport, they protect against atherosclerosis through multiple mechanisms. They prevent LDL oxidation by carrying antioxidant enzymes such as paraoxonase-1 (PON1), reducing inflammation and limiting immune cell activation. HDL also enhance endothelial function by promoting nitric oxide (NO) production, which helps blood vessels relax. In addition, HDL support the repair and renewal of the endothelium.

Through these combined effects, HDL particles help maintain healthy blood vessels and lower cardiovascular risk.

so, what is the risk factor?

Excess LDL-C is a key driver of plaque formation in arteries, but cardiovascular risk is influenced by more than just LDL-C levels. Both the **cholesterol content within LDL particles** and the **number of**

---

6 *This process is facilitated by ABCA1 (ATP-binding cassette transporter A1), which moves cholesterol from cell membranes to nascent HDL.*

A CLOSER LOOK

is HDL always protective?

DR KOSTNER

HDL (the high-density lipoprotein particle) is generally considered cardioprotective but occasionally this is not the case. Surprisingly, in some situations, HDL may increase cardiovascular risk.

A standard HDL-C measurement in a lipid panel does not indicate if HDL is 'beneficial', 'detrimental', or 'indifferent'. Similarly, a low HDL level does not always indicate increased risk.

HDL exists in different forms that vary in size, density, and function. The smallest lipid-poor forms, such as pre-β HDL, act as precursors, collecting cholesterol from tissues. As HDL matures, it transforms into HDL-3, a denser form involved in early cholesterol transport, and then into HDL-2, which carries more cholesterol and is generally considered the most protective.

HDL particles are highly dynamic, constantly changing shape and composition. As they accumulate lipids, discoidal HDL evolves into spherical HDL, facilitating reverse cholesterol transport – a process that removes excess cholesterol and supports cardiovascular health.

However, not all HDL is beneficial. Under certain conditions, HDL can become dysfunctional and may even contribute to atherogenesis. Factors such as oxidative stress, inflammation, and metabolic disorders can impair HDL function, making it pro-inflammatory and pro-oxidant. Instead of protecting blood vessels, dysfunctional HDL may promote LDL oxidation and contribute to cholesterol build-up.

In conditions like diabetes and chronic inflammation, HDL's role in reverse cholesterol transport can be compromised. Some small, dense HDL particles may also become trapped in plaques or fail to interact effectively with receptors, further reducing their protective function.

This is why focusing solely on HDL-C levels in a standard lipid panel can be misleading. More advanced lipid testing (currently still at the research stage) – including assessments of HDL function, cholesterol efflux capacity, and HDL subtypes – is beginning to offer a clearer picture of HDL's true impact on cardiovascular health.

LDL particles contribute to atherosclerosis, with size and density also influencing their atherogenicity.

To complicate matters, while higher LDL-C generally suggests more LDL particles, this relationship isn't always linear. Additionally, other atherogenic lipoproteins – such as VLDL and IDL – also play a role in plaque build-up, further increasing cardiovascular risk.

Since all these atherogenic particles contain ApoB-100, **measuring ApoB levels provides a more accurate picture of the total number of particles contributing to atherosclerosis**. **Elevated ApoB-100** is strongly linked to increased cardiovascular risk, making it **one of the most important markers** to consider.

IMPORTANT POINTS ✓

LIPOPROTEINS EXPLAINED

- Lipoproteins are complex particles that transport hydrophobic lipids, including cholesterol, through the bloodstream.
- They are categorised into several types depending on their density and function:
    - chylomicrons, derived from the intestines after absorption of dietary fats and lipids
    - very-low-density lipoproteins (VLDL), made by the liver
    - intermediate-density lipoproteins (IDL), made from VLDL as the VLDL offload TG around the body
    - low-density lipoproteins (LDL), remnants of VLDL metabolism as IDL release more TG and become more cholesterol-dense
    - high-density lipoproteins (HDL), made by the liver mainly, and intestines, they have a key role in reverse cholesterol transport, taking cholesterol back to the liver for reprocessing or excretion.

continued next page

IMPORTANT POINTS

LIPOPROTEINS EXPLAINED

from the previous page

- LDL / HDL is the lipoprotein carrier, while LDL-C or HDL-C is the cholesterol being transported by the respective lipoprotein particle in the bloodstream.
- Impaired clearance or excessive production of LDL can cause LDL-C levels to build up in the bloodstream. This increases cardiovascular risk.
- While LDL-C is measured in a lipid profile, cardiovascular risk is influenced significantly by **both** the number of LDL particles and the amount of cholesterol they carry.

Next, we explore how plaque forms – and why it matters.

chapter 5

PLAQUE FORMATION: A SLOW, HIDDEN PROCESS

Plaque build-up is a slow, complex process that can begin early in life and remain unnoticed for decades. It starts silently, often long before any symptoms appear. A small, seemingly harmless deposit of cholesterol within an artery wall can, over time, trigger a cascade of events that narrows blood vessels, reduces blood flow, and can lead to a heart attack or stroke.

What causes this build-up? Why do some people develop dangerous plaques while others do not? Understanding how and why plaque forms is crucial for preventing CVD and managing risk before it becomes a life-threatening emergency.

The basics of plaque formation tell us that cholesterol and other substances accumulate within artery walls, the body reacts and over time, this complex process can lead to blockages and ruptures. Different forms of plaque exist and not all are equally dangerous. However, there is much more to this.

complexities

Not all cholesterol behaves the same way, and plaque differs in its risk. Some plaques remain stable for years, while others rupture unpredictably, triggering sudden cardiac events.

Raised cholesterol levels do not always mean a person will develop plaque. In our practices, we see patients who have:

- elevated cholesterol and significant plaque build-up in their arteries;
- elevated cholesterol but surprisingly little or no plaque;
- average-to-low cholesterol but with severe arterial disease, and
- low or average cholesterol with healthy arteries.

Clearly, the relationship between cholesterol levels and arterial health is more complex than 'high cholesterol equals bad arteries' and 'low cholesterol equals good arteries'. While some people with high cholesterol do not develop CAD or CVD, it is far more common for elevated cholesterol levels to lead to plaque formation, heart attacks, and strokes.

To unravel this mystery, let's look more closely at plaque deposition and build-up – and where this process might lead.

We will examine this sequentially:

- the site – the coronary arteries
- the problem – plaque
    - how it develops
    - its consequences
- the role of cholesterol.

coronary arteries

When a baby is born, its new, healthy arteries are plaque-free. A healthy artery consists of (diagram right, from the top):

- an **inner layer** of endothelial cells,
- a **middle layer** of smooth muscle cells, and
- an **outer layer** of collagen.

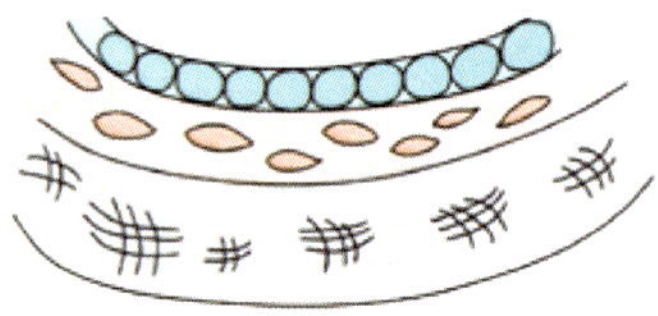

The **inner layer** (*tunica intima* – meaning inner coat) is a smooth lining made from sheets of cells called the **endothelium** (*endo* – inside; *thelium* – skin). This unique layer of cells is coated by the **glycocalyx**, a carbohydrate-rich layer that acts as a protective shield and helps ensure the blood's contents run smoothly through the artery without sticking or clumping to the side walls. Together, the glycocalyx and endothelium function as a 'Teflon lining', with the endothelium also responding to stress within the artery, communicating with the muscle layer of the artery to influence relaxation or contraction.

The **middle layer** (*tunica media* – middle coat) is made up predominantly of muscle cells. These are special muscle cells called smooth muscle. They are different from the muscles in your leg, which are skeletal muscles (or, in your heart, for that matter, which is cardiac muscle). Nerves do not control smooth muscles in the way they control skeletal muscles, but smooth muscle responds to the automatic regulatory systems of the body. (You find smooth muscle in the wall of the stomach, gut, bladder, and ureters.)

If you were to be frightened, the body's autonomic (automatic) nervous system (ANS) would go into overdrive, pumping adrenaline into the bloodstream, as well as activating the special nerves of the ANS, leading to stimulation of the artery's smooth muscle. As the smooth muscle contracts, it narrows the artery. Blood pressure (BP) increases as the same amount of blood is pumped through narrower arteries. So, this layer of the artery has a significant influence on BP regulation. (Dr W.: Oversimplified, but this conveys the basic idea.)

The **outer layer** (*tunica adventitia* – outside coat), the main scaffold of the artery, consists of collagen, the tissue that binds together almost all tissues in the body. The outer walls of the major arteries are, and must be, very tough to deal with years of pulsating blood being forced through the body. Interestingly, the stretch and recoil of the walls of those big arteries act as a secondary pump for the body, maintaining the flow between heartbeats.

how does plaque develop?

Plaque formation is a site-focused process that begins early, potentially starting in adolescence. It is closely linked to areas in the arteries that experience constant wear and tear such as the proximal regions (closer to the aortic root) and branch points. This makes **aging** the most significant **non-modifiable risk factor** for atherosclerosis. To some degree, atherosclerosis can be viewed as the body's response to this wear and tear - *a form of healing*, if you will.

It is important to understand that mechanical stress on arterial walls puts physical strain on the cells of the artery, triggering an inflammatory response. This response is part of the body's natural healing process, aimed at repairing damage. However, when LDL and other risk factors are present, this healing process can be disrupted, leading to the formation of unstable plaques that may block arteries or rupture, accelerating CVD progression.

cholesterol

LDL (the particle), LDL-C and Lp(a) play central roles in this process. **The greater their concentration in areas of arterial damage, the higher the likelihood of adverse plaque development.** Conversely, lowering LDL-C and, if possible, Lp(a) slows plaque progression.

While LDL is central to the development of atherosclerosis, LDL-C is the key modifiable factor influencing both the extent of plaque build-up and its potential to cause harm. It also raises an intriguing question: Could CAD begin not as a disease at all, but as a healing process that, when exposed to factors like raised LDL-C and Lp(a), goes awry?

inflammation

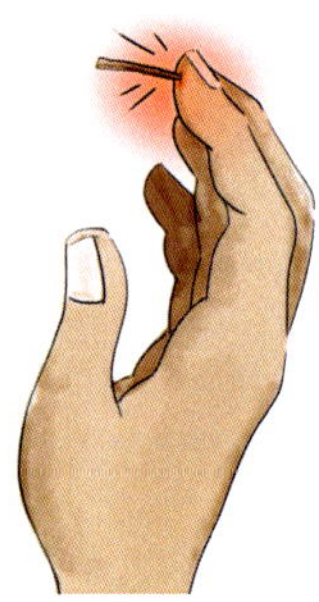

Consider a common scenario: a splinter in your finger. This simple event helps illustrate the complex process of inflammation and cholesterol build-up. When an injury occurs, the body launches an inflammatory response. Damaged cells release chemical signals that attract white blood cells, which rush in to clean up debris and begin repair. Macrophages, a type of immune cell, consume cellular waste, clearing the way for healing. The influx of blood to the area causes redness, warmth, swelling, and pain as inflammatory chemicals flood the site.

A similar process occurs in the arteries. Plaque formation begins when the inner lining of an artery, the endothelium, is injured or becomes dysfunctional. This can result from high blood pressure, smoking, diabetes, poor diet, physical inactivity, or the normal mechanical stress from blood flow as we have already discussed.

When the endothelium is injured, **LDL** particles penetrate the artery wall, contributing to an immune response. Some may become oxidised, forming the more atherogenic oxidised LDL (oxLDL).

The body recognises oxidised LDL as a foreign substance and sends in monocytes, which transform into **macrophages**[1]. These macrophages

1 *Monocytes are a type of white blood cell that circulate in the bloodstream, ready to respond to injury or infection. When they reach damaged tissue, such as an injured artery wall, they transform into macrophages. These larger, specialised cells engulf harmful substances*

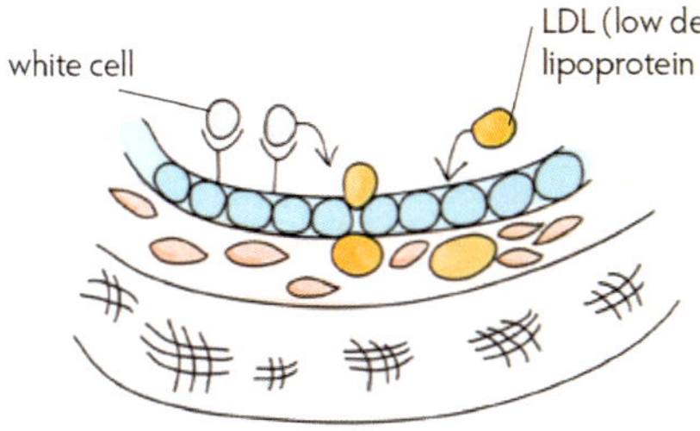

at the site of damage to endothelium

White cells and cholesterol (LDL) are drawn into the artery at the site of damage or trauma to the endothelium.

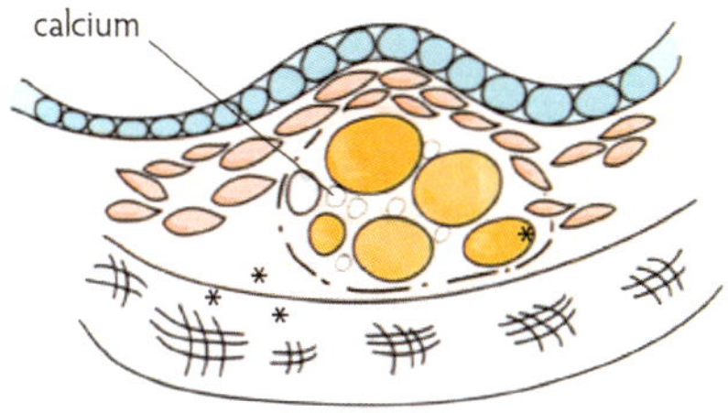

development of plaque

White cells and cholesterol collect in plaque as macrophages and lead to scarring. Calcium moves into scarred areas of plaque.

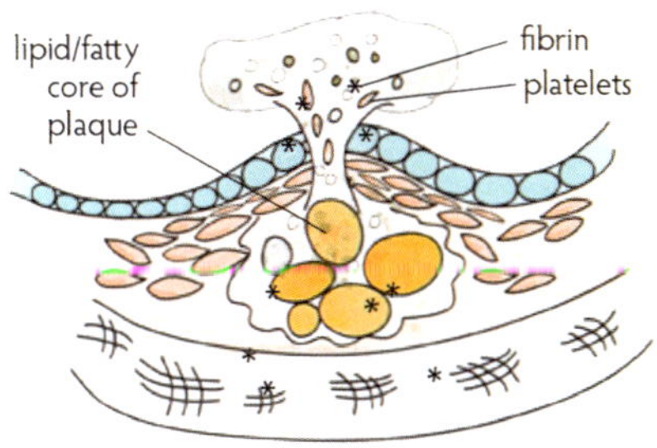

rupture of plaque and formation of clot (thrombosis)

Blood contents react with the contents of the plaque when it ruptures. A clot forms.

engulf the oxidised LDL and transform into **foam cells**, which accumulate and contribute to the growth of a **fatty, non-calcified plaque.**

At first, this process is protective – a natural repair mechanism. But over time, as more foam cells accumulate, die, and spill their contents, the plaque grows larger and more unstable. The mix of cholesterol, cellular debris, enzymes, collagen and fibrin scaffolds, and calcium are the basis of atherosclerosis. As this process evolves, plaques begin to differ in how they behave based on the body's healing process and the presence or absence of associated risk factors (the more risk factors, the more dangerous they become). **Not all plaque is equally harmful.** Some plaques – rich in calcium and encased by a thick fibrous cap – remain stable for years (especially if people are on cholesterol therapy), posing little immediate risk. Other plaques, however, are thin-capped, cholesterol-rich, and highly vulnerable to rupture.

---

like oxidised LDL, playing a key role in both immune defence and the development of fatty plaques in atherosclerosis.

When a plaque ruptures, its contents spill into the bloodstream, triggering a clot that can suddenly block an artery and cause a heart attack or stroke. This helps explain why some individuals with significant plaque but only minimal plaque narrowing can suffer major events, despite being asymptomatic.

Interestingly, a narrowed artery isn't always the biggest danger. Many heart attacks occur when non-obstructive plaque ruptures unexpectedly, leading to a complete arterial blockage. This is why even individuals with moderate cholesterol levels and no prior symptoms can still be at risk.

Ironically, it may all begin as a **healing process**. This focal inflammation explains why CAD is a patchy process – why one person may have only a single plaque that leads to a fatal event. It also underscores why blood cholesterol levels alone do not precisely predict cardiovascular risk. **The real danger lies in the interplay between how much cholesterol is present and where and how inflammation occurs in the arteries.**

IMPORTANT POINTS

PLAQUE FORMATION

- A healthy coronary artery consists of an inner 'Teflon-like' layer of endothelial cells, a middle layer of smooth muscle cells, and an outer layer of collagen.
- The build-up of plaque begins with inflammation (the body's response to damage or attack), and is accelerated by increased LDL and oxidation. This is a process that starts early and develops over many years.
- The formation of plaque, ironically, likely begins as a process to heal, yet can end in death.

You are now equipped with the basics of inflammation and plaque build-up. Let's drill down into the interesting detail that begins to explain some of the cholesterol controversy.

chapter 6

PLAQUE DEVELOPMENT: A PATCHY PROCESS

Atherosclerosis – the build-up of plaque (cholesterol, fatty substances, cellular waste, and calcium) in the arteries – is patchy in that there is no specific area in which it might manifest. This is important as it means that **focal factors** in the artery **must** play an **essential role** over and above the traditional risk factors that we think about in the setting of CAD.

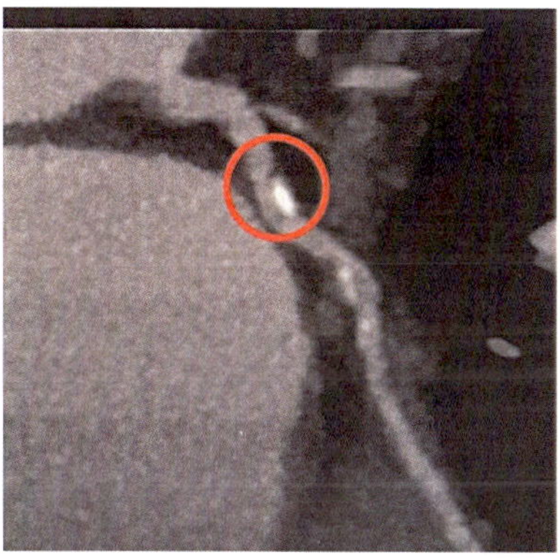

image 1

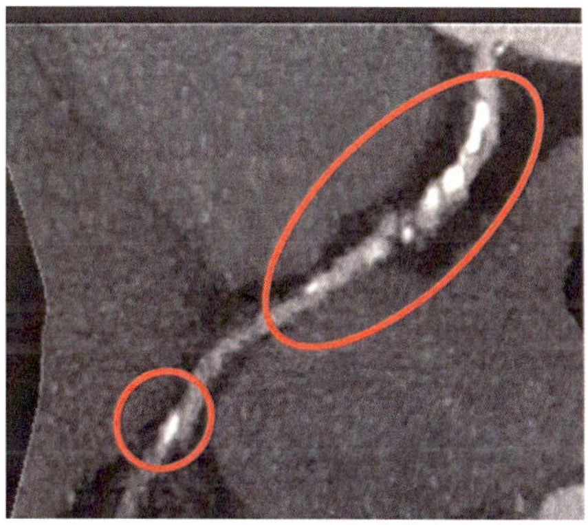

image 2

These images show the right coronary artery (image 1) and the circumflex artery (image 2) in the same patient. You can see the affected parts of each artery circled by red rings. You can also see parts of the artery are not affected.

In this patient, the cholesterol levels, blood pressure, exercise undertaken, diet, age, smoking status, diabetes or prediabetes (if applicable) – essentially all the risk factors – would be equally represented along the arteries. Yet, they result in uneven plaque distribution.

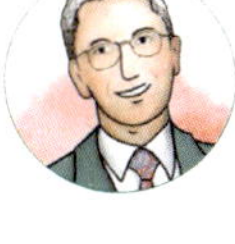

Pause and think about this for a moment. What comes next is important.

If cholesterol were primarily central to the process and had the same concentration throughout the bloodstream – which it does – then the deposition of cholesterol through the artery **should** be uniform. Yet, it isn't. Rather, while each of the above-mentioned risk factors can contribute, the process must be focal and local.

shear stress

Within an artery, a significant mechanism for damage will arise from the shear stress generated by a combination of blood pressure, the viscosity of the blood, and the shape of the artery.

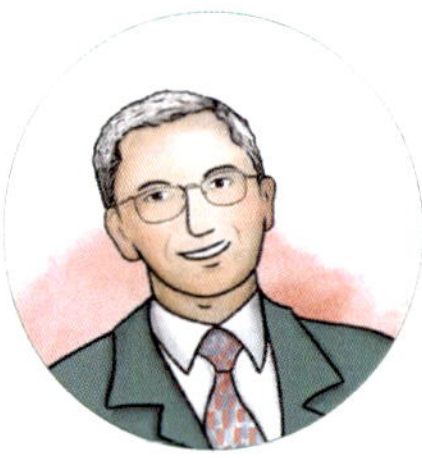

Interestingly, this pattern of injury and repair is central to what's known as the clotting hypothesis of atherosclerosis (still unproven) – the idea that tiny, repeated injuries to the vessel wall trigger small clots as part of the healing process. Over time, these layers of clot material – mainly fibrin and platelets – can become incorporated into the artery wall, contributing to the growth of atherosclerotic plaque.

shape

Think of the complex area of flow dynamics. A meandering river provides an example (see right). At a bend in the river, the water flow along the inside of the bend is slower than the water along the outside of the bend. Debris is deposited along the inside of the bend by the slower-moving water, while the faster-moving water will undercut the land along the other bank. This interplay of deposit and shear stress plays out in the arteries in a way well beyond the scope of this text. However, we want you to appreciate the complexity of the process.

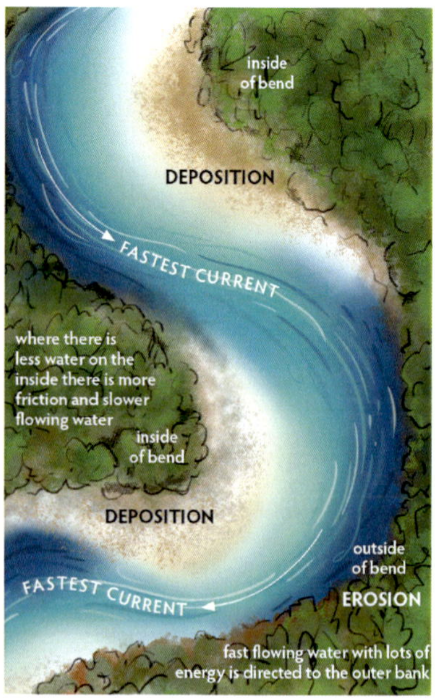

volume

While the shape of the river impacts flow, so does the volume of water in the river. After rain, for example, with more water moving more rapidly, the bank suffers greater scouring by the water moving through the outer curve of the bend, causing erosion of the bank.

Coronary arteries have the same fluid dynamics (haemodynamics), with faster and slower blood flow related to the outside and inside of the curve within the artery. Wear and tear, deposition and erosion, are similarly driven by the amount of blood and its pressure as it flows along the artery.

Clinically, this is the **heart rate** and, very importantly, **blood pressure**. These differences in shear stress within the arteries help us understand CAD's focal nature.

are all LDL-C levels the same?

Why is there an apparent difference in the propensity to deposit plaque in the arteries between individuals with similar LDL-C levels? This variance leads to confusion and contributes to the cholesterol controversy.

(lipoprotein) particle size

Particle size comes up frequently and is considered by some to be central to explaining the presence or absence of plaque in a person's arteries. We are about to consider what particle size means. However, from the outset, we want to make it clear that we believe **ALL LDL-C increases the risk of plaque build-up and CVD.**

In recent years, cholesterol research laboratories have identified that LDL can vary in size, density, and composition: **large and fluffy**, or **small and dense** particles.

This is important.

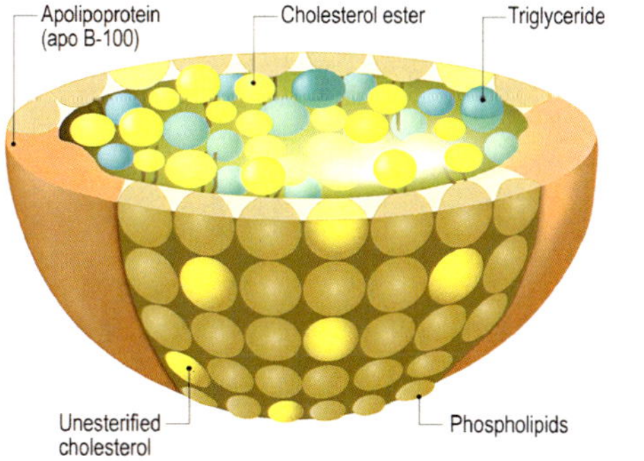

low-density lipoprotein (LDL) structure

Two individuals may have

the same LDL-C levels but very different particle numbers, with the greater particle number conveying the greater risk.

The theory is that smaller particles can pass more readily through the fenestrae, which are pore-like holes found on the internal wall (endothelium) of the artery. These small, dense particles end up within the wall of the artery and so contribute to the formation of the plaque. While this sounds plausible and holds some truth, the small, dense particles tend to be linked to other potential risk factors such as elevated TG levels, reduced HDL-C levels, and increased insulin levels (generally in prediabetic and diabetic patients).

That a small, dense particle can enter through the endothelial openings more readily than a large fluffy particle is a persuasive concept and one to which many 'Google research' patients cling. While it is not a 'fat' lie, neither is it the unifying truth.

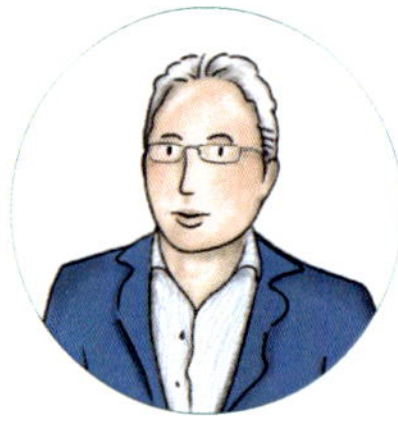

Furthermore, the presence of small, dense particles in an individual's lipid profile is almost negligible if the TG-to-HDL ratio is 1.0:1.3 or lower.

Let's scale it up to something to which we can relate. Imagine that

- a fenestra (hole on an endothelial cell) is the size of a basketball ring,
- the large, fluffy LDL particle is as big as a basketball,
- the small, dense particle is the size of a volleyball.

Imagine standing on the free throw line and tossing both balls at the hoop. You will likely shoot more volleyballs into the ring. However, plenty of basketballs will drop as well. They are the right size, after all.

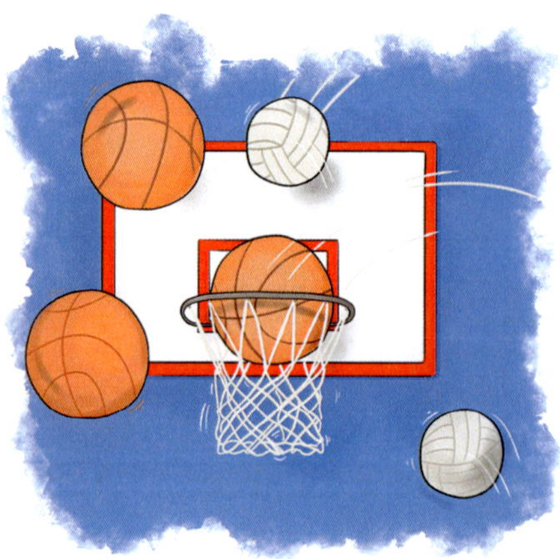

MAKE NO MISTAKE: both large and fluffy AND small and dense LDL particles will pass through a fenestra.

(lipoprotein) density

Density measures mass per unit volume – how much matter is packed into a specific space (in this case, an LDL particle). A small change in sphere diameter – like the difference between a basketball and a volleyball – can significantly impact density. Remember, density relates to the radius (half the diameter) raised to the power of 3, so a **small radius change** results in a **significant density change**. Hence, some small, dense and large, fluffy particles are surprisingly close in size.

this is important

Some proponents of the particle size theory, especially in popular and social media, suggest that 'large, fluffy' LDL particles are protective and only 'small, dense' LDL particles are harmful. **This is simply not true**. Having 'large, fluffy' LDL is certainly better than 'small, dense', as particle size is directly related to metabolic health. Small, dense LDL are linked to raised TG, low HDL-C, and elevated insulin levels (diabetes and prediabetes) – each a factor of significantly increased cardiovascular risk.

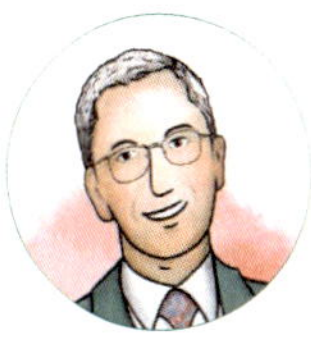

Remember, given enough attempts and time, plenty of basketballs will also pass through the ring!

I, Dr K., see many families with genetically very high cholesterol levels – familial hypercholesterolaemia (FH) – which we will explore in more detail in chapter 20. Most of them develop CAD. This is not a matter of 'if' but 'when'.

We also see seemingly fit and healthy adults having coronary events prematurely, men in their 40s to 50s and women a decade later. Many of these individuals do not have high levels of small, dense LDL particles, yet their overall LDL burden is so high that excessive particle numbers overwhelm the endothelial fenestrae, allowing more to penetrate.

So, while cholesterol levels and particle numbers are important, there's another layer of complexity: the inherent characteristics of the particles themselves.

IMPORTANT POINTS

PLAQUE DEVELOPMENT

- Plaque build-up within coronary arteries is a focal and patchy process.
- Localised factors are significant in consideration with CAD's traditional risk factors.
- Shear stress – generated by a combination of blood pressure, blood viscosity, and artery shape – is a significant mechanism for damage of the artery walls.
- LDL particle size can be very misleading in the cholesterol conversation as **all** LDL-C, Lp(a), and ApoB-containing particles are 'bad' and a significant risk factor.

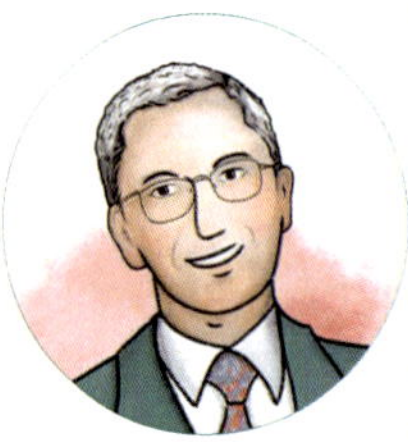

Before we conclude our discussion on plaque development, we would like to mention there are several other unproven hypotheses. Professor Vladimir Subbotin, for example, proposes that atherosclerosis may originate – not from lipid entry through the arterial lumen – but from the outer arterial layers via the vasa vasorum (small blood vessels), particularly in response to low oxygen levels in a thickened arterial wall. Importantly, whether plaque forms from the inside out or the outside in, it is accelerated by increased LDL particles.

Particle size is interesting, but not the whole story. Next, we look at inherited traits that influence how lipoproteins behave.

chapter 7

CARDIOVASCULAR RISK: FACTORS YOU CAN'T CONTROL

By now, it is clear that LDL is the primary lipoprotein that concerns us. As a remnant of VLDL off-loading its TG, LDL continues to carry cholesterol from the liver throughout the body, serving as the source of cholesterol in the arteries. As described in the previous chapter, this particle can be big and fluffy or small and dense. While we have already looked at some of the details of the almost incomprehensible complexity of these particles, let's dive a little deeper.

proteins (apolipoproteins)

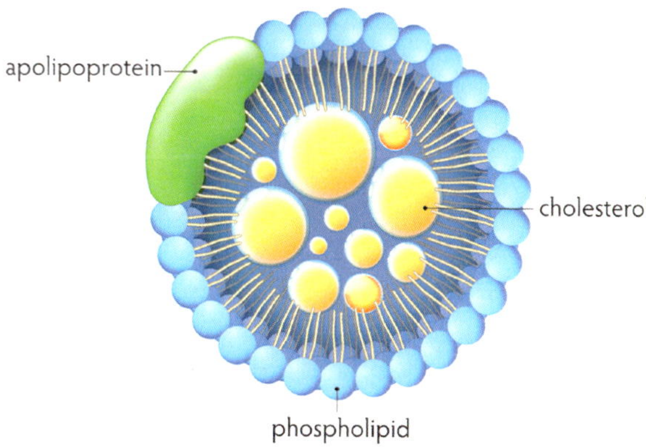

We have examined the structure of **lipoproteins**, those wonderfully intricate miniature Ferrero Rocher-like spheres of apolipoproteins, phospholipids, cholesterol, cholesteryl esters, and TG that carry the cholesterol in the bloodstream, giving it to the tissues as needed.

Now, let's focus on the proteins with these particles: the **apolipoproteins**[1].

All proteins are based on each person's unique DNA, received from parents, and made through a two-step process.

1 *Remember, apolipoproteins are proteins that combine with lipids to form lipoproteins. They play a crucial role in lipid metabolism and transport, particularly in the bloodstream. These proteins are involved in regulating the movement of cholesterol and other lipids throughout the body.*

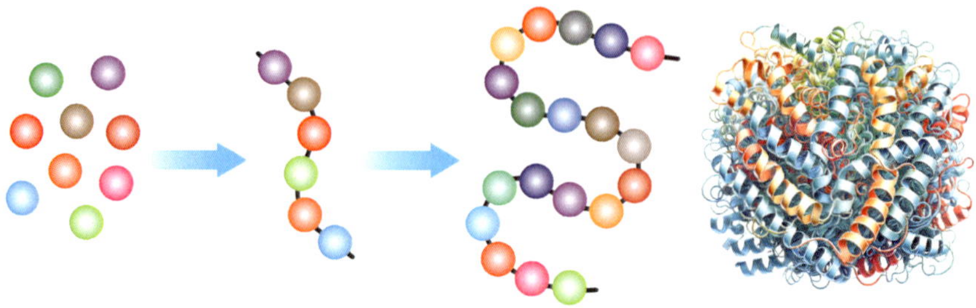

Inside the cell's nucleus, a specific section of DNA is copied into a molecule called messenger RNA (mRNA)[2]. Then, this mRNA leaves the nucleus and goes to a ribosome[3] in the cell's cytoplasm[4]. The ribosome reads the mRNA sequence and assembles amino acids[5] in the correct order, linking them together to form a chain called a peptide[6]. As the peptide chain grows, it eventually folds into a specific shape, becoming a functional protein (see above). This process ensures that the proteins, which are essential for various body functions, are created based on the instructions from our DNA.

Think of siblings in a family. They have the same genetic parents yet the sex, hair colour, height, personality, and other attributes differ from one to another. The proteins in lipoprotein particles are the same; they, too, have different attributes.

---

2 *Ribonucleic acid (RNA) is a pivotal molecule in cellular biology, involved in a range of critical functions including the coding, decoding, regulation, and expression of genes. It plays a key role in the transfer of genetic information from DNA to protein synthesis, essential for cellular function and growth.*

3 *A ribosome is a small structure within cells that plays a crucial role in making proteins. It acts like a factory, reading the genetic instructions carried by messenger RNA (mRNA) and linking together the correct sequence of amino acids to form a protein. Ribosomes are essential for translating the genetic code from DNA into functional proteins that the body needs for various functions, such as building tissues and regulating processes. They can be found floating in the cell's cytoplasm or attached to another structure in a cell called the endoplasmic reticulum.*

4 *The cell's cytoplasm is the gel-like substance inside the cell membrane that surrounds the cell's nucleus and other organelles. It is mostly made up of water, salts, and proteins. The cytoplasm provides a medium for chemical reactions to take place and helps to support and protect the cell's organelles. It also plays a role in transporting materials within the cell and maintaining the cell's shape. Essentially, the cytoplasm is the environment where most of the cell's activities occur.*

5 *Amino acids are the basic building blocks of proteins. There are 20 different amino acids in the human body, each with a unique structure and properties.*

6 *When two or more amino acids link together, they form a peptide. A peptide is a short chain of amino acids.*

So, small genetic differences in the amino acid sequences of the proteins on the surface of lipoproteins influence how the proteins function – and, therefore, how the lipoproteins behave. A **genetic variance** that makes it easier for a particle to be taken up by the cells into the tissues may increase susceptibility to plaque formation within a family or even among individuals within that family.

Let's consider the **electrical charge** of lipoproteins. Changes in the amino acid composition of apolipoproteins can alter the overall charge of the lipoprotein particle, affecting how it interacts with the artery wall. This becomes relevant when the lipoprotein passes through a fenestra and moves through the connective tissue that includes collagen within the layers of the artery wall.

Collagen has a negative charge. A lipoprotein particle with an amino acid sequence yielding a net positive charge is more likely to 'stick' as it passes through the collagen. In contrast, a lipoprotein particle with an amino acid sequence with a net negative charge is more likely to be repelled by the collagen and, so, less likely to 'stick'.

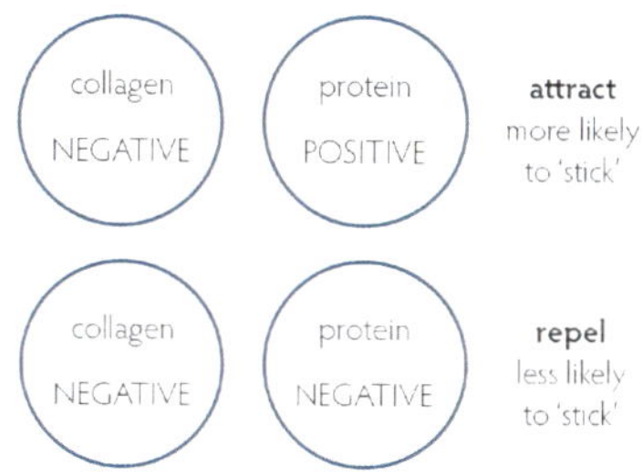
collagen
NEGATIVE
protein
POSITIVE
attract
more likely
to 'stick'
collagen
NEGATIVE
protein
NEGATIVE
repel
less likely
to 'stick'

opposites attract

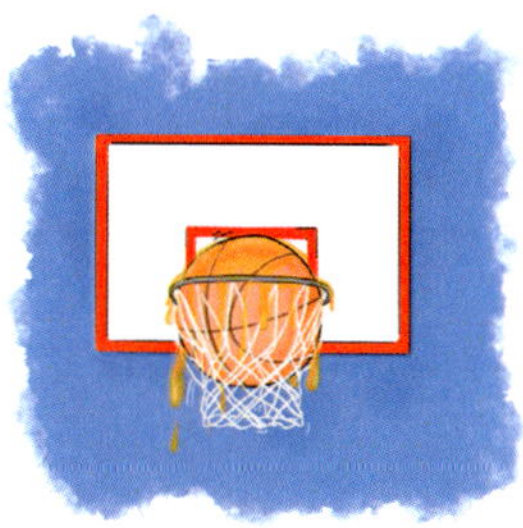

Imagine again our basketball ring. Think of the net under the ring as the collagen, the structural tissue that the lipoprotein particle passes through. If we were to cover the basketball with a lubricant oil, it would slip straight through. So, there would be no accumulation of balls. What if we covered our basketball with honey? The ball becomes stuck in the net, hindering other balls from passing through.

So it is with the lipoprotein passing through the collagen:

- the **number** need not have changed,
- the **size** of the particle need not have changed, yet,
- the **inherent properties** of the particle's surface and how it **interacts** with its surroundings become central to the process.

This difference in amino acid sequence – reflecting individual and family variance because of DNA sequencing – allows us to begin to understand that we have **little chance** of looking at someone on the outside and predicting with any accuracy what's going on at a cellular and molecular level inside. And that is without considering the variation that could occur in the collagen.

Yes, eating well, exercising, good blood pressure, and controlling your weight are all desirable and will **influence** how your genetics play out. Yet, on their own, they cannot guarantee a plaque-free existence.

So, how do we know who will be at risk?

risk

Currently, the application of a population based risk calculator to the individual continues to be a clinical challenge – as we discuss – that needs to be dealt with by your doctor in consultation with you.

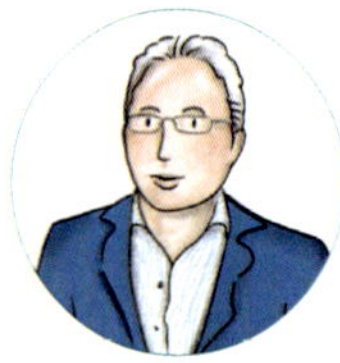

In discussing issues of risk factor assessment concerning CAD, it is extremely important to be clear about the difference between association and causation.

association or causation

As cardiologists, we regularly need to explain to patients that they have cholesterol build-up in their arteries. Often, they reply,

"But Doctor, my cholesterol is fine."

"But Doctor, I exercise regularly."

"But Doctor, I eat healthy food and keep my weight down."

These patients are expressing a belief that is **broadly accepted but universally misleading**: that factors such as high cholesterol, lack of exercise, poor diet, or excess weight are the **direct causes** of CAD. Rather, they are risk factors that contribute to its development.

They are **not causes**; they are **associations**.

Alcohol is associated with an increased incidence of car accidents. **Alcohol does <u>not</u> cause the car accident**; it does not drive the car. Yet, alcohol can impair the driver's reflexes and assessment, and **contribute** to that driver having an accident. The actual **cause** of the accident may be approaching a sharp bend too quickly, another car stopping unexpectedly, the driver losing concentration, or a dog running on to the street.

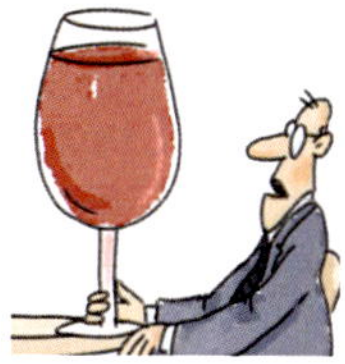

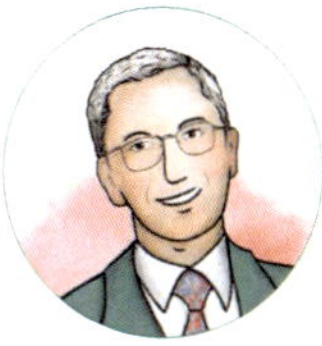

We are not saying that minimising alcohol consumption is not important. It is – for all aspects of health. However, there are other factors that alcohol amplifies.

understanding

Our **understanding** of CAD remains **incomplete**

- for an individual,
- in a particular artery,
- at a particular location within the artery.

Our science around CAD is based on the science of **observation**, ***not*** the science of **mechanism**. The science of observation leads to better understanding of association while the science of mechanism leads to a clearer understanding of cause.

what if?

Accepting their significance, but for the moment putting aside the lack of evidence-based trials, **what if** we could identify patients who were going to have a heart attack soon and started primary prevention therapy before they had their coronary event? **What if** we could identify those patients with plaque but who were also asymptomatic? This would require us to be far more precise in our evaluation of the individual, and far less reliant on the risk of that individual within a population. **What if,** in an intermediate-risk population – a group in which 15 people out of 100 will have an event in a 10-year period – we were able to find those 15 and start primary prevention therapy before their events?

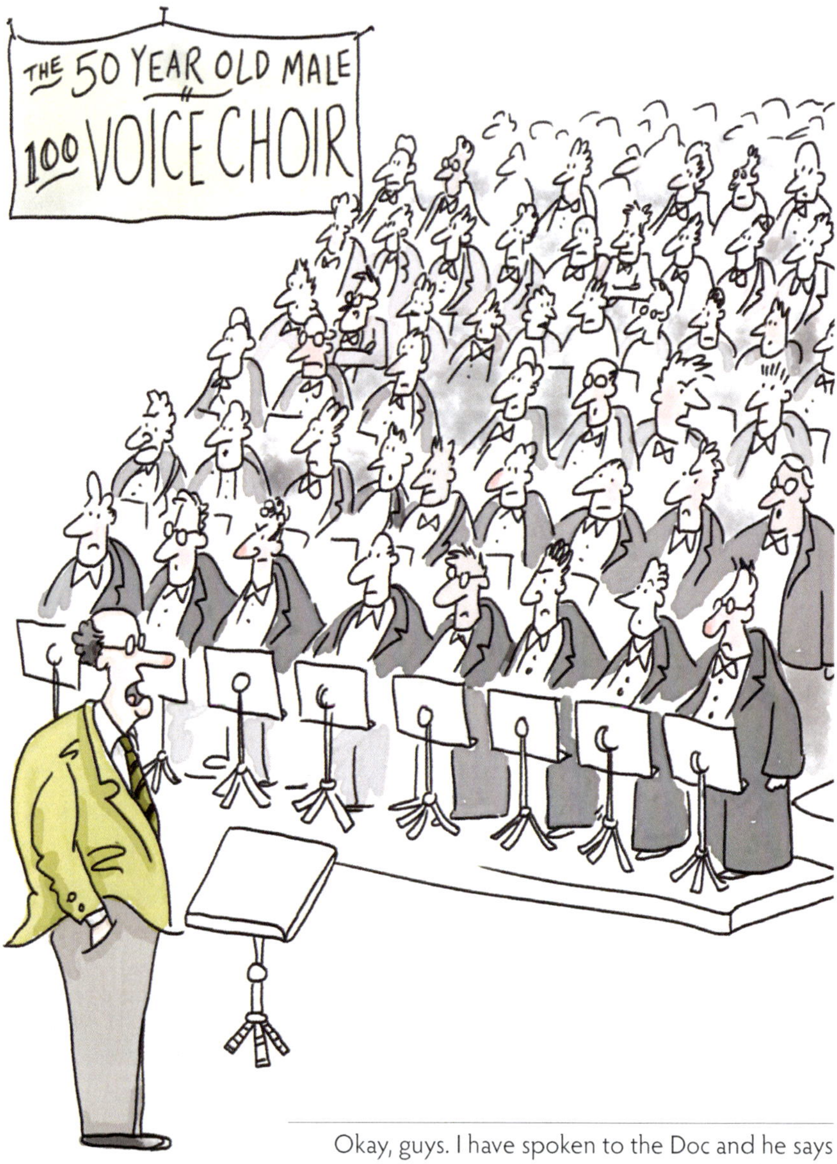

Okay, guys. I have spoken to the Doc and he says 10 to 15 of you will have a heart attack in the next 10 years. Could I just ask that it is not all the tenors?"

While no formal, randomised study like this has been done (so it is an evidence-free zone), we put to you that, logically, **if** we can improve the way we find high-risk people before they become high risk, then there is every chance we can make a **meaningful difference**.

expertise

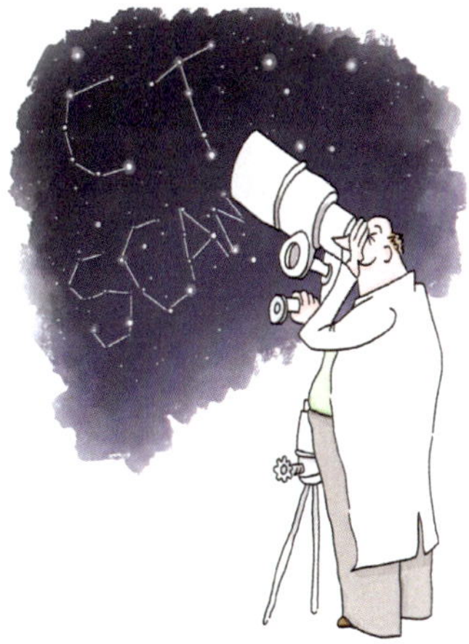

An experienced medical practitioner evaluates the patient and that person's particular needs. Then, knowing and being familiar with the **evidence base** and **clinical experience** from other individuals, the practitioner comes to a **conclusion** that leads to an appropriate **management** plan.

I, Dr W., try to explain this to my patients in a way that paints doctors a little like astronomers. We look out into the universe that we do not fully understand, nor do we fully know its boundaries. Within that universe, there are constellations, stars, and moons. These are fixed points about which we have some certainty. Imagine those fixed points as our studies, the trials that provide the 'evidence base'. When faced with an individual patient, it is our role to try to most appropriately fit our knowledge to that universe of information for the individual. For a certain patient we align the stars of knowledge into the Big Dipper. For another patient, those stars of knowledge may rearrange to a different constellation, perhaps Capricorn, Aquarius, or Orion.

Dr K., however, approaches this slightly differently. He considers genetics, lipid levels, family history, other cardiovascular risk factors, and imaging results, in a structured decision-making process (an algorithm) to determine the appropriate level of treatment for the patient.

critical

Awareness of where the evidence base lies is absolutely critical for appropriate care. It is also absolutely critical to be aware that the application of that evidence base has **limitations** and **boundaries**. Our role as clinicians is to **understand** and **navigate** those boundaries of medical knowledge in association with the **nuances** of the patient's situation to try to find the **best** solution, the **best** answers, and the **best** care for that person. The reason for highlighting this is that there is a **substantial gap** between association and causation. This gap is what we will shed light on in subsequent chapters.

A CLOSER LOOK

defining risk

The risk of a coronary artery event is assessed as **low, intermediate,** or **high**. In reality, it lies on a **continuum** shaped by many factors, including LDL-C years, the cumulative effect of high LDL-C over time. (See pages 102-104.)

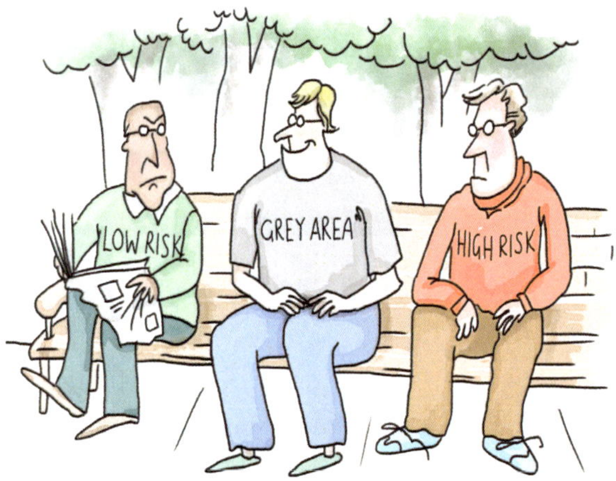

Low risk is considered less than 10 per cent chance of a coronary event within 10 years. **High risk** is considered a greater than 20 per cent chance of an event within 10 years. So, **intermediate risk** is between 10 and 20 per cent of an event within 10 years.

This means that, if we were to take a group of 100 people who were high-risk and follow them for 10 years, 20 or more of those people would have a coronary event or symptom. If we introduced aspirin and cholesterol-lowering medication to reduce the risk of an event in this group of 100, then, statistically, we would be treating up to 80 people who were not going to have an event and did not need treatment.

This has a significant impact on the way the effectiveness of that intervention is assessed. The statistical significance of assessing the effectiveness of primary prevention in this group is diluted by the people within the population who were not destined to have an event.

Similarly, if we were to take a group of 100 people with low risk of an event and follow them for 10 years, up to 10 of those individuals could have a coronary event, and 90 would remain without any symptom or sign. Here again, the problem is: how do we appropriately treat the 10 but not over-treat the 90?

The way that we evaluate and calculate risk in individuals is based on **observational** data. This means that, over the years, databases have been established of features and factors found in individuals who have had CAD. The occurrence of those features and factors then lends weight to their being used as **predictors** for people before they have an event. This simply means that observational data collected on a large number of patients who have had heart attacks indicate that factors such as increasing age, being male, increased blood pressure, diabetes, and smoking all feature as **associations** to having had a coronary event.

This type of risk modelling, using **multiple associations with observed outcomes**, was first widely published and used by the Framingham Group. This Framingham-type risk modelling, which began in 1948, continues to form the basis of our current risk assessment in **primary prevention**.

The interesting thing about this, of course, is that these factors are **associations** and **not causations**. This means that there can be people who are high-risk based on factors such as age, sex, and cholesterol levels, and yet have never had an event. Conversely, there are people who would appear to be well and who would score low on these risk calculators but still manage to have a problem.

The other important concept is, if your doctor does a 'risk' calculation, it is the rate of event in 100 people with your characteristics when you want to know if **your event rate** over the next 10 years will be zero or 100 per cent.

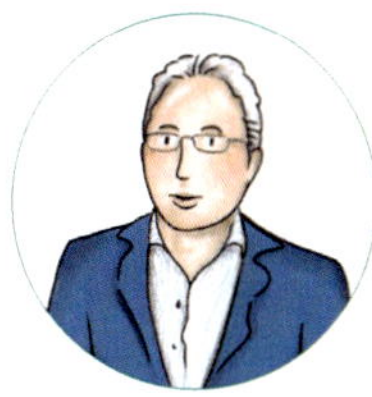

We both use risk calculators in our practices but recognise their limitations. A low five or 10 year risk for a 30-year-old man becomes almost meaningless when we consider plaque formation as a lifelong process related to cumulative LDL-C exposure, wear and tear (age) and the impact of other risk factors. That 'low risk' assessment at 30 will not be reliable in protecting the patient in his early 60s. Think of CVD risk as a lifetime journey.

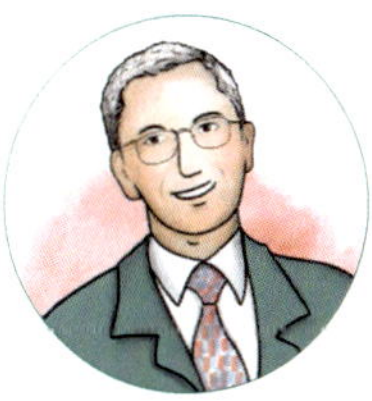

Australian and New Zealand risk calculators

If you wish to find the rate of event **within the population** in which you sit, you can access the Australian risk calculator here:

www.cvdcheck.org.au

IMPORTANT POINTS

CARDIOVASCULAR RISK

- Apolipoproteins (proteins that combine with lipids to form lipoproteins) play a crucial role in lipid metabolism and transport of lipids within the bloodstream. While LDL particles vary in size and density, all are 'bad'. Genetic factors also influence their complexity.
- Slight genetic differences in the amino acid sequences of proteins on lipoprotein particles can impact their function and influence the likelihood of plaque forming.
- Understanding the distinction between associations (e.g., high cholesterol) and causations (e.g., specific mechanisms causing CAD) is fundamental when evaluating and managing individual risk, and in any cholesterol discussion.
- Risk of CAD is categorised as either low, intermediate or high based on observational data and factors such as age, elevated cholesterol levels, sex, blood pressure, diabetes, and smoking status. But it is a continuum that is also influenced by the cumulative exposure of the arteries to 'bad' cholesterol.

Understanding inherited risk is important – but just as important is knowing what you can control. That's where we go next.

chapter 8

CARDIOVASCULAR RISK MANAGEMENT: WHAT YOU CAN CONTROL

Cholesterol management is a conversation we have frequently with patients. Occasionally, patients will have done their research (commonly Internet-based). As we speak one-on-one, we can respond very specifically to that person's situation and questions, and this works well.

However, in 2018, I, Dr W., created a Facebook group, *Know Your Real Risk of Heart Attack*, to provide reliable information for patients and anyone interested. I hoped that it would be a resource that could inform and educate patients about medical issues related to the heart to improve their questions, their understanding of their own condition, and thus improve their outcome.

Although the group started looking at heart attack prevention, it soon covered many other topics related to the heart. A favourite one became cholesterol and statins. A few members had very strong views about cholesterol and its role in heart disease and statins ('satans') and their role *or not* in preventing heart disease. A difficulty arose because some of the members had such fixed opinions that there was no opportunity for discussion. They were clearly polarised and clearly passionate about their position. They were adamant cholesterol was not important in heart disease and that statins did not work. Worse, they maintained the unacceptable side effects were anything from loss of memory to cancer and depression.

Jeff

One member, Jeff, who had dedicated much of the past decade of his life to looking into heart disease after an unfortunate experience through another healthcare system, was an active contributor, posting over and over – and over again – similar material. His position was that cholesterol was not important in the development of CAD and that statins were of no benefit.

And so, the burning question:

> **When we know that the current convention – supported by a *large* body of literature and guidelines – is to lower cholesterol by using statins for people with CAD or CVD, how can there be such polarised opinion within the community?**

Both of us accept – and think it's important – that people search for information beyond their conversations with their medical practitioners. Yet, how can such diligence lead to such divergence?

In Jeff's case, it was a failure to understand the **differences** between **association** and **causation** and **primary** and **secondary prevention**.

association or causation – again

Some people argue that cholesterol doesn't cause heart attacks – and they're partly right. As we have seen, cholesterol is an **association**: it **increases** the risk, but **doesn't guarantee** the outcome.

Let's return to alcohol and car accidents. Alcohol impairs judgement and slows reaction time, making an accident **more** likely – but it doesn't **cause** the crash every time. Other factors might be involved, or the accident might not happen at all.

It's the same with cholesterol. High levels **increase** the chance of plaque forming and rupturing, especially over time. But **not everyone with high cholesterol will have a heart attack** – and people with low or average cholesterol still might have an event.

Understanding this difference – between something that **contributes to risk,** and something that **directly causes the event** – is essential when deciding how best to manage that risk.

high risk

So how does this play out in life – especially for people at higher risk?

Let's take a closer look at high-risk individuals, where the benefits of cholesterol-lowering treatment are clear and well supported by the evidence.

We'll move beyond cholesterol and consider people who are **known** to be at high risk because **they have had an event** from a build-up of plaque within their arteries – our secondary prevention population. **People at high risk will benefit from lowering their cholesterol levels using medications.** There is no question within the literature and our experience that has accumulated over the last 30 to 40 years.

low risk

What's not so clear is the situation of low-risk patients who may have no other issue except elevated cholesterol. We know that treating those people may not necessarily lead to a significant improvement in their outcomes – and it is here where some of the confusion lies.

primary and secondary prevention

Throughout this book, the message is clear: **prevention is central**. The aim is either to prevent a first problem from occurring, **primary prevention**, or to prevent further issues once CAD has shown itself, **secondary prevention**. Both situations are important, although they call for different strategies and levels of urgency.

Primary prevention aims to avoid the first event. Preventing chest pain and the complications of a heart attack is the holy grail of preventive cardiology. The challenge lies in addressing **what has not yet been revealed**: deciding on treatment before symptoms appear, weighing a person's risk factors, and estimating the likelihood of an event. We believe that current practice has scope for re-evaluating how we assess risk in individuals before disease becomes apparent.

Secondary prevention focuses on those who have already experienced a cardiovascular event, such as a heart attack, stroke, or the need for a stent or bypass surgery. Here, the path is clear: treatment, and close management of risk factors are essential to prevent further events and to support better long-term outcomes.

Understanding where you sit – in primary or secondary prevention – not only guides today's treatment, it also frames the long-term approach to your heart health.

effect of cumulative LDL-C on RISK OF HEART ATTACK

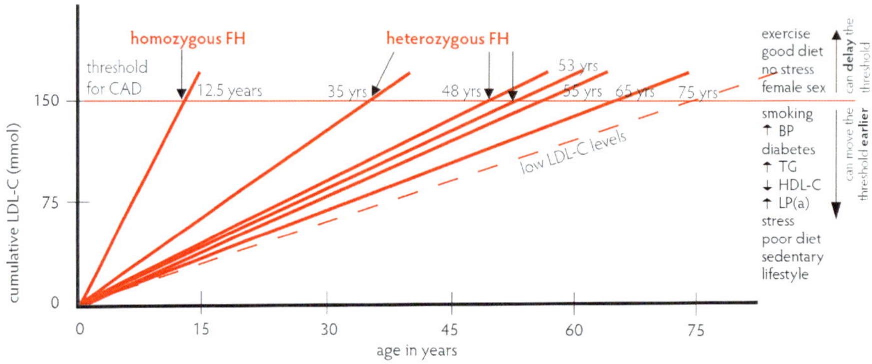

effect of cumulative LDL-C on PROGRESSION OF PLAQUE in the arteries

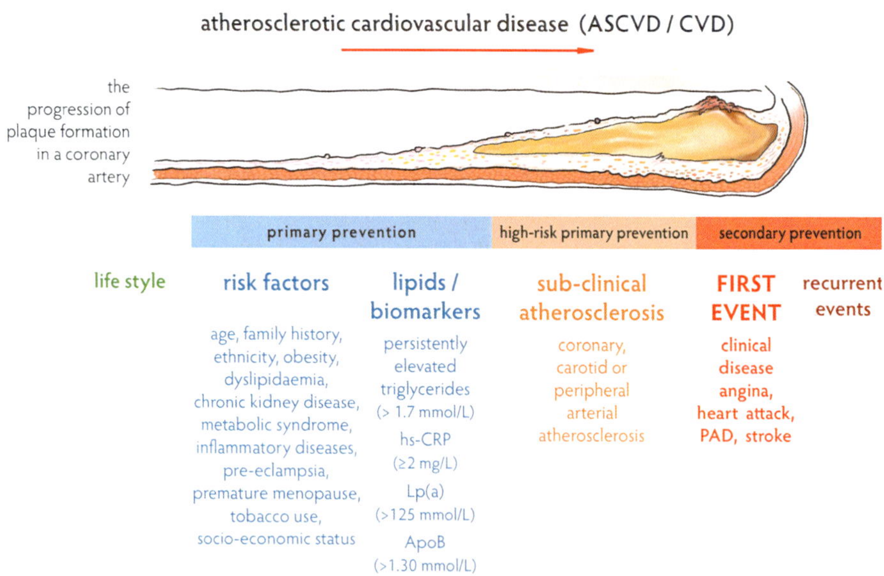

top: The graphic shows how cumulative LDL-C exposure influences the timing of heart attack risk, with the red horizontal line being the threshold for heart attack; higher LDL-C levels accelerate the cumulative effect while lower levels slow it down.

above: This graphic demonstrates how atherosclerosis progresses over time, mirroring cumulative LDL-C exposure.

treatment

So, when considering possible treatment for lowering cholesterol, we need to take into account:

- whether the patient's care is primary or secondary prevention,
- if primary, whether the patient is high risk or low risk,
- how long the patient has had high LDL-C,
- how high the LDL-C level is,
- the targets to which we are treating,
- other risk factors that the individual might have including living with high blood pressure, being a smoker, having diabetes, being physically inactive, having a poor diet, and
- risk-benefit of treatment.

LDL-C years

A key treatment consideration is a person's **cumulative exposure** to LDL-C over time: the concept of LDL-C years. Much like pack-years in smoking, it recognises that both the **level** of LDL-C and the **duration** of exposure determine the **burden** on the arterial wall.

For example, a young man with moderately elevated cholesterol from his twenties is likely to accumulate far more arterial damage by middle age than someone whose cholesterol rises only later in life. This cumulative load helps explain why CAD can appear early in patients with familial hypercholesterolaemia, where lifelong exposure begins at birth.

Clinically, LDL-C years highlight the importance of early detection and sustained lowering of LDL-C. Short-term reductions are valuable, but the greatest benefit comes from lowering cholesterol as **early** and **consistently** as possible, thereby reducing total exposure across the lifespan.

This concept:

- strengthens the argument for early intervention in high-risk individuals,
- supports the use of intensive therapy in familial and secondary-prevention settings, and

- provides a framework for patients to understand why 'normal for age' is not always protective.

It also shifts the focus from cholesterol levels at a single point in time to the overall trajectory of exposure – a perspective that can guide both public health strategies and individual treatment plans.

LDL-C years is an especially important consideration in familial hypercholesterolaemia (FH), where cholesterol has been high since birth.

So, if you have had a heart attack, a stroke, a stent, or bypass surgery – in other words, if you are a high-risk patient – then the evidence is very clear and reassuring: **lowering your cholesterol *will improve* your outcome**, no matter what your cholesterol level is when treatment begins.

Medicines are very safe, highly effective, and proven to deliver long-term benefits.

high cholesterol only

If you have high cholesterol only and you are otherwise fit and well without other risk factors and without any family history, the situation can be less clear. Key factors include how long your LDL-C has been elevated, how high it is, if your Lp(a) level is elevated, and any other risk factors.

Guidelines from major cardiology societies around the world recommend that **very high cholesterol levels should be treated** to reduce the long-term CVD risk, **even in the absence of other risk factors.** We recommend you discuss it with your GP, or preferably a cholesterol specialist, a lipidologist, or a preventive cardiologist.

Further testing could help clarify the situation.

You may be a suitable candidate for a **cardiac scan** that looks at the health of your coronary arteries. This will show if there is a build-up of plaque within the arteries. If there is, then treating cholesterol – a component of that plaque – makes sense. If there's not, the discussion returns to how best to tackle the cholesterol – medications, lifestyle changes, nutraceuticals – to achieve the best long-term outcome.

a time-critical consideration: ACS

There is another critical, but often overlooked, consideration when it comes to cholesterol treatment: the **management of acute coronary syndrome** (ACS).

While secondary prevention guidelines are well established, a persistent and concerning **shortfall exists in the care of patients who are hospitalised** with ACS. ACS refers to a range of life-threatening conditions – including heart attacks and unstable angina – that result from a sudden drop in blood flow to the heart. This treatment gap exists not only in Australia but worldwide.

Patients hospitalised following a heart attack or stroke or other CAD event are at **high risk** – not only of imminent death or serious complications, but also of **future events.** This makes it **imperative** to initiate cholesterol-lowering therapy and broader risk factor control as soon as possible (ideally from the person's arrival at the hospital). In some cases, genetic risk factors such as Lp(a) can be assessed, and family screening can be initiated.

Data sets are clear: **early intervention improves outcomes.** Yet numerous studies show that **too few patients** receive **optimal care after discharge**. This not only increases the burden of illness for patients and their families, but also imposes avoidable costs on the wider health system.

Cardiologists, trainees, junior doctors, coronary care unit nurses, and cardiac rehabilitation coordinators all have a vital role to play in maximising inpatient care **and** planning for long-term management. After discharge, general practitioners are essential in continuing – and if needed, intensifying – the goals and strategies set in hospital to ensure sustained progress and reduced risk.

The medical classification refers to 'low risk' as up to a 10 per cent chance within 10 years and does not consider treatment. This could be expressed as a one per cent chance per annum of having a major event. Would you find the same risk acceptable if applied to air travel?

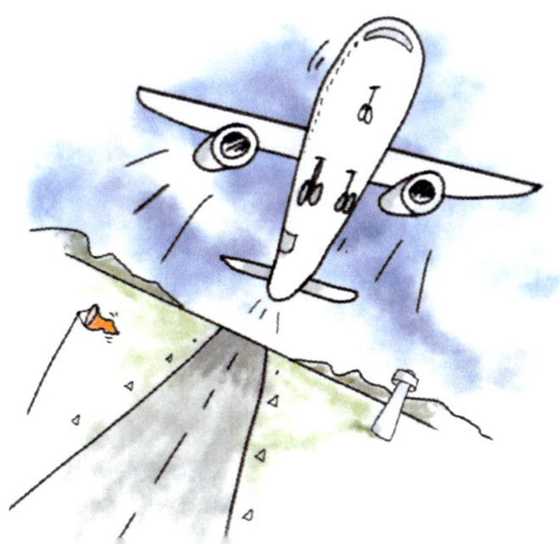

IMPORTANT POINTS

CARDIOVASCULAR RISK MANAGEMENT

- It is crucial to understand the difference between associations and causes, as well as between primary and secondary prevention, when evaluating the risk of CAD.
- High-risk patients – those people with a history of coronary events, including CAD, peripheral vascular disease, cerebrovascular disease, diabetes, and/or familial hypercholesterolaemia (FH) – benefit significantly from lowering their cholesterol levels through medication.
- For low-risk patients, treatment benefits are less clear.
- Consideration of individual risk factors, including blood pressure, smoking status, and diabetes, is also required for personalised cholesterol management.
- Imaging can be helpful in assessing risk.
- While the concept of LDL-C years is an especially important consideration in familial hypercholesterolaemia (FH), treating cholesterol early and over the long term brings benefits.
- Very high cholesterol levels should be treated even in the absence of other risk factors in otherwise well individuals.
- A cholesterol treatment gap exists worldwide in the care of patients who are hospitalised with acute coronary syndrome (ACS). For high-risk patients, cholesterol-lowering treatment should be started as soon as possible.

Clinical assessments benefit from the precision offered by cardiac CT imaging.

chapter 9

CARDIOVASCULAR IMAGING: SEEING HIDDEN DANGER

By now, you know that if you have had any cardiovascular event, significantly lowering your cholesterol will benefit you in terms of minimising further events. *Secondary prevention.* This extends to any vascular event, for example, a stroke.

In the *primary prevention* setting, there's no doubt that treatment of individuals with familial hypercholesterolaemia (we will discuss this in the book's next section) will pay dividends in terms of reduced rates of event, improved quality of life, and the aspirational goal of normal life expectancy.

What is the situation, however, if:

- your cholesterol level is high or at least elevated, and yet there is no family history of premature CAD (an event before 55 years of age for men and 60 for women, in a first-degree family member), or
- your cholesterol is in the normal range, yet your family history is 'terrible' for premature CAD?

precision

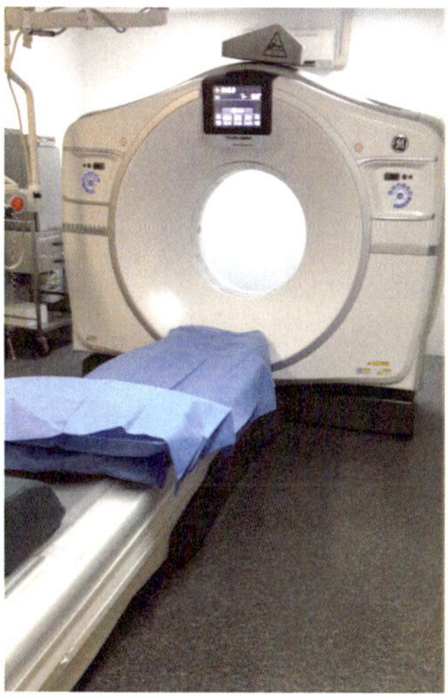

A way to bring precision to our decision-making is to consider **imaging** the coronary arteries to determine if plaque is present or not. Imaging the coronary arteries using computed tomography (CT) scanning is a non-invasive, safe way to discover the health of coronary arteries in an asymptomatic person. Imaging shows an individual's **specific circumstances** rather than basing management on a population trend. This is called **precision medicine**.

cardiac CT imaging

Although technology that captures a beating heart is now broadly available, cardiac CT (computed tomography) imaging[1] is currently **not** a guideline recommendation in many parts of the world, including Australia. This lack of support exists even though numerous reassuring published position papers exist, particularly papers concerning patients at intermediate risk of heart disease.

In this patient group, imaging provides insight into whether the patient is more high risk or more low risk, thus informing the best way to care for the person.

CT imaging can also be helpful in managing patients:

- with high cholesterol levels who want clarity about what's going on in their arteries before starting therapy;
- who are apprehensive about therapy, or
- with a perceived unremarkable or low risk of CAD based on traditional risk factors but with a 'terrible' family history.

In primary prevention for people without symptoms, the most commonly used CT imaging test is a coronary artery calcium (CAC) scan, which provides a score. For people with symptoms such as chest pain, coronary CT angiography (CCTA) is used.

radiation

CT imaging uses x-ray radiation, but the exposure is well within the range considered reasonable for prevention (similar to a breast screening mammogram). Modern machines further reduce this to very small doses, generally less than a year's exposure to natural background radiation.

---

1 *Two types of cardiac CT scans are available, each serving a distinct purpose.* ***Coronary artery calcium (CAC) scoring*** *measures the amount of calcium in the coronary arteries to help* ***assess cardiovascular risk.*** *No dye or contrast is used.*

Coronary CT angiography (CCTA) *uses dye to visualise the coronary arteries in more detail to detect blockages or narrowings and is, at times, an alternative to invasive coronary angiography.*

calcium

Central to comprehending this scanning, we must first understand that a build-up of cholesterol within the arteries *generally* leads to **associated deposits of calcium** in the artery. So, calcium is used as the **indicator** of plaque build-up.

For about 100 years, observations have been made, primarily by radiologists in the early years, that calcium could build up in the arteries, although there were different opinions about its significance. It was not until the 1980s – when a technology called **electron beam computed tomography** (EBCT) became available – that interest was again ignited in trying to evaluate the health of an individual's coronary arteries. These early scanners were large and extremely expensive and only a few machines existed in the world.

In 1996, pathologist J. A. Rumberger established the clear relationship between calcium and cholesterol within the structure of plaque, showing that calcium moved into the wall of the artery following the deposition of cholesterol.

Calcium serves as a **marker**[2] of the process with which we are concerned – the presence of atherosclerotic plaque in the arteries. However, **calcium itself is not the issue**; it is simply an indicator. The real concern is the build-up of plaque within the coronary arteries. Calcium is a bystander – relatively inert in the arteries, where it can remain. Our focus is on addressing the underlying process that leads to its presence.

---

2 *A surrogate marker is a substitute measure used in clinical trials and medical research to infer the effect of a treatment when direct measures of clinical outcomes are not available. These markers are often biological or biochemical indicators that can be easily and accurately measured and are believed to reflect the underlying clinical outcome of interest.*

coronary artery calcium score

Regardless of a patient's cholesterol levels, the amount of exercise he or she undertakes (or not), or how healthy the person claims his or her diet is, I, Dr W., want to know the **health** of **that individual's** arteries. I do not want to know the risk that a population of people with the same characteristics may have. We obtain the most information by using a scan to look directly into the arteries.

To begin this investigation, we obtain a coronary artery calcium (CAC) score with a specialised, non-invasive scan. It is a sensitive and reliable indicator of plaque in the coronary arteries.

The CAC score is expressed as an **absolute number** (the amount of calcium in the arteries) and as a **percentile** (that compares this score to others of the same age and sex). Importantly, the calcium score percentile, which reflects the propensity of an individual to develop plaque compared

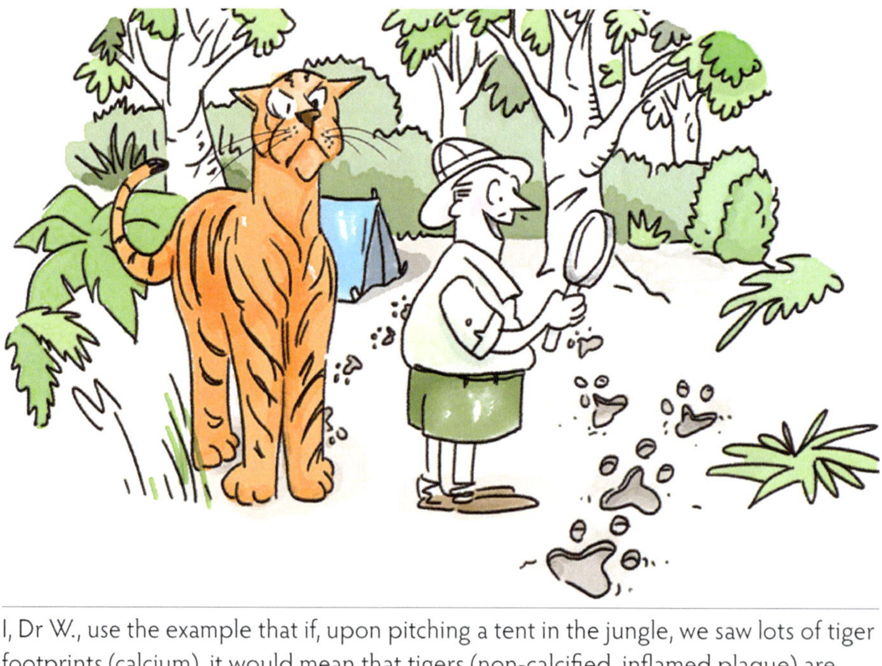

I, Dr W., use the example that if, upon pitching a tent in the jungle, we saw lots of tiger footprints (calcium), it would mean that tigers (non-calcified, inflamed plaque) are around and it might not be a great place to pitch the tent. Not seeing tiger footprints doesn't mean that there are no tigers in the vicinity, nor does it mean that they might not come later, but it certainly makes it a better place to pitch a tent than if the footprints are present.

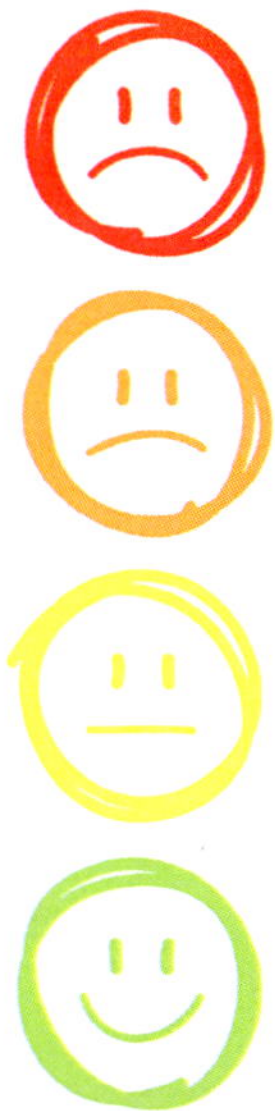

300 +
secondary prevention

100 +
therapy suggested

1-100
intermediate risk

0
low risk

The coronary artery calcium score is an absolute number that is used in conjunction with other factors to help determine treatment strategies. Recent research says that a score of 300 or above should be treated as secondary prevention although the test is used in primary prevention situations only. Importantly, the calcium score as a percentile can be used to guide individualised care.

to 100 age and sex matched equivalents, is also a valuable guide to future risk. The higher the percentile the greater the risk, with percentiles over 75 per cent often triggering intervention[3].

The CAC scan is a **primary prevention test only**. The **intermediate-risk group will receive the most benefit** as the scan result will move them to either low risk or high risk.

A wealth of research supports the premise that higher CAC scores are associated with an increased likelihood of future cardiovascular events, making it a valuable tool for stratifying risk and guiding clinical decisions. Importantly, a score of zero can provide reassurance of low short-term risk, while progressively higher scores warrant more aggressive risk factor management. An elegant study by Dr Matthew Budoff[4] showed that **a CAC**

3 *For further information on CAC scores, scans and percentiles, please refer to Dr Bishop's book,* Have You Planned Your Heart Attack?

4 *Budoff, M, Kinninger, A, Gransar, H. et al. When Does a Calcium Score Equate to Secondary Prevention?: Insights From the Multinational CONFIRM Registry. J Am Coll Cardiol Img. 2023 Sep, 16 (9) 1181–1189. https://doi.org/10.1016/j.jcmg.2023.03.008*

A CLOSER LOOK

when a CAC scan is not helpful

For young people, plaque may be forming in the arteries, but may not YET have had time to calcify. This is especially important for those with familial hypercholesterolaemia (FH), where early detection of vascular changes can be crucial in guiding treatment to reduce long-term cardiovascular risk. Using an ultrasound technique can be the solution in this situation.

carotid ultrasound

Carotid ultrasound is a valuable tool as it can detect **plaque formation and arterial narrowing <u>before</u> calcium appears or symptoms arise**.

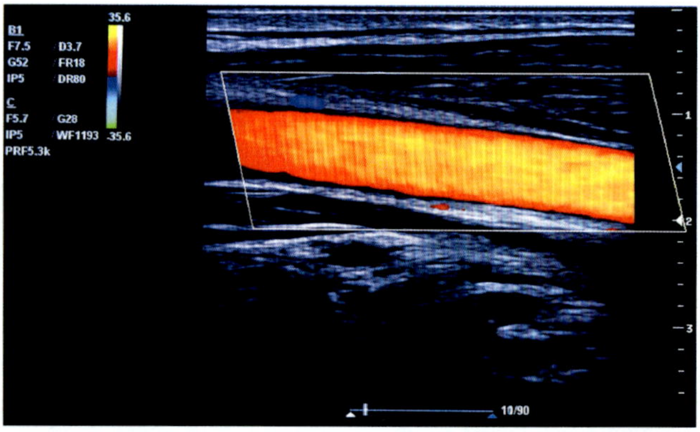

If plaque is detected, it underscores the need for aggressive lipid-lowering therapy to prevent progression. Even if no plaque is found, the scan can offer reassurance while reinforcing the importance of lifelong cholesterol management.

intima-media thickness (IMT)

Measuring carotid intima-media thickness (IMT) provides **insight into the earliest stages of atherosclerosis, even <u>before</u> plaque forms**. For young FH patients, IMT can detect subtle early thickening of the arterial walls, which reflects long-term exposure to high LDL-C levels and may indicate an increased risk of future CVD.

While IMT is more commonly used in research and preventive cardiology rather than routine clinical practice, it can help track the impact of lipid-lowering therapies over time. However, IMT alone does not diagnose significant arterial disease, and its findings may not always lead to immediate changes in treatment. In young FH patients, it is best used as a supplementary measure rather than a stand-alone decision-making tool.

score of equal to or greater than 300 carried the *same risk as someone who had suffered an event*. This means that **we should be treating CAC scores equal to or greater than 300 as we would treat secondary prevention.**

As we have already discussed, calcium is not the problem but it is an indicator of a potential risk. The problem is the plaque build-up[5].

Calcium scoring has become a prominent and sensible marker in risk assessment. Observational data in relation to people with zero calcium score is robust. This makes coronary calcium scoring a very powerful **negative predictive test** (meaning the condition, in this case, plaque, is not present).

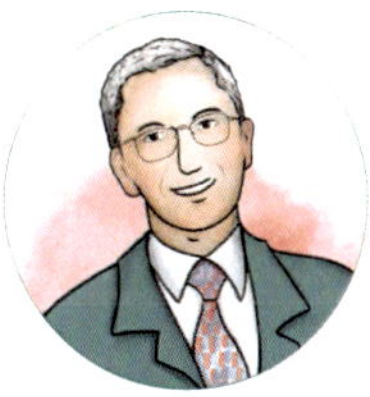

Currently, in Australia, cardiac CT testing – coronary artery calcium (CAC) score – incurs an out-of-pocket cost of several hundred dollars as it is not covered by a Medicare rebate. However, when considered against the cost of servicing your car, the scanning represents exceptional value to look after the most important engine in your life.

finding high-risk patients in the crowd

The approach to CAD, historically, has been driven by **responding to symptoms late in the process** or has been guided by risk calculators that have limitations to their application. From a pragmatic point of view, the objective is to be **ahead of the game** so that we know who has a significant atherosclerotic plaque burden and who might be at significant risk **before** a CAD event. Our objective in trying to reduce risk for individual patients is to prevent them from having an out-of-hospital CAD event[6] that leads to death

5 *Scavenger cells (macrophages) try to clean up the cholesterol and, in so doing, can become so full that they burst and spill. The spilled contents include digestive enzymes that in turn cause scarring in the artery wall. The build-up of cholesterol, macrophages, scar tissue* **and** *calcium in the wall is the plaque.*

6 *A reminder of what CAD events are: angina stable or unstable (chest pain due to reduced blood flow to the heart), heart attack (complete blockage of a coronary artery, causing heart muscle damage and sometimes death), cardiac failure (the heart can't pump blood effectively), arrhythmias (irregular heartbeats due to impaired blood supply), sudden cardiac arrest (a severe electrical disturbance that stops the heart and mostly causes death).*

or substantial damage to the heart muscle; outcomes that are irreversible, costly, and potentially avoidable.

We want to stabilise the plaque to prevent rupture and slow its progression. Interestingly, the CAC score will often increase with aggressive lipid-lowering therapy. This does not necessarily mean the disease is worsening; rather, it often reflects a transition towards more stable, calcified plaque that is less likely to rupture.

If we screen and identify potential high-risk individuals, and if we initiate cholesterol-lowering and other[7] therapies, then, instead of having a catastrophic heart attack, the patient may never present. If the person does present, it is (hopefully) with a more stable situation, such as chest pain on exertion or shortness of breath. Having been educated as part of the process of being identified as a high-risk patient, the person knows to present immediately, which has its own positive prognostic benefit.

By initiating lipid-lowering therapy *and* other therapies in the high-risk group, we have the potential to **reshape** the course of CAD in patients. This could notably decrease the incidence of acute heart attacks and other problems, thereby alleviating both the emotional and financial burdens on individuals and the community.

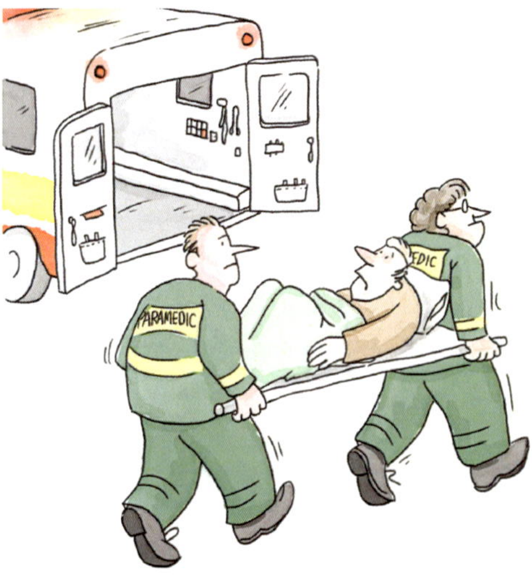

7 *'Other' may include aspirin, blood pressure therapy, diabetic medication and further specific interventions based on the individual patient.*

case study JACK

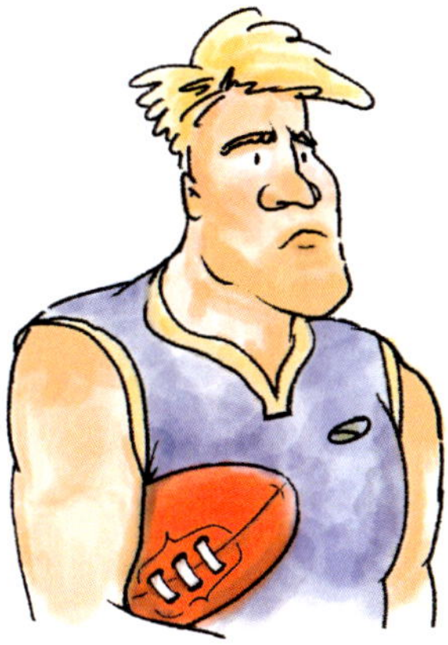

JACK is a former prominent AFL player with a long and distinguished career. He was in his mid 40s when he became a patient of mine, Dr K.

Even after his active playing days, he had maintained his fitness.

He had had an elevated LDL-C level (5.2 mmol/L) for many years but because he was superfit, had a very good diet, no other risk factors and no related problems, he was not started on any medication for his elevated LDL-C.

He had no early family history of heart disease but did not know his father's family history as his father had been adopted.

We did a cardiac CT scan which revealed significant non-obstructive plaque[1] in two of his major coronary arteries and a calcium score of 399. This score put him into the top one per cent of males his age with regards to calcified plaque in his arteries.

I started Jack on a combination of a statin and ezetimibe, and made plans to reassess his LDL-C in three months. We also discussed the use of aspirin as it is supported by a CAC score higher than 300. If the score remains unacceptably high, I will explore the Pharmaceutical Benefits Scheme criteria for the possible prescription of an injectable PCSK9 inhibitor.

I also advised him to have his children checked for elevated LDL-C as there is a 50 per cent chance they could have inherited this from him. Effective therapies are available from an early age.

---

1 *Non-obstructive plaque refers to the build-up of atherosclerotic plaque in the arteries that does not significantly block blood flow. These plaques are usually less than 50% of the artery's diameter and may not cause symptoms under normal conditions. However, they can still be dangerous because they may rupture, leading to blood clot formation and potentially causing heart attacks or other cardiovascular events. So, even plaques that do not limit blood flow are clinically important. They identify high-risk individuals.*

case study **MARGARET**

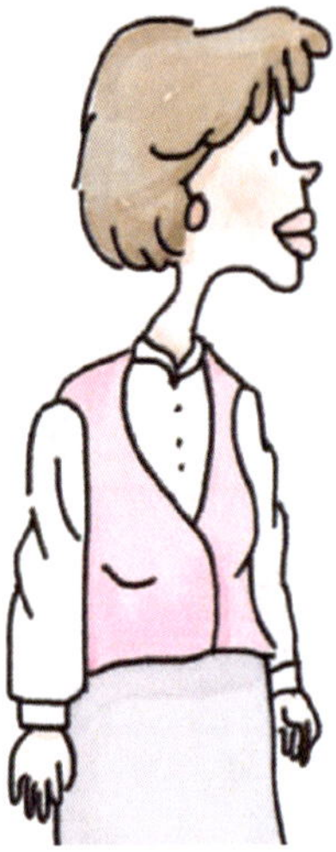

MARGARET was a 60-year-old woman who came to see me, Dr W., for cardiovascular risk stratification.

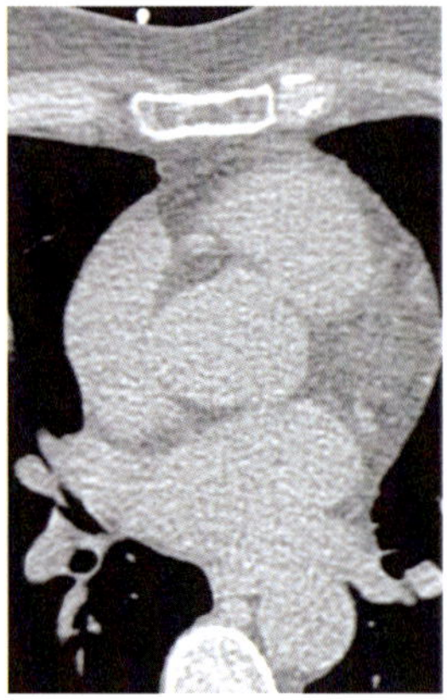

She was generally fit and well, not on any regular medication, and her family had no history of premature CAD.

This is Margaret's scan (right). Her lipid profile is below.

total cholesterol (TC)	9.1	ideally < (less than) 5.2 mmol/l
triglycerides (TG)	2	ideally <2.0 mmol/l
high-density lipoprotein cholesterol (HDL-C)	2.1	ideally > (greater than) 1.0 mmol/l
TC to HDL-C ratio	4.3	ideally <4.0 ratio
non HDL-C	7	ideally <4.0 mmol/l
low-density lipoprotein cholesterol (LDL-C)	6.1	ideally* <3.4 mmol/l (*ideally refers to the general, healthy population. Importantly, lower targets may be indicated based on an individual patient's clinical situation.)

Her coronary calcium score was zero. Despite her elevated cholesterol levels, there was no evidence of plaque build-up. We did not undertake any further evaluation.

Margaret experienced fantastic relief. Her general practitioner's desire to have her on a cholesterol-lowering tablet, despite the side effects she had suffered, had stressed her, catching her between the fear of an event and the side effects of medication.

Based on her scan result, I reassured her that the available research suggested that a zero calcium score represented a very low risk – a risk of an event of less than one per cent in five years (all things being equal).

While discussing a management plan, I suggested a gentle lipid-lowering treatment regime, as her cholesterol really was high. It is better to avoid plaque than wait until it appears, and then try to play 'catch-up'.

Margaret was not keen.

Eventually, we agreed that, as there was no evidence of plaque, taking a statin or aspirin was not an immediate priority. However, we acknowledged that the literature's suggestion of a very low five-year event risk might not apply in her case because of her higher-than-average cholesterol level.

So, to err on the side of caution, we decided to repeat the scan in four years and reconsider treatment based on that result.

A demonstrated low risk of an event informed the immediate medication decision. A plan for ongoing surveillance supported this action. Margaret was happy with this outcome, as was I.

IMPORTANT POINTS

CARDIOVASCULAR IMAGING

- Imaging the coronary arteries moves evaluation from being population-based to patient-specific, providing a clear picture. This is called precision medicine.
- Calcium, a component of plaque build-up, is used as a marker (indicator) of plaque in the arteries. It is not the problem.
- Coronary artery calcium (CAC) score is reported as an absolute number and a percentile. A high absolute score indicates a significant plaque burden, while a high percentile suggests a strong propensity to develop plaque, highlighting potential future risk. The score is obtained through a CAC scan, a specialised cardiac CT scan.
- At least one study has clearly shown that a CAC score of 300 or more carries the same risk as a person who has had an event; treatment should be aimed at secondary prevention targets.
- In high-risk patients (plaque build-up can be seen in the arteries), cholesterol-lowering and blood-thinning therapies can be started before the first event (most likely a heart attack), thus lowering the person's risk.
- A carotid ultrasound and intima-media thickness (IMT) tests can be useful for young people.
- Associated education on recognising and responding to symptoms as they arise also helps improve the patient's future health outcomes.

The proof of the 'pudding' is in the studies.

chapter 10

CHOLESTEROL STUDIES: THE EVIDENCE BEHIND TREATMENTS

Research interest in cholesterol and its interplay with atherosclerosis has been around for more than 100 years. Russian pathologist and scientist Nikolai Anitschkow (Anichkov) and colleagues undertook pioneering work in the early 20th century (and later) on the role of cholesterol in atherosclerosis. Experiments in 1913 showed that feeding rabbits a diet enriched with cholesterol led to the development of atherosclerosis.

A raft of activities after World War II, including:

- observational studies that started pointing to lipids – and in particular, cholesterol – as being central, as an association, and
- the advancement of knowledge associated with atherosclerotic cardiovascular (heart blood vessels) and cerebrovascular (brain blood vessels) diseases

drove growth in the number of major trials trying to offer greater understanding in this area. American President Dwight D. Eisenhower's heart attack in 1955 galvanised not only the medical fraternity but that nation into an interest and investment in cardiovascular health leading to significant advancements in research, development, treatment and care.

clinical trials

For a new drug to gain treatment approval, it must undergo extensive testing through clinical trials involving thousands of patients. This process begins with Phase I trials, followed by Phase II, III, and IV trials. Each phase assesses different aspects of the drug's safety and effectiveness. Substantial financial investment, often totalling millions of dollars, is involved before it can be approved for use in countries like Australia. This rigour ensures that the drug is effective and safe for public use. In Australia, it also needs to be cost-effective to be included in the Pharmaceutical Benefits Scheme (PBS), which provides subsidised prescription medicines to Australian residents. The whole trial process can take 15-20 years. (Dr K. has been involved in more than 50 clinical trials over many years.)

Framingham Heart Study

The Framingham Heart Study is one of the first, best-recognised, and longest-running studies in cardiovascular research. Starting in 1948, it enrolled 5209 participants from Framingham, Massachusetts, USA.

Set up as a longitudinal cohort study[1], it tracked the natural history of certain diseases within the participants. The study aimed to identify potential risk factors associated with the development of CVD. It explored potential risk factors that might be identified as associations, thus establishing links with the occurrence and progression of those diseases.

Unbelievably, and to the researchers' credit, the study continues today – with third generation participants.

This study was instrumental in setting the scene for our modern risk calculators. The ability to collect multiple data sets on individuals within a population and track their outcome over time allowed risk calculation that yields the rate of an event or disease within a **population** based on the characteristics of that population. It linked cholesterol levels (particularly the total cholesterol [TC] to HDL-C ratio) to heart disease.

This research, however, was without the strong statistically significant data the medical profession likes to see before formulating management guidelines and/or changing practice. There wasn't a double-blind randomised controlled trial demonstrating that the intervention of cholesterol reduction made a difference to outcomes. (In the midst of this data vacuum, the 'cholesterol wars' which originated in the United Kingdom were in full swing. See p 257.) This changed in 1994[2].

However, before then, a class of compounds, HMG-CoA reductase inhibitors (commonly known as statins), was developed by a large American multinational pharmaceutical company, Merck, Sharp & Dohme (MSD).

---

1 *A longitudinal cohort study follows a group of individuals (cohort) over time, tracking exposures and outcomes to identify associations, such as risk factors for disease.*

2 *The main results of the 4S trial (about to be discussed) were published in the Journal of the American Medical Association (JAMA) on November 22, 1994.*

MSD's first patent was for lovastatin, which received FDA approval as the first commercial statin in September 1987. Simvastatin, was its second. Other pharmaceutical companies became involved. Pravastatin followed in 1991, fluvastatin in 1994, atorvastatin (1997), cerivastatin (1998, withdrawn in 2001), rosuvastatin (2003)[3], and later pitavastatin (still in clinical use).

Scandinavian Simvastatin Survival Study (4S)

The publication of the Scandinavian Simvastatin Survival Study (4S study) in 1994 represents an inflection point and the beginning of the therapeutic cholesterol-lowering journey, setting a new course for the management of high-risk cardiovascular patients.

The 4S study started in 1988 and enrolled 4444 patients who had angina or had survived a myocardial infarction (heart attack). So, all patients were in a **secondary prevention** setting. Patients[4] (definitely high risk and proven to develop plaque in their arteries) were placed randomly into one of two groups. One group received simvastatin (treatment), the other, a placebo (no treatment). The dose of simvastatin was started at 20 mg and adjusted up or down depending on tolerability.

At the time, statins were not yet part of routine secondary prevention, so simvastatin was added to standard care, which focused on symptom control, blood pressure management, and lifestyle advice.

With advances in research, we now consider the cholesterol levels used in that research (see footnote 4) to be on the high side. ALSO OF NOTE, only about 35 to 40 per cent of the patients were on aspirin and 25 per cent were, at the time, smokers. These figures are low and high, respectively, for the modern Western world.

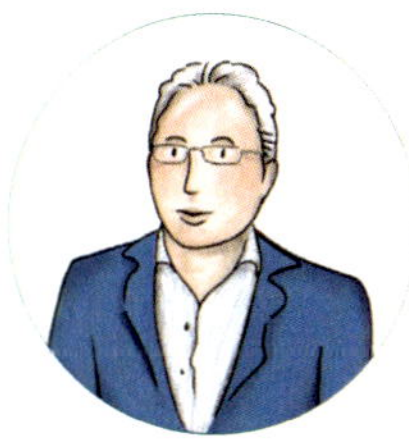

3 *Hajar, R. (2011). Statins: Past and Present. Heart Views: The Official Journal of the Gulf Heart Association, 12(3), 121-127. https://doi.org/10.4103/1995-705X.95070*

4 *Participants had an entry total cholesterol level over 5.5 and less than 8 mmol/L, while the average for both arms of the study (the treatment arm and the placebo arm) was 6.7 mmol/L.*

By the end of six months:

- approximately 40 per cent of participants had increased their dose to 40 mg,
- approximately 60 per cent had remained on 20 mg, and
- less than one per cent experienced a dose reduction to 10 mg daily.

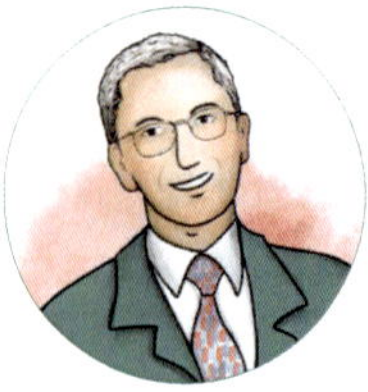

It would be fair to say that these doses are only modest in the current era. Doses of atorvastatin or rosuvastatin at 40 or 20 mg, respectively, would be routine and significantly more effective than the 40 or 20 mg of simvastatin in the 4S trial. This suggests that the 4S trial under-represented the benefits of the intensity of the cholesterol-lowering we would consider routine in current practice.

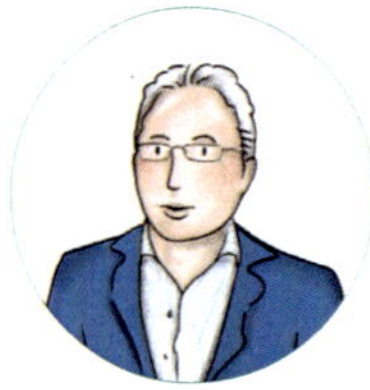

Overall, findings from the trial for those patients on simvastatin were:

- a 25 per cent average reduction of total cholesterol,
- a 35 per cent reduction of LDL-C, and
- an eight per cent increase in HDL-C.

One hundred and eighty-two deaths were recorded within the treatment group and 256 deaths were recorded within the placebo group, at eight per cent and 12 per cent event rate, respectively, over 5.4 years. These figures demonstrated an absolute reduction of four per cent in the treatment group.

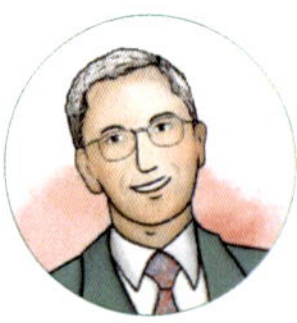

This was all-cause mortality – from any cause, not only heart attack. Impressive!

The numbers became even more compelling when all-cause mortality was changed to coronary deaths: 111 deaths in the simvastatin group and 189 deaths in the placebo group, meaning a relative risk of 0.58 or a 42 per cent reduction within the treatment group, with a 95 per cent confidence interval.

To put this into context, the four per cent absolute reduction for all-cause mortality means that by treating 100 people you would prevent four deaths. This signified that 25 people need to be treated to save one life.

The study went beyond saving lives. It demonstrated a significant reduction in coronary events, including coronary death (fatal outcomes from CAD), heart attacks (both silent and symptomatic), and resuscitated cardiac arrest, with 19 per cent occurring in the treatment group and 28 per cent occurring in the placebo group. This is an absolute reduction of nine per cent in the treatment group, meaning that only 11 patients needed to receive the intervention to prevent one event.

Although the dosages would be considered less than optimal in our current world, aspirin was used sparingly, and there was still plenty of smoking happening. This was a clear and statistically significant outcome, showing cholesterol-lowering use of simvastatin had mortality benefit – in a double-blind randomised controlled trial.

cholesterol dawn

Cholesterol-lowering and statins had arrived.

The results of the 4S trial led to an explosion of activity; the efficacy of statins improved and studies flourished.

Atorvastatin, which was developed by the large American pharmaceutical company Pfizer, was followed by **rosuvastatin**, developed by the British-Swedish pharmaceutical company, AstraZeneca. These drugs achieved far greater LDL-C reductions, reliably and safely, than the earlier statins, and continue to underpin modern cholesterol management today.

The studies that also followed examined both secondary and primary prevention settings.

secondary prevention

The secondary prevention trials included the CARE trial, LIPID trial, GREACE trial, TNT trial, AVERT trial, and IDEAL trial. Each demonstrated a clear benefit from using lipid-lowering drugs for the high-risk patient.

Three more recent secondary prevention trials have shown major progress in preventing further heart problems by combining new lipid-lowering medications with statin treatments to lower LDL-C levels. They are:

- IMPROVE-IT trial (Improved Reduction of Outcomes: Vytorin Efficacy International Trial), started in 2005 and published in 2015;
- the FOURIER Trial (Further Cardiovascular Outcomes Research with PCSK9 Inhibition in Patients with Elevated Risk), started in 2010 and published in 2017, and
- the ODYSSEY Trial (Odyssey Outcomes Study), started about 2012 and published in 2017.

The **IMPROVE-IT** trial investigated whether adding **ezetimibe** (a novel lipid-lowering drug) to simvastatin (a statin) would offer additional cardiovascular benefits compared with simvastatin alone in patients with recent acute coronary syndrome (ACS)[5]. This combination therapy led to a lower incidence of major adverse cardiovascular events, such as heart attacks and strokes, highlighting the benefit of using ezetimibe in addition to statin therapy. (Ezetimibe blocks cholesterol absorption in the small intestine, while statins lower cholesterol production in the liver.)

The **FOURIER and ODYSSEY** trials focused on **PCSK9 inhibitors**. PCSK9 inhibitors block the PCSK9 protein, which normally reduces the liver's ability to remove LDL-C. By inhibiting this protein, more LDL-C is cleared from the bloodstream, lowering cholesterol levels.

The *FOURIER* trial evaluated the efficacy of the PCSK9 inhibitor, **evolocumab**, in reducing cardiovascular events in patients with a CVD history who were already on statin therapy. Compared with statin therapy alone, the combined therapy showed significant risk reductions for events such as heart attacks, strokes, and cardiovascular death.

The ODYSSEY trial assessed the impact of another PCSK9 inhibitor, alirocumab, on cardiovascular outcomes in patients with a history of CVD who were receiving statin therapy. It significantly reduced the risk of CVD, including heart attacks and strokes, compared with a placebo, highlighting the benefits of PCSK9 inhibition in secondary prevention.

5 *Acute coronary syndrome (ACS) refers to conditions caused by a sudden reduction in blood flow to the heart, often due to a ruptured plaque and clot formation in the coronary arteries (unstable angina, heart attack). ACS is a medical emergency requiring urgent treatment.*

These trials marked significant advancements in secondary prevention, confirming the benefit of LDL-C lowering regardless of the agent used. Several other trials, including MIRACL, PROVE IT-TIMI 22 and STATIN STEMI, contributed to better patient outcomes.

primary prevention

Important trials that investigated statins in the primary prevention setting included WOSCOPS, AFCAPS/Tex CAPS and the JUPITER trial.

Against this strong background of evidence, researchers began to ask a more nuanced question: Could statins help people who didn't meet the usual cholesterol thresholds but still carried hidden cardiovascular risk? The earlier trials such as WOSCOPS and AFCAPS/TexCAPS focused on people with raised LDL-C. But many heart attacks still occur in those whose LDL-C appears 'normal', suggesting other processes – particularly inflammation – might be at play.

This is when the **JUPITER** trial (2008) became so influential.

The Justification for the Use of Statin in Prevention: an Intervention Trial Evaluating Rosuvastatin (JUPITER) trial[6] set out to answer an important question: Could statins help people who have average LDL-C levels but signs of underlying inflammation? High-sensitivity C-reactive protein (hs-CRP) is a blood marker of low-grade inflammation, and higher levels predict a greater risk of heart attack and stroke. Statins lower LDL-C, but they also lower hs-CRP, so researchers wondered whether both effects together might reduce risk in people who looked 'healthy' by cholesterol criteria.

More than 17,800 men and women who had LDL-C below 130 mg/dL (3.4 mmol/L) but hs-CRP of 2 mg/L or higher were randomly assigned to **rosuvastatin** 20 mg daily or placebo. None had known CVD. Participants were followed for major cardiovascular events, including heart attack, stroke, arterial revascularisation, hospitalisation for unstable angina, or cardiovascular death.

After a median of 1.9 years, the trial was stopped early because the

6 *Ridker PM, Danielson E, Fonseca FAH, et al. Rosuvastatin to prevent vascular events in men and women with elevated C-reactive protein. N Engl J Med. 2008;359(21):2195–2207. DOI: 10.1056/NEJMoa0807646*

benefits were so clear. Rosuvastatin lowered LDL-C by about 50 per cent and hs-CRP by 37 per cent. Compared with a placebo, it reduced the risk of the primary outcome by 44 per cent. Heart attack risk almost halved, stroke dropped by about 48 per cent, and the need for revascularisation or treatment for unstable angina was cut nearly in half. There was no significant increase in muscle problems or cancer, although slightly more cases of physician-reported diabetes were seen in the rosuvastatin group.

JUPITER was the first large study to show that people with average LDL-C but raised hs-CRP can benefit from statin therapy. It reinforced two key ideas that shape modern prevention strategies: cardiovascular risk is driven by more than cholesterol alone, and inflammation plays a significant role. JUPITER opened the door to understanding how reduction of both LDL-C **and** inflammation impact atherosclerosis.

Building on the foundations laid by previous primary prevention studies, the **VESALIUS-CV** trial (published in November 2025) explored if even more intensive LDL-C reduction could prevent first events in people already receiving optimal therapy.

The VESALIUS-CV (Effect of Evolocumab in Patients at High Cardiovascular Risk Without Prior Myocardial Infarction or Stroke) study[7] examined more than 12,000 people with atherosclerosis (CAC >100) or diabetes but no prior heart attack or stroke. Participants received the PCSK9 inhibitor **evolocumab** in addition to **statins** and **ezetimibe**.

The study showed a 25 per cent relative reduction in the risk of a composite outcome of coronary heart disease death, heart attack, or ischaemic stroke (3-point MACE), and a 19 per cent reduction in a broader composite that also included any ischaemia-driven arterial revascularisation (4-point MACE). Importantly, the substantial LDL-C lowering achieved with evolocumab also reduced heart attack risk by 36 per cent.

Among those enrolled in the lipid sub-study, the median on-treatment LDL-C fell to 45 mg/dL (1.16 mmol/L) compared with 109 mg/dL (2.8 mmol/L) in the placebo group.

---

7 *Bohula E. A., Marston N. A., Bhatia A. K., et al. Evolocumab in Patients without a Previous Myocardial Infarction or Stroke. N Engl J Med. Published online 8 November 2025. doi:10.1056/NEJMoa2514428.*

This landmark trial reinforces a clear message: lowering LDL-C reduces cardiovascular events in people without established disease, mirroring what we see consistently in secondary prevention.

Dr K. was a primary investigator and contributed more than 35 patients to the study.

The combination of this range of secondary and primary prevention cholesterol-lowering trials, mediated by statin therapy, continues to consolidate the evidence base for cholesterol's central role in CVD.

With many thousands of patients treated (and millions of patient-years), an extraordinary amount of data collected, and outcomes recorded, the statistical analysis allowed complex interpretation of the results with greater insights. For example, one evaluation of the data by S. Yusuf (2004) that included 170,000 patients and 26 randomised primary and secondary trials, concluded that for every millimole per litre reduction in LDL-C, there would be a 20 per cent reduction in risk of major vascular event.

This is compelling: For every 1 mmol LDL-C reduction, a 20 per cent relative risk reduction is achieved.

can we shrink plaque?

Beyond events, could we see disease change?

In another fascinating development, imaging studies such as the ASTEROID and GLAGOV trials have shown that **reducing cholesterol to very low levels *stops* plaque from *progressing*** and, in some instances, ***reduces* the *amount* of plaque** in the arteries.

ASTEROID

The ASTEROID (A Study to Evaluate the Effect of Rosuvastatin on Intravascular Ultrasound-Derived Coronary Atheroma Burden) trial[8] was a clinical study that assessed whether intensive statin therapy could reduce coronary atherosclerosis. Conducted across 53 centres in the United States, Canada, Europe, and Australia, the trial involved 507 patients with

8 *Effect of Very High-Intensity Statin Therapy on Regression of Coronary Atherosclerosis (The ASTEROID Trial) Steven E. Nissen, MD; et al JAMA. 2006;295(13):1556-1565. doi:10.1001/jama.295.13.jpc60002 https://jamanetwork.com/journals/jama/fullarticle/202629?utm*

A CLOSER LOOK

advanced artery scanning techniques

INTRAVASCULAR ULTRASOUND (IVUS) is a highly accurate and detailed imaging technique used to assess and measure plaque in the coronary arteries. By providing detailed cross-sectional images of the artery's interior (see below), IVUS enables precise evaluation of atherosclerosis, offering invaluable insights into CAD progression and the effects of treatment.

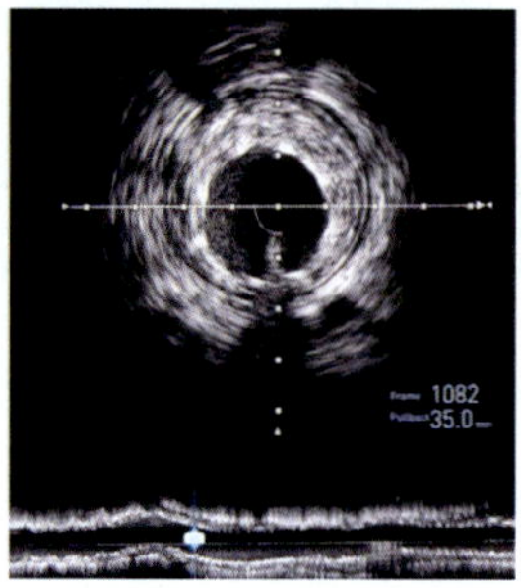

IVUS is an invasive procedure that uses a catheter-mounted ultrasound probe inserted into the artery. The probe emits sound waves to produce high-resolution images of the arterial wall and plaques. This allows for measuring plaque burden – the percentage of the artery's cross-sectional area occupied by plaque – and identifying different types of plaques.

IVUS has been used in clinical trials (e.g., ASTEROID, GLAGOV) to monitor the impact of therapies like statins or PCSK9 inhibitors on plaque volume and regression. Unlike coronary angiography, which visualises only the arterial lumen (the inner space of the artery), IVUS also assesses the vessel wall and can detect early plaque build-up before significant narrowing occurs. Despite its benefits, because IVUS is invasive, it carries procedural risks. Additionally, it cannot fully evaluate the biochemical composition of plaques, for which complementary imaging techniques may be required.

While IVUS primarily provides structural data, advanced techniques like **INTRAVASCULAR ULTRASOUND – VIRTUAL HISTOLOGY** (IVUS-VH) offer better insights into plaque composition, helping to identify vulnerable plaques that are more prone to rupture and cause heart attacks.

OPTICAL COHERENCE TOMOGRAPHY (OCT) offers high-resolution imaging to visualise the detailed structure of coronary plaques (see right). It is especially useful for identifying thin fibrous caps and microstructures, aiding in assessing plaque vulnerability and optimising stent placement.

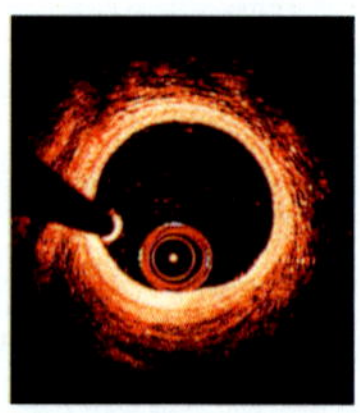

NEAR-INFRARED SPECTROSCOPY (NIRS) complements these techniques by detecting lipid-rich plaques in coronary arteries through chemical composition analysis, helping to assess the risk of plaque rupture.

established CAD. Participants received 40 mg of rosuvastatin daily for 24 months. Intravascular ultrasound (IVUS) imaging (see previous page) was used to measure changes in plaque volume within coronary arteries.

The results were significant.

- **LDL-C reduction:** LDL-C levels decreased by 53.2 per cent; from an average of 130.4 mg/dL to 60.8 mg/dL (3.37 mmol/L to 1.55 mmol/L).
- **HDL-C increase:** HDL-C levels increased by 14.7 per cent; from an average of 43.1 mg/dL to 49.0 mg/dL (1.05 mmol/L to 1.30 mmol/L).
- **Plaque regression:** There was a mean reduction of 0.98 per cent in percentage atheroma (plaque) volume (PAV) across the entire vessel and a decrease of 6.1 mm^3 on average in atheroma volume within the most diseased 10 mm segment.

These findings demonstrated that aggressive lipid-lowering with high-dose rosuvastatin not only improved cholesterol profiles but also led to the regression of coronary atherosclerosis. The trial provided compelling evidence supporting **the use of intensive statin therapy to manage and potentially reverse CAD.**

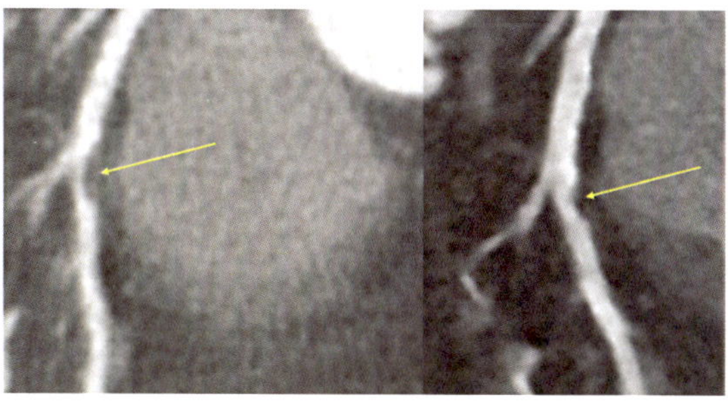

This is the same left anterior descending artery (LAD) – a scan taken in 2019 before treatment (left) and then in 2024 after treatment. The change – a marked decrease in the amount of 'fatty' or non-calcified, inflamed plaque (unstable) – is clearly visible.

GLAGOV

The GLAGOV (Global Assessment of Plaque Regression with a PCSK9 Antibody as Measured by Intravascular Ultrasound) trial[9] evaluated the impact of adding the PCSK9 inhibitor, **evolocumab**, to statin therapy

9 *Effect of Evolocumab on Progression of Coronary Disease in Statin-Treated Patients (The GLAGOV Randomized Clinical Trial) Stephen J Nicholls, Rishi Puri et al. JAMA. 2016;316(22):2373-2384. doi:10.1001/jama.2016.16951 https://jamanetwork.com/journals/jama/fullarticle/2584184?utm*

on coronary atherosclerosis. This double-blind, placebo-controlled study involved 968 patients with established CAD who were already on statins. Participants were randomised to receive either monthly injections of evolocumab (420 mg) or a placebo alongside their ongoing statin treatment, over 76 weeks.

Key findings from the trial included:

- **LDL-C reduction:** The evolocumab group achieved a mean LDL-C level of 36.6 mg/dL (or 0.9 mmol/L), compared with 93.0 mg/dL (2.4 mmol/L) in the placebo group, marking a significant reduction;
- **mean plaque regression:** Patients receiving evolocumab experienced a mean decrease of 0.95 per cent in percentage atheroma volume (PAV - a measure of plaque burden in the coronary arteries), indicating regression of coronary plaque, whereas the placebo group showed a slight increase of 0.05 per cent in PAV, and
- **greater proportion of patients with regression:** Plaque regression was observed in 64.3 per cent of evolocumab-treated patients, compared with 47.3 per cent in the placebo group.

These results show that adding evolocumab to statin therapy can significantly lower LDL-C levels and promote **regression of coronary atherosclerosis**, offering impressive benefits for patients with CAD.

intensive vs moderate if high risk

The PROVE IT–TIMI 22 (Pravastatin or Atorvastatin Evaluation and Infection Therapy–Thrombolysis in Myocardial Infarction 22) trial[10] was a pivotal study that assessed the effects of intensive versus moderate lipid-lowering therapy in patients who had recently experienced acute coronary syndrome (ACS). Conducted between November 2000 and December 2001, the trial enrolled 4162 patients across Australia, Europe, and North America.

Participants were randomised to receive either intensive therapy (atorvastatin 80 mg daily) or moderate therapy (pravastatin 40 mg daily).

10 *Pravastatin or Atorvastatin Evaluation and Infection Therapy: Thrombolysis in Myocardial Infarction 22 - PROVE IT/TIMI 22 - Lipid Lowering Results American College of Cardiology (2004) (http://bit.ly/4eZMYow)*

Additionally, in a 2 × 2 factorial design[11], patients were assigned to a 10-day course of the antibiotic gatifloxacin or a placebo to evaluate the potential impact of infection therapy on cardiovascular outcomes. Gatifloxacin was chosen as it is broad spectrum, works within cells, and is effective against *chlamydia pneumoniae*, a bacterium thought to be implicated in atherosclerosis.

The key findings were:

- **LDL-C reduction:** The atorvastatin group achieved a median LDL-C level of 62 mg/dL (1.60 mmol/L), while the pravastatin group reached a median of 95 mg/dL (2.46 mmol/L);
- **primary endpoint:** The composite endpoint – including all-cause mortality, myocardial infarction (heart attack), unstable angina requiring rehospitalisation, revascularisation, and stroke – occurred in 22.4 per cent of the atorvastatin group compared with 26.3 per cent of the pravastatin group, representing a 16 per cent relative risk reduction ($p = 0.005$);
- **secondary endpoints:** All-cause mortality was 2.2 per cent in the atorvastatin group and 3.2 per cent in the pravastatin group ($p = 0.07$). Unstable angina requiring rehospitalisation occurred in 3.8 per cent of the atorvastatin group compared with 5.1 per cent in the pravastatin group ($p = 0.02$), and
- **safety profile**[12]**:** Elevations in alanine aminotransferase (ALT) levels greater than three times the upper limit of normal were observed in 3.3 per cent of patients in the atorvastatin group and 1.1 per cent in the pravastatin group ($p < 0.001$).

The PROVE IT–TIMI 22 trial demonstrated that intensive lipid-lowering therapy with high-dose atorvastatin significantly reduced the risk of adverse cardiovascular events compared with moderate therapy. This supports the strategy of more aggressive LDL-C reduction in high-risk patients to improve clinical outcomes. The antibiotics arm of the trial produced no significant difference between the two groups.

---

11 *A 2 × 2 factorial design is an experimental setup that examines the effects of two independent variables, each with two levels, on an outcome. This design allows researchers to assess the individual impact of each variable and the combined interaction on the dependent variable.*

12 *Alanine aminotransferase (ALT) levels were monitored as a safety measure to assess potential liver toxicity associated with statin therapy.*

IMPORTANT POINTS

CHOLESTEROL STUDIES

- The foundation stone for our understanding of cholesterol and heart disease was laid in the early 1900s, with many studies conducted throughout the 20th century.
- Soon after statins were discovered in 1976, pharmaceutical companies began developing and registering statin patents.
- The Scandinavian Simvastatin Survival Study (4S Study) established the beginning of the therapeutic cholesterol-lowering journey. Many studies followed.
- Newer studies involving novel drugs – the IMPROVE-IT, FOURIER, and ODYSSEY trials – have advanced treatment strategies for secondary prevention.
- Numerous primary prevention trials have contributed markedly to better patient outcomes and an improved knowledge base.
- Imaging studies using advanced scanning techniques have shown that very low LDL-C levels can stop plaque progression, reduce the amount in an artery, or stabilise unstable plaque.

What do you know about triglycerides, the most common fat in the body?

chapter 11

OTHER LIPIDS: WHY TRIGLYCERIDES MATTER TOO

Lowering LDL-C has transformed cardiovascular prevention and reduced events across a wide range of patients. Yet CVD continues to occur, even in well-treated individuals. This shifts attention toward other lipid fractions, including triglycerides (TG) and triglyceride-rich lipoproteins, and their contribution to residual risk.

A high TG level (hypertriglyceridaemia) is an independent risk factor for CVD and is often associated with:

- lipid and particle changes
  - TG-rich and remnant lipoproteins
  - lower HDL-C levels
  - increased numbers of small, dense LDL particles;
- body fat distribution
  - central adiposity (excess weight around the abdomen)
  - visceral adiposity (dangerous fat around organs such as the liver, heart, and intestines), and
- metabolic and vascular effects
  - raised blood pressure
  - prediabetes and type 2 diabetes
  - increased inflammation and blood viscosity (thicker, stickier blood), adding cardiovascular stress

These conditions can also increase the risk of blood clots. They often coexist and exacerbate each other.

complex system

Recalling what we have already learnt, TG are the body's main energy storage unit. They consist of three fatty acids attached to a backbone of glycerol (a three-carbon molecule with hydroxyl groups [-OH] attached to each carbon).

TG metabolism is more complex than cholesterol metabolism.

The body produces TG from dietary fats, oils, and carbohydrates (such as oils, butter, animal fats, and processed foods). These fats are

- broken down in the small intestine. There, bile salts help break dietary TG into fatty acids and monoglycerides (a single fatty acid chain attached to a glycerol molecule). They are then 'repackaged' in the intestinal lining, absorbed, and released into the lymphatic system, transported in chylomicrons (lipoproteins);
- chylomicrons move through the lymphatic system into the bloodstream and eventually reach the liver. There, TG are processed into VLDL, which can then be metabolised into IDL particles, and finally, into LDL particles.

Fat (adipose) cells store energy as TG, which can be broken down into glycerol and free fatty acids (FFA). The FFA can then be taken up and used by muscle cells as a source of energy.

heart health

Although TG are not found in plaque, they contribute to plaque formation through being present in TG-rich lipoprotein remnants. TG associations, including low HDL-C levels, smaller and more dense LDL particles, also point to underlying processes and the person's overall metabolic health.

Triglycerides are important in heart health as they:

- are a marker of metabolic health,
- correlate with other lipid abnormalities,
- play a role in energy storage and use,
- impact blood viscosity and clotting, which may trigger pancreatitis, and
- have implications for certain genetic disorders.

Let's look at these indicators more closely.

Triglyceride levels are a key **indicator of metabolic health**. High TG levels are a major component of metabolic syndrome, a cluster of conditions that significantly increases the risk of heart disease, stroke, and type 2 diabetes.

Metabolic syndrome includes high TG, high blood pressure, high blood sugar, excess body fat around the waist, and abnormal cholesterol levels. These interconnected conditions collectively heighten risk; managing TG and their associations is essential.

Elevated TG levels **often accompany other lipid abnormalities**. They typically correlate with higher levels of small, dense LDL particles and lower levels of HDL-C. This lipid profile is particularly concerning because it increases the risk of atherosclerosis. Moreover, high TG levels link to increased inflammation in the body, which can further contribute to CVD.

Triglycerides also play a crucial role in **energy storage and utilisation.** As we already know, they are the body's main form of stored fat. An excess of TG often indicates an imbalance between energy input and output. This imbalance can lead to obesity, which is a significant risk factor for heart disease.

Additionally, high TG levels often accompany **liver disease**, recently renamed **metabolic dysfunction-associated steatotic liver disease** (MASLD)[1] . This condition is linked with risk of CVD. Thus, managing TG levels helps maintain a healthy energy balance and prevents obesity-related heart issues.

Another important aspect is the effect of TG on **blood viscosity and clotting**. Elevated TG levels can make the blood more viscous (thicker and stickier), impairing blood flow and increasing the risk of clot formation.

In the most extreme cases, raised TG levels can 'clog up' the arteries of the pancreas and lead to pancreatitis[2], a life-threatening condition. Blood clots

---

1 *Steatotic is the term used to describe something related to or characterised by steatosis, which is the abnormal retention of lipids within a cell.*

2 *When TG levels are very high, fatty deposits can form in the pancreas. These deposits can cause inflammation and damage the pancreatic cells, resulting in pancreatitis. Additionally, the breakdown of TG into free fatty acids can be toxic to the pancreas, further contributing to inflammation and pancreatitis.*

can lead to severe cardiovascular events such as heart attacks and strokes. Therefore, keeping TG levels in check is vital for maintaining smooth blood flow and reducing the risk of these potentially life-threatening events.

Finally, certain **genetic disorders**, such as familial combined hypertriglyceridaemia and familial chylomicronaemia, can cause extremely high TG levels. Individuals with these conditions have a higher risk of developing pancreatitis and, in some cases, CVD. Recognising and managing this genetic predisposition is crucial for preventing severe health outcomes.

management

Managing TG levels is imperative for cardiovascular health because it helps address these associated risks and conditions.

Triglycerides generally respond more readily to lifestyle changes and nutraceuticals than cholesterol does. Managing elevated TG **always begins with lifestyle modifications,** particularly dietary changes and exercise.

A diet that is low in saturated fat, limits alcohol and sugars, and incorporates omega-3 fatty acids is a key strategy, often complemented by nutraceuticals. While medications may be used, addressing the secondary factors – such as diabetes, alcohol intake, thyroid disease, and hormone levels (including oestrogen and testosterone) – is essential for effective management.

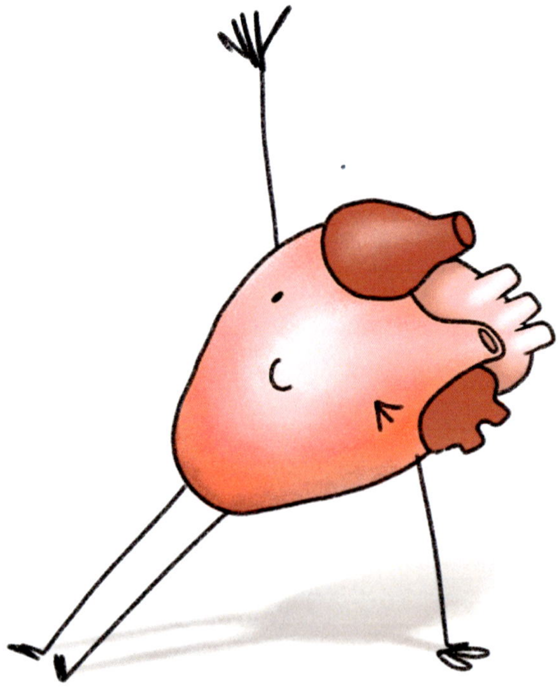

The next section of the book will examine these elements, including the usefulness of therapies such as fish oil.

IMPORTANT POINTS

OTHER LIPIDS: TRIGLYCERIDES

- Triglycerides (TG) are common lipids (fats) that the body uses for energy. They are the main energy storage unit within the body, and are the body's main form of stored fat.
- They originate from dietary sources as well as being produced in the body.
- A high TG level is called hypertriglyceridaemia and is associated with several other conditions that often co-exist with and exacerbate each other. These conditions can also include the increased risk of blood clots.
- Lowering TG through lifestyle changes and nutraceuticals is generally easier than lowering cholesterol using the same approach.
- TG levels reflect metabolic health and independently contribute to CAD risk.

YOU have control. Now discover how to effectively take charge of your heart health with medications, proactive lifestyle changes, and targeted treatment strategies – with the help of your GP and specialist.

cholesterol curiosities

metabolic dance partners

Triglycerides and cholesterol are metabolic dance partners – sometimes cooperating, sometimes competing, yet always influencing each other!

travelling companions, but ...

TG and cholesterol travel together but dislike each other chemically. Although cholesterol and TG are both lipids, but they are chemically incompatible with water in different ways. They have to be packaged together in lipoproteins (e.g. VLDL, LDL, HDL), but the ratio matters. High TG actually 'dilute' the cholesterol content of these particles, which is why calculated LDL-C becomes unreliable when TG exceed 4.5 mmol/L (400 mg/dL+).

triglycerides are not a single substance

TG are a *family* of molecules made from different fatty acids, which influence how they behave in the body.

and, what's more ...

Eating fat raises TG temporarily; eating sugar raises them chronically. A fatty meal spikes TG for three to six hours, but excess carbohydrates, especially fructose, cause the liver to synthesise new TG from scratch leading to chronically elevated levels.

AND

Statins lower cholesterol efficiently but TG reluctantly. Fibrates flip the script. They tackle TG head-on while nudging cholesterol as an afterthought.

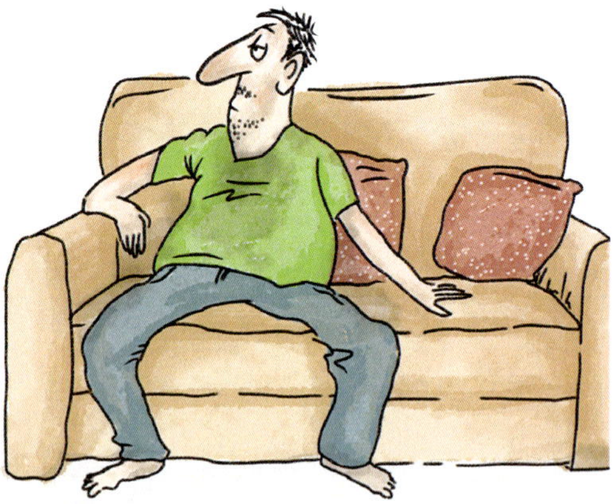

Managing elevated TG always starts with lifestyle modifications, especially dietary changes and exercise. Although medication may sometimes be necessary, it's essential to address secondary factors, such as diabetes, alcohol consumption, thyroid disorders, and hormonal imbalances, to achieve effective long-term control.

TAKING CHARGE OF CHOLESTEROL LEVELS

medications treatments

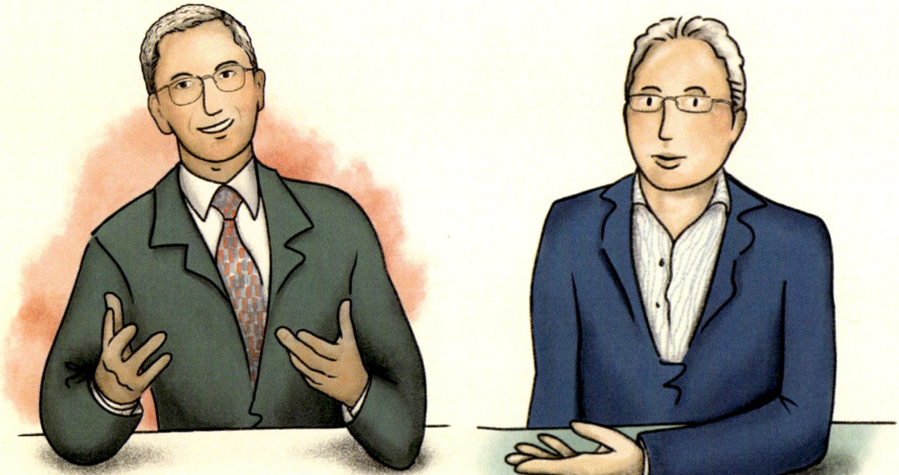

chapter 12

LIPID-LOWERING INTERVENTIONS: TREATING THE LIPID PROFILE

This section is 'where the rubber hits the road' – where theory transforms into practical implementation. This signifies the critical juncture where we transition from understanding the principles to applying effective treatments. In the following chapters, we delve into the strategies for managing high cholesterol levels, aiming not only to reduce risks but also to maintain, or even improve, your heart health.

The objective is to significantly reduce LDL-C, especially for people identified as high risk (such as those who have a genetic risk, dyslipidaemia, or diabetes or who have had an event). Several treatment options are available. However, it is essential to understand that treatment plans will vary based on individual health factors, and **all decisions** should be made in consultation with healthcare professionals, including your cardiologist and general practitioner. **For optimal cholesterol management, medication is essential** alongside lifestyle changes and, if appropriate, nutraceuticals.

options

statins: Statins are the most commonly prescribed class of medications to lower cholesterol. They inhibit the production of cholesterol in the liver. They are highly effective and safe and are used in accordance with the recommendations of drug regulating authorities around the world.

medications other than statins: These include

- **ezetimibe,** which reduces the absorption of cholesterol in the small intestine. It is often prescribed in combination with statins or as an alternative for those who do not tolerate high doses of statins;
- several newer and developing medications target specific proteins in the body. These include:

- **PCSK9 inhibitors** (such as evolocumab and inclisiran), which block the PCSK9 protein, thus increasing the number of LDL receptors;
- the **MTP inhibitor** (lomitapide), which blocks lipoprotein assembly;
- the **ANGPTL3 inhibitor** (evinacumab), which aids fat clearance, and
- the **ATP citrate lyase inhibitor** (bempedoic acid), which reduces cholesterol production in the liver.

• **bile acid sequestrants**, **niacin**, and **fibrates** were historically important but now are used infrequently.

omega-3 fatty acid supplements: Fish oil supplements, rich in omega-3 fatty acids, may have a modest impact on lowering TG and improving overall heart health.

plant sterols and stanols: These are naturally occurring substances found in certain plant foods. They can be added to the diet through fortified foods or supplements and may help lower LDL-C levels.

soy: Soy protein consumption may help lower LDL-C levels.

fibre supplements: Soluble fibre, such as psyllium, may help lower cholesterol levels. It works by binding to cholesterol and preventing the absorption of cholesterol in the intestines.

regular cholesterol monitoring: Regular blood tests to monitor cholesterol levels are essential for assessing the effectiveness of treatment and making adjustments as needed.

You may ask: What about diet, exercise, and weight? While vital for heart health, these lifestyle changes have little effect on lowering LDL-C, except in mixed dyslipidaemia or raised TG.

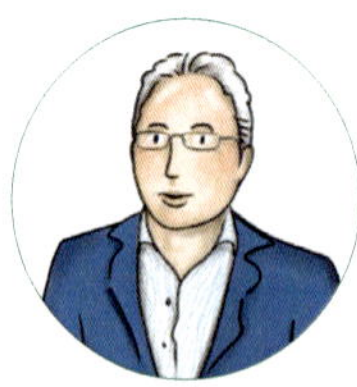

Finally! A closer look at statins – through a deep dive into the first and most important LDL-C lowering option.

chapter 13

STATINS: THE CORNERSTONE OF CHOLESTEROL LOWERING

Statins are the go-to group of drugs to lower cholesterol. HMG-CoA reductase inhibitors, they are safe and effective. Their use is supported by an abundance of data from trials and by drug regulators around the world.

Statins work by blocking an enzyme in the liver called beta-hydroxy-beta-methylglutaryl coenzyme A reductase (HMG-CoA reductase), which reduces cholesterol production, particularly that found in LDL particles. While it might seem that the key effect is inhibiting cholesterol synthesis, the real benefit comes from what happens next: the drop in liver cholesterol triggers the liver to increase the number of LDL receptors (LDLR) on its surface. These receptors pull more LDL out of the bloodstream, resulting in a significant reduction – often up to 50 per cent – in LDL-C levels.

This group of drugs was developed about 50 years ago after its discovery by Japanese biochemist Akira Endo (1933-2024), whose work centred on the relationship between fungi and cholesterol biosynthesis. The first statin was mevastatin, also known as compactin. Although this did not become an approved drug, the mevastatin derivative, pravastatin, did. Lovastatin was the first commercial statin. Others followed: pravastatin, simvastatin, fluvastatin, atorvastatin, rosuvastatin and pitavastatin.

statin LDL-C reduction table

statin	approximate LDL-C reduction (%)
Atorvastatin (10-80 mg)	30-55%
Rosuvastatin (5-40 mg)	45-60%
Simvastatin (10-40 mg)	25-45%
Pravastatin (10-40 mg)	20-35%
Fluvastatin (20-80 mg)	20-35%
Lovastatin (10-40 mg)	20-40%
Pitavastatin (1-4 mg)	30-50%

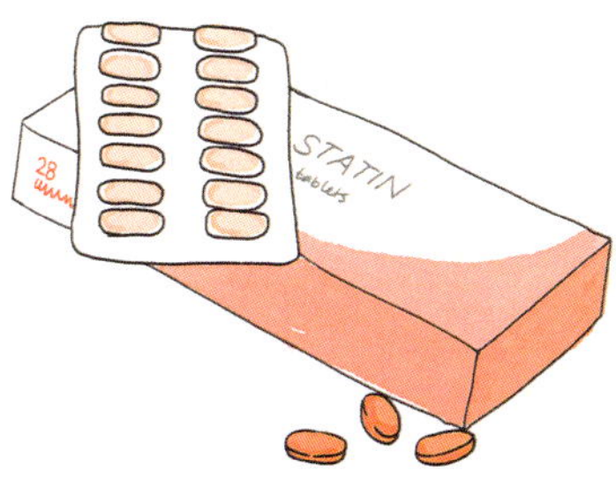

Each agent has a different potency and some differences in chemical qualities. For example, atorvastatin is lipo**philic** (loves fat), meaning that it moves into fatty tissue, while rosuvastatin is lipo**phobic** (doesn't like fat), meaning that it stays in the blood plasma. **Atorvastatin** and **rosuvastatin** are the most potent of the drugs and the most prescribed today. Numerous published trials support their efficacy and safety in reducing events.

Easy access to the Internet means that everyone can consult 'Dr Google', and so patients come to us 'well informed', and with 'a plan'. Many patients have great questions, legitimate concerns and genuine wants.

"I want to manage my cholesterol with diet and exercise."

"What effect will lowering cholesterol have on my memory?"

"What about the effect of lowered cholesterol on hormones?"

"I don't want to take a tablet unless I have to."

"I've tried a statin before, and it didn't agree with me."

risk vs benefit in primary prevention

There are no medications without possible side effects and all patients will have a variable potential benefit. So, we discuss the risks of the medication versus the benefits that the individual will gain from taking the medication. If a patient has borderline cholesterol and (at an older age) no

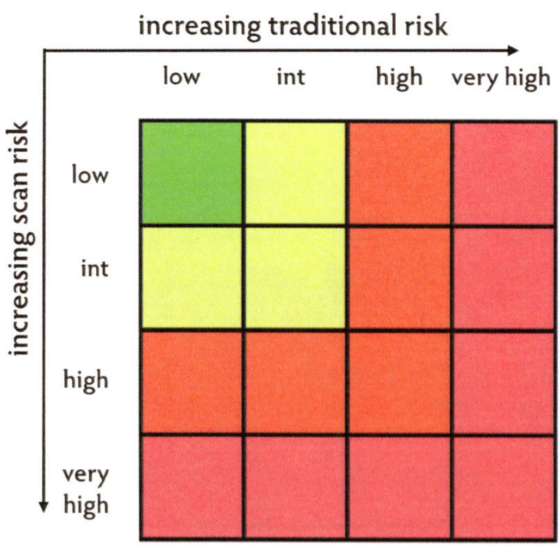

Dealing with risk in any situation is dealing with the weakest link in the chain or the greatest risk situation. When it comes to cardiovascular risk, treatment is required if the traditional risk factors are high or if the scan demonstrates high risk or a combination of both.

evidence of plaque build-up in the arteries, then taking a statin is a potential **side effect risk *without* benefit**. It might be hard to justify the patient taking the medication in this situation.

Conversely, if the artery shows a significant build-up of plaque, then taking a statin is a potential **side effect risk *with* benefit**. The important point to understand (and remember) in the cholesterol story is that using blood cholesterol levels to predict if somebody is at risk of heart disease can be **inaccurate in the individual**. However, if we do further testing (scans) and find that an individual has CAD or high-risk atheroma (plaque) burden, or associated risk factors, then the literature says that treating those individuals with a statin **will reduce the risk of an event.**

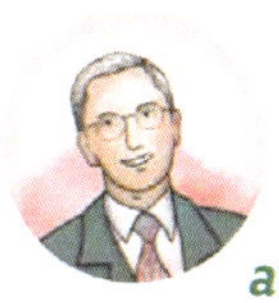

*I (Dr W.) use the term **coronary atheroma burden** to describe plaque in the arteries of a patient who is otherwise well. It is a description for the extent of plaque formation within the coronary arteries as demonstrated on imaging before the development of a disease. (In other words, a **primary prevention** setting.)*

With the widespread availability of statins and a **misdirected belief** that **all** cholesterol is a problem, many patients are taking cholesterol-lowering medication in a primary prevention situation when they **may** have no build-up of cholesterol – no plaque – in the arteries. So, they could be taking a medication, with possible side effects, and see no beneficial outcome.

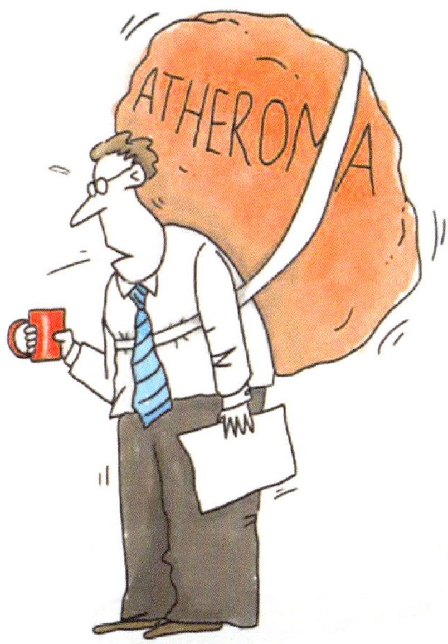

This is when cardiac CT imaging can clarify the condition of the coronary arteries and help weigh risks and benefits. By knowing a patient's **artery health**, we can then be clear about the benefit that person will obtain from taking a statin (or not), with its risk of side effects.

side effects

Statins are, collectively, the most studied and most prescribed medication in history. Although their side effects are well documented, side effects are infrequent and usually mild. Statin-related rhabdomyolysis, when muscle becomes damaged, is severe and occurs in about one in 70,000 statin-takers. Serious liver toxicity occurs at a similar rate. Statin-associated muscle symptoms (SAMS) – encompassing any muscle-related symptoms including muscle pain, weakness, cramps, and fatigue – affect approximately one in 20 patients, with the majority able to continue their therapy. An increase in the blood sugar (glucose) level is important for people who have prediabetes. Such an increase leads to diabetes in about one in 500 patients.

When asked, I, Dr W., often say that the side effect we are hoping for is longevity. Jokes aside, though, I have to say that, as a general rule, I don't tell patients what side effects may arise from the medication, not to be paternalistic, but, I'm aware of the power of suggestion and nocebo[1]. I've learned that if I warn patients a medication *may* cause slight dizziness or blurred vision, 50 per cent of patients will feel it before leaving my office! Helpful pharmacists also provide pages of side effect information. In theory, this educates, but patients often give them to me, highlighted to show every side effect they've 'experienced'.

I'm not being dismissive of side effects. It is **critical** to be aware of **tolerability**, particularly when the patient may be on the medication long-term. Yet, I see little point in running a high chance of evoking a side effect-through-expectation. (The SAMSON trial is covered in chapter 14.) What I say to patients is that some people will be allergic, and this is completely unpredictable, like reacting to peanuts. Some patients may have trouble, but only a trial of the medication will let us know this. **The vast majority**

1 *The nocebo effect occurs when a patient experiences adverse or side effects from a treatment or intervention, not because of the treatment itself but due to an expectation of harm; the opposite of a placebo. There will be more about this in the chapter on statin intolerance.*

of people take them *without* a problem. That is why these drugs have been rigorously evaluated by the Therapeutic Goods Administration (Australia) and other regulators worldwide, and why doctors are authorised to prescribe them.

Having said that, the most **commonly reported** side effects are muscle aches and pains. As mentioned on the previous page, on very rare occasions, this can be severe, causing muscle damage, and is called rhabdomyolysis. It occurs especially in people who are taking immune suppressant drugs, are dehydrated, older, and/or have impaired renal function. Rhabdomyolysis always increases creatinine kinase (CK) levels (confirming muscle damage). While this severe reaction is seen once for every 70,000 patients on a statin, it is important to remember that **we are treating a severe condition that kills approximately one in four people.** The development of aches and pains is variable and will be patient-specific. And, as we are giving these medications to patients who are mostly over 50 years of age, separating aches and pains caused by medication from getting a bit older and stiffer is difficult. I, Dr W., suspect statins are occasionally blamed when ageing, arthritis and a busy day in the garden may be closer to the cause.

We look more closely at side effects in chapter 14
STATIN INTOLERANCE: WHAT THE SCIENCE TELLS US

let's be clear

When considering taking a statin, what is always important is to be clear about the risk and benefit and to work with them. Patience is often required.

- If the patient has a low-risk atheroma burden, then persisting with the medication with side effects makes little sense.
- If the patient has known CAD, or a high-to-very-high risk atheroma burden, then it is important to find a solution. This patient **will benefit** from the medication, so the side effects need to be managed. In this situation there are several options:
    - Most importantly, **be certain that it *is* the statin that is causing the side effects**. This should be evaluated under medical supervision and will require the withdrawal of the medication and re-challenge. This may need to be repeated.

- **Try a different statin**. As we have learned, some of the statins are lipophilic, and some are lipophobic. It is worth changing from one to the other to see if that makes a difference, or try alternate day dosing.
- Another option is to **lower the dose** to a level that doesn't cause the side effects. The doctor and patient will need to have a 'tolerance conversation' and then work closely adjusting (titrating) the dose of the best-tolerated statin to find a dose that suits the individual. Dr W. and Dr K. have patients taking half a tablet of the lowest dose of statin twice a week without problems. Any more than this and side effects impact their daily well-being. In this situation, a little is better than none.
- Today, **non-statin** cholesterol-lowering drugs are available that can work synergistically with the statin.

For more guidance on statin-associated muscle symptoms, please review the NPS Medicinewise Algorithm[2] written by leading Australian lipidologists, including Dr K.

effectiveness

Statins are preferably **taken at night** when cholesterol production is at its peak. Over the past 20 years, we've seen a shift in CAD, with improved patient outcome. Those started on cardioprotective agents like statins after their first event often remain remarkably stable. Other health changes may be confounders. Risk factors, such as lipoprotein(a) and diabetes, also affect outcomes. For high-risk patients or those with significant vulnerable atheroma (fatty, cholesterol-rich build-up) on imaging, LDL-C-lowering statins remain the most **efficient**, **cost-effective**, and **measurable** part of management. Even without trial data, for the right patient, statins **reduce** CAD events, strokes, and vascular dementia (the most common dementia in Australia and other Western countries).

Statin **choice** depends on patient response, medical history, and potential side effects

2 *Statin-associated muscle symptoms (SAMS), NPS Medicinewise, 17 June 2017 (https://www.nps.org.au/professionals/managing-lipids/statin-associated-muscle-symptoms-sams)*

A CLOSER LOOK

important conversations

DR BISHOP

Some patients report difficulty tolerating statins or are hesitant to restart them due to past side effects. These conversations matter. Doctors should adopt a straightforward, reassuring approach that respects concerns while aiming for effective treatment. Most issues are not true allergies or rare reactions, so the focus can usually shift to improving tolerance and finding a workable solution.

ALLERGIC REACTIONS The first and most serious type of medication reaction is an allergic or anaphylactic response, which is extremely rare. These reactions are immune-driven and can include symptoms such as swelling, hives, and difficulty breathing. An example would be a severe response to peanuts or a bee sting. If someone has experienced an allergic reaction to a statin, reintroduction would not be considered. The risks are too great.

IDIOSYNCRATIC REACTIONS This second type of reaction is one that is clearly caused by the drug, but is both *unpredictable* and *unexplained*. A well-known example arose during the COVID-19 pandemic when the AstraZeneca vaccine, although effective, triggered blood clots in a small number of people. These kinds of reactions cannot be anticipated, and for this reason, rechallenge is generally not appropriate. The same principle applies to statins: if someone has had an idiosyncratic response, reintroduction would not be advised.

TOLERANCE Statin-related side effects also fall into a third category – **the most common**, and importantly, the **most manageable** response. People respond differently to the same substance. A helpful illustration is alcohol: one person may feel tipsy after a glass of sherry, while another may tolerate several pints of beer without noticeable effect. Some of this may be due to biological variation; some to conditioning. But in both cases, the concept of tolerance explains the wide variation in response.

With statins, each intolerant person has a threshold: above it, symptoms begin; below it, they remain comfortable. The goal is to identify and stay beneath that point. This might mean starting with a very low dose once or twice a week, then gradually increasing the dosage if tolerated. At the other end of the spectrum, a person might take a moderate dose most days with no trouble.

I encourage patients to self-titrate. As we work together, they feel ownership in the healing and prevention process.

Framing this as a spectrum can help patients see that a gradual reintroduction is safe and often effective. It respects their past experiences and gives them control over the pace of reintroduction. Most importantly, it helps balance two vital goals: living as long as possible and living well.

DOING IT NATURALLY Many patients express a strong preference to 'do it naturally' rather than take medication. This is a valid and admirable desire. Still, it is important to step back and consider the bigger picture: the human body, as remarkable as it is, wasn't designed by nature to live well into old age.

the limits of evolution Our DNA – the biological blueprint that governs repair, recovery and resilience – was shaped millions of years ago on the African plains. Back then, living into one's 20s was already a success in evolutionary terms. Natural selection prioritised early survival and reproduction, not long life. We did not evolve to live into our 70s, 80s, and 90s. Thanks to modern medicine, better hygiene, nutrition, and safety, we are now living far beyond what our DNA was designed to support. But the blueprint hasn't changed. Our genes have not evolved in step with our extended lifespan.

outsmarting our blueprint So when someone wants to 'do it naturally', it's helpful to recognise that nature never expected us to live this long. If we want to remain healthy, mobile, and independent into older age, we are, in effect, pushing against our natural limits. That means we must be smart – and sometimes that means using every advantage available, including modern medicine. This isn't about 'giving in' to the big pharmaceutical companies. It's about doing everything we reasonably can – with lifestyle, with medications when appropriate, with science – to support healthy ageing and long-term health.

REFRAMING THE CHOICE When people are reluctant to take medication, especially after previously experiencing side effects, it can help to revisit the types of reactions (allergic, idiosyncratic, or tolerance-based). If the issue is one of tolerance, a carefully considered reintroduction may be possible. And if the issue is philosophical – a desire to remain 'natural' – then the key message is this: We are no longer living in a natural world. If our aim is to live not just longer, but better, we may need to work smarter than our DNA intended.

CUSTOMISING CARE: a practical solution for Paul

It was a weekend of very out-of-the-ordinary heart palpitations that led me to be sitting anxiously in front of Dr Bishop discussing the results of a treadmill heart stress test. Dr Bishop was easy to talk with and thorough in his explanation of my good results. I left the appointment feeling greatly relieved. Further episodes of the palpitations a few months later saw me back. A nightly tablet prescribed at this visit worked well so I was quite looking forward to my next review appointment so I could pass on the good news.

It was during this appointment that Dr Bishop suggested I consider having a CT scan to get a far more detailed picture and understanding of my heart, particularly plaque levels and the condition of my heart arteries. I was very happy to have the scan as up until my palpitations started I had been a typical Aussie male and hadn't given much thought to my heart. I considered that I consumed a healthy diet, was quite active and didn't have any family history of concern.

To my surprise and subsequently I realised later, thankfully, the scan revealed a coronary artery calcium (CAC) score of 327, which Dr Bishop said carried an unacceptably high future risk for me if left untreated.

He prescribed a statin medication and low dose aspirin, with one tablet of each to be taken daily. This preventive approach made sense as I've always believed that prevention is far better than cure when options exist.

After a week or so I started to notice some muscle aches and pains, which continued to increase over subsequent weeks. I ceased taking the tablets to relieve the side effects. At my next review appointment, Dr Bishop prescribed a different statin and also suggested I experiment with the dosage to see what worked best for me.

To ensure I could keep a reliable track of my 'experiment' I printed off a yearly calendar and developed a simple method for showing what tablets I took and when. Initially, I started taking the new medication on every second day. Eventually, I settled on a dosage of three tablets per week.

As this provided good relief, I felt I should also re-try my original tablets for comparison. I noticed a further reduction in pain so I continued for a further few months until my next review.

I was very pleased to see that my cholesterol levels were 'on target'. Dr Bishop was happy for me to continue with my three-tablet-per-week routine, with a subsequent follow-up review.

PERSONALISED PREVENTION: Jane's pathway

I have had 'high' cholesterol for as long as I can remember. However, while my LDL-C was high, so, too, was my HDL-C, giving a total cholesterol (TC):HDL-C ratio that was within the acceptable range. There was never any pressure, or even suggestion, from GPs over the years to take medication.

In 2013, I became Dr Bishop's patient for a matter unrelated to cholesterol. During testing, it was found that I had a zero CAC score. So, I was one of those people with high cholesterol yet no plaque in the arteries. Five or six years later, when the test was repeated, a smidgen of plaque was found in the proximal left anterior descending artery (not the best place for it to be).

I've followed Dr Bishop's Healthy Heart Network for some time, including his podcasts, and am familiar with concepts such as 'LDL-C years'. So when two sets of blood tests showed that my lipid profile was deteriorating, I asked my GP whether I could try a statin – understanding that this was in a primary prevention setting – to lower cholesterol levels and reduce the risk of plaque build-up.

He prescribed one rosuvastatin tablet, 10 mg daily. I was in the fortunate position that if I suffered side effects, then I could stop taking the statin without concern.

I took the tablets with good regularity between July 2023 and February 2024. For much of that time I was walking regularly and trying to improve my eating habits.

I had another (fasting) blood test in mid-February 2024, and the results were – well, you can see for yourself:

	test 1	test 2	
total cholesterol (TC)	7.2	4.9	ideally < (less than) 5.2 mmol/l
triglycerides (TG)	1.2	0.9	ideally <2.0 mmol/l
HDL-C	1.9	2.1	ideally > (greater than) 1.0 mmol/l
TC to HDL-C ratio	3.8	2.3	ideally <4.0 ratio
non HDL-C	5.3	2.8	ideally <4.0 mmol/l
LDL-C	4.7	2.4	ideally* <3.4 mmol/l (*ideally refers to the general, healthy population. Importantly, lower targets may be indicated based on an individual patient's clinical situation.)

Needless to say, I was – and remain (2025) – thrilled with those and more recent results. Staying on the statin gives me peace of mind, knowing I'm actively taking steps to protect my heart health.

Side effects? If they exist, they've been subtle enough to blend into the usual ups and downs of daily life. Any stiffness or soreness I feel seems more linked to long days sitting at the computer or gardening or walking than the medication. Even if there were mild side effects, the overwhelming benefit of lowering my cholesterol and reducing my risk of future heart issues makes it entirely worthwhile.

Prevention is the best strategy. I look forward to my next blood test as continuing reassurance that I'm on the right path.

IMPORTANT POINTS

STATINS

- Statins are the most important drugs for cholesterol management.
- They are safe, effective and cheap.
- They block the production of cholesterol in the liver.
- Any drug taken has the potential to produce side effects. Any side effects must be weighed against the benefit of taking the drug for each individual.
- Statin side effects are generally mild and infrequent.
- Statins can be combined with other medications for enhanced LDL-C lowering.
- Statins reduce CVD events in high-risk patients. No doubt.

Statins and their side effects often attract negative attention but are these concerns genuine, or are they amplified by the influence of media exaggerations?

chapter 14

STATIN INTOLERANCE: WHAT THE SCIENCE TELLS US

Yes, statin intolerance does exist. However, Dr K. observes in his practice that statin intolerance is infrequent and rarely leads to discontinuation of therapy. And recent studies suggest it may not be as common as widely believed. We want to share these fascinating results with you.

This book emphasises that for those who can tolerate them, statins are highly efficient and effective in lowering cholesterol. Yet, patients often present saying that they suffer aches and pains as a consequence of taking them, especially at high doses. We need to be clear. **Any drug can induce side effects in certain patients.** Our bodies respond differently to various chemicals. Tomatoes may trigger arthritis in certain people. The allergic reaction to peanuts can be severe enough to be fatal for some.

alirocumab trial

Let's look firstly at a paper, Efficacy and safety of alirocumab in statin-intolerant patients over 3 years: open-label treatment period of the ODYSSEY ALTERNATIVE Trial (conducted by the pharmaceutical company Sanofi).

Alirocumab[1], a monoclonal antibody PCSK9 inhibitor[2], is one of the new agents that works through a completely different pathway to statins – the PCSK9 pathway (proprotein convertase subtilisin/kexin type 9).

The trial involved a statistically significant number of **patients** who were said to be **statin intolerant**. Before being selected, participants underwent rigorous screening for statin intolerance.

Participants had a four-week run-in, during which researchers gave them

1 *Alirocumab was discontinued in Australia in 2024 for commercial reasons.* *See p 167 – evolocumab and footnote 4 – for further information,*

2 *For more information on PCSK9 inhibitors, see p 166.*

a sugar pill to ensure no previous treatment residue remained in their bodies at the start of the trial. During that four-week sugar tablet run, 6.4 per cent of patients reported statin-intolerant symptoms and withdrew.

This result is particularly interesting because these people were not on any medication, only a sugar pill. Therefore, any aches and pains could NOT have been related to a statin.

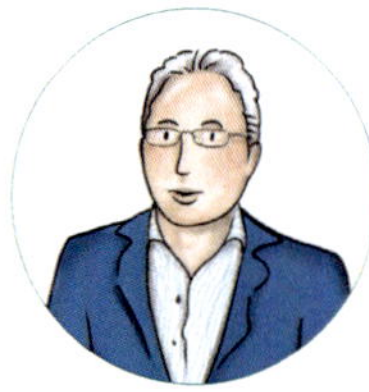

After the initial four weeks, the participants were given 20 mg of atorvastatin (probably the most used statin, generally given at the maximum dose of 80 mg) for 24 weeks. At the end of that time, 46 per cent, or almost half, reported some form of statin-associated muscle symptom (SAMS).

Of the 46 per cent, about half (22 per cent) discontinued the trial because the symptoms were too severe.

And, from a practical perspective, that's what should happen. If you are taking medication and it gives you intolerable side effects, you should not take it.

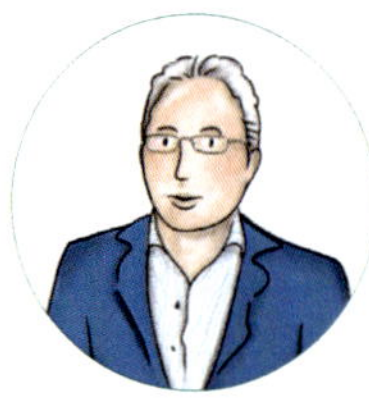

That meant 24 per cent could continue because their aches and pains were mild. So, after 24 weeks, if 46 per cent had some symptoms, 54 per cent had no problem.

These figures are extremely interesting. Fifty-four per cent – half of the people who **thought they were statin intolerant** and had persuaded their specialists to believe they were statin intolerant – had **no symptoms**. Of the 46 per cent who had some symptoms, about half could continue. So that extra 24 per cent, plus the 54 per cent who did not have any symptoms, means that **78 per cent** of patients **could take** the medication. Yet when they entered the study, **100 per cent** believed they **could not tolerate statins!**

Not only is this extremely interesting, but it is also incredibly important.

If you – as a patient – believe that you cannot tolerate statins, could you be **one of the 78 per cent missing out on a potentially life-saving therapy?**

If – as a cardiologist, clinical lipidologist, endocrinologist, diabetologist, or primary care physician – we **unquestioningly accept** that 100 per cent of people who claim statin intolerance are genuinely intolerant, then we **may be doing our patients a disservice**, hindering their best possible future care.

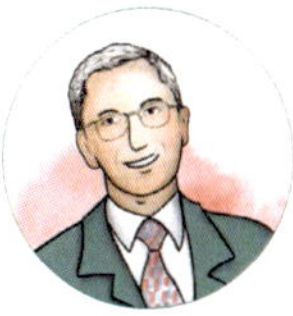

Our comments here have focused on the reliability of a person's claim of statin intolerance. The outcome of the trial was that alirocumab was well-tolerated and consistently reduced LDL-C over three years. You will find more information about PCSK9 inhibitors in chapter 15.

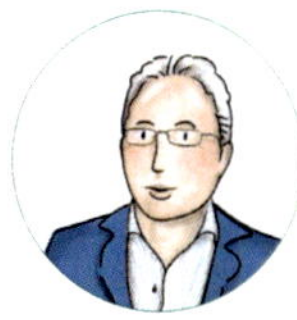

The highly regarded Cleveland Clinic (USA) undertook a similar observational study through its clinics. It concluded that **72 per cent of people who self-reported as statin intolerant were able to take the medication without any problems** if **blinded** to the therapy.

why?

This begs the question, Why?

We can't ignore today's extensive use of social media and the Internet more generally, all of which prime people for the possibility that these statins **might** cause problems. This phenomenon is concerning.

When we look at this in more detail, if we double-blind people to alirocumab, ezetimibe, and atorvastatin, musculoskeletal side effect rates are respectively about 16 per cent, 20 per cent, and 22 per cent. These are not significantly disproportionate, but they indicate that people **may anticipate** problems. When we moved to open label alirocumab, which had a reported statin-associated muscle symptoms (SAMS) of nearly 16 per cent, reported problems dropped to two per cent. This information signals the nocebo effect.

nocebo effect

The nocebo effect occurs when a patient experiences adverse or side effects from a treatment or intervention, not because of the treatment itself but due to an **expectation** of harm; the opposite of a placebo.

I, Dr W., could give a patient a sugar pill and say that it is the best headache treatment therapy available, that it is new and expensive and that it has been tested around the world. About 50 per cent of the time, that pill will have a positive placebo effect. The nocebo effect is the opposite; that anticipation of a negative outcome will give a negative outcome.

personal approach

This brings us to the Self-Assessment Method for Statin side effects Or Nocebo (SAMSON) trial, undertaken in the United Kingdom and funded by the British Heart Foundation. In an attempt to gain more depth, the SAMSON trial took a personalised approach to understanding more about the side effects people experience while taking statins.

Between June 2016 and March 2019, researchers recruited 60 patients. Each personalised trial ran for 12 months. The participant received four lots of three bottles: one bottle was empty; one contained sugar pills; one contained identical-looking pills but with an active ingredient (the statin, atorvastatin at a dose of 20 mg). The bottles were used in a specified random order, one per month over the 12 months. The researchers also provided the participants with a phone app to record their symptoms daily from zero (no symptoms) to 100 (worst symptoms) even on no pill days. If the symptoms became too severe, they were able to stop taking the tablets for that month. Forty-nine of the 60 participants completed the 12 months of their trial.

The results are amazing. For no treatment (empty bottle) months, the mean symptom intensity (the average severity or strength of symptoms experienced by a group of individuals) was 8.0. This figure nearly doubled to 15.4 for placebo months and then went to 16.3 during statin months. Amazing. This tells us that a considerable component of the reported side effects in this cohort was **driven by the *anticipated* side effects they *might* experience.**

The results of the study were four-fold:

- 90 per cent of the symptoms that people reported while taking a statin were also experienced while they were taking a placebo;
- people experienced more symptoms when they were taking a tablet (either statin or the placebo) than when they were not taking a pill;
- participants were just as likely to temporarily stop taking their placebo tablets due to side effects as they were with statins, and
- after participants received an explanation of their results at the end of the study, half of them successfully restarted their statin.

some responses

researchers

Professor Darrel Francis, Primary Investigator, SAMSON[3]

> "This research showed many of the very real side effects of taking a statin were the result of knowing that you are taking a tablet, not the result of the statin inside the tablet."

James Philip Howard, PhD, MB, a fellow at Imperial College in London (a presenter at the American Heart Association Scientific Sessions 2020[4]*)*

> "SAMSON certainly leaves no doubt that patients really do get side effects from statin tablets, but what SAMSON shows us is that 90% of their symptomatic burden is elicited by placebo tablets, too. Because this trial design has built-in no-tablet periods, participants could see as clearly as we could the surprisingly powerful magnitude of the 'nocebo' effect, and this led to half of our patients happily restarting statins.

---

3 *quoted in Can a personalised approach help get people back on statins? 17 November 2020; N Engl J Med 2020; 383:2182-2184 DOI: 10.1056/NEJMc2031173 © 2020, Massachusetts Medical Society*

4 *'Nocebo' effect explains 90% of symptoms in patients who quit statins because of side effects (article in association with the American Heart Association Scientific Sessions 2020, presented virtually 13-17 November 2020): https://www.ccjm.org/page/aha-2020/noceba-statins N Engl J Med 2020; 383:2182-2184 DOI: 10.1056/NEJMc2031173; © 2020, Massachusetts Medical Society*

"The most important message from SAMSON is that side effects from statin tablets are very real, but they are mainly caused by the act of taking the tablets, not by the statin that is contained within them."

Discussant[5] Francine K. Welty, MD, PhD, associate professor of medicine, Harvard Medical School, Boston, replied:

"In practice, many patients develop symptoms later than 2 weeks, so these findings cannot be generalised to them, and limiting enrolment (sic) to those who developed symptoms within 2 weeks of starting a statin could have biased the findings toward a nocebo effect.

"Because statin stoppage increases the risks of stroke, myocardial infarction, and total mortality, management of side effects to permit treatment persistence is important. Supplementing patients with vitamin D whose vitamin D level is below 30 mg/mL has been shown to improve statin tolerance.

"The Cleveland Clinic experience supports alternate dosing (i.e., 2 to 3 times per week), she noted. In patients treated with alternate dosing, total mortality was 2% at 8 years, and similar to daily dosing, compared with 7% in those who discontinued statins (P = .08).

"In those who awaken at night with cramps, try morning dosing because the cramps may occur during the day and may be less likely to affect lifestyle."

participants

One of the participants in SAMSON was Janice Richardson, a retired nurse from West Yorkshire, UK. Janice was originally prescribed statins in 2015 but stopped taking them several times due to developing various aches and pains, which she was convinced were caused by the statins. Her results showed that she experienced the same symptoms when taking the placebo as she did when taking a statin[6].

"I was so surprised that my aches and pains were not due to the statins themselves – you can convince yourself of anything! I'm now very happy to be taking my statins again. Looking back, I walk a lot in

5 *ibid.*

6 *op. cit. (Can a personalised approach ...?)*

the valley where I live and have plenty of stairs in my home that I go up and down multiple times a day. No wonder my body was feeling these pains!"

closer to home ...

We see patients who are adamant they can't tolerate statins. As I'm writing this, I, Dr W., remember a patient who very clearly articulated that statins were causing him side effects. I'll let Jim share his own experience.

Jim

A routine check-up in 1997, when I was aged about 47, found that I had high cholesterol. I was prescribed statins by my treating practitioner. After using them for a short time, I experienced significant side effects. These included thigh muscle pain and occasional nausea. After consulting with my GP and trying different brands and agents, I stopped taking the statins after about three months.

In 2017, I experienced unstable, shortness of breath, and left-sided chest pain on exertion. While I avoided a myocardial infarction, I underwent emergency quadruple bypass surgery.

Post-operatively, I was again prescribed statins and again experienced the side effects of thigh muscle pain and nausea. When I considered stopping the statins again, my GP referred me to Dr Bishop, who explained the importance of the medications for maintaining healthy cholesterol levels.

As the side effects persisted, Dr Bishop's investigations took on a wider approach. During one of my consultations with him, I told him I had a back injury from many years earlier. He immediately examined my legs, found irregularities in power and reflexes, and went on to order an MRI of my spine. He sent me to a neurosurgeon who treated me with a laminectomy and decompression, which relieved my leg pain.

Thanks to Dr Bishop's broader, holistic approach to my cardiac health, I am free of leg pain and able to take my statins with no ill effects. Now aged 74, my cholesterol is the best it has been for a very long time.

We need to recognise that statins are often wrongly accused. Of course, this doesn't mean everyone tolerates them – they can't. Remember our tomatoes and peanuts at the beginning of this chapter. However, medical practitioners should look beyond the obvious and ensure we're not missing something amenable to other therapies, such as Jim with his spine problems.

IMPORTANT POINTS

STATIN INTOLERANCE

- While there will always be some patients who suffer side effects, many patients will be affected by the anticipated side effects they might suffer.
- Medicos should both respect and question the claim of side effects.
- Both patients and medicos need to be prepared to look beyond the obvious and to seek alternative explanations and solutions.

While statins are the current 'pharmaceutical guardians' for lower LDL-C, newer alternative agents are now available.

chapter 15

NON-STATIN THERAPIES: ALTERNATIVE LIPID CONTROL

Beyond the well-established use of statins like atorvastatin and rosuvastatin, other medications have now emerged to help lower cholesterol and TG levels and improve cardiovascular outcomes. Each therapy works in a different way, targeting specific steps in how cholesterol is absorbed, produced, transported, or cleared. They can:

- reduce cholesterol absorption or synthesis *(lowering the supply)*
  - **ezetimibe** reduces cholesterol absorption in the intestines;
  - **bempedoic acid** reduces the liver's production of cholesterol by inhibiting ATP citrate lyase;
  - **bile acid sequestrants** bind bile acids in the intestines, increasing cholesterol excretion and stimulating hepatic cholesterol use;
- reduce PCSK9 activity, which lessens LDL receptor degradation allowing more LDLR on the cell surface *(improving LDL uptake from the blood)*
  - **evolocumab** (PCSK9 inhibitor) blocks the PCSK9 protein;
  - **inclisiran** (siRNA therapy) reduces PCSK9 protein production;
- lower LDL -C independently of LDLR *(important for very high-risk or genetic conditions)*
  - **evinacumab** (ANGPTL3 inhibitor) lowers LDL-C by blocking a protein that interferes with lipid clearance, even when LDLR are limited or absent;
  - **lomitapide** (MTP inhibitor) blocks lipoprotein assembly in the liver and intestine, reducing LDL production at its source;

- primarily target triglycerides *(in metabolic and TG-focused therapies)*
  - **fibrates** lower TG and can modestly raise HDL-C;
  - **omega-3 fatty acids**, prescribed in highly purified forms, lower TG and are used in selected high-risk settings;
- have an historical or diminishing-role in therapies
  - **niacin** (vitamin B3) was an early, versatile option. While no longer favoured, it retains a niche role for selected patients.

reduced cholesterol absorption or synthesis

ezetimibe

Ezetimibe is a **cholesterol absorption inhibitor** (the only drug in its class) and works in the intestine blocking cholesterol reabsorption.

Available since the early 2000s, ezetimibe, primarily targets a protein called Niemann-Pick C1-like 1 (NPC1L1) found in the small intestine. This protein reabsorbs cholesterol before it is excreted through bile and faeces. By inhibiting NPC1L1, ezetimibe reduces the reabsorption of dietary cholesterol, lowering blood cholesterol levels.

Most of the drug stays in the small intestine, with little reaching muscles or organs. As such, side effects are rare, so that it is well tolerated. Occasionally, however, it can cause mild gastrointestinal symptoms such as reflux or bloating. Although recommended to be taken at night when the body's cholesterol production peaks, it can be taken any time and works for 24 hours.

in combination

When used alone, ezetimibe can reduce cholesterol levels by up to 20–25 per cent in some people. Its greatest benefit, however, comes when it is **combined with a statin**, producing high-end reductions of 60-70 per cent. This combination is **powerful** because it targets both cholesterol absorption/reabsorption (ezetimibe) and production (statins). People who are genetically high absorbers of dietary cholesterol (around 20 per cent of the population) tend to see greater LDL-C and total cholesterol reductions than those who are good producers of cholesterol.

As ezetimibe only blocks reabsorption, it is **not a substitute for statins** unless the patient cannot tolerate them. For convenience and cost, several fixed-dose combination preparations are available.

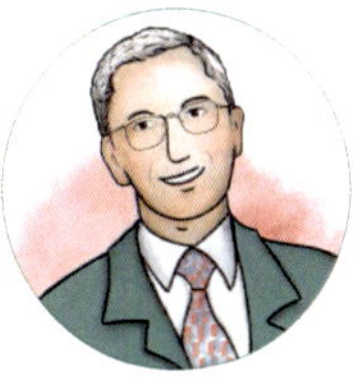

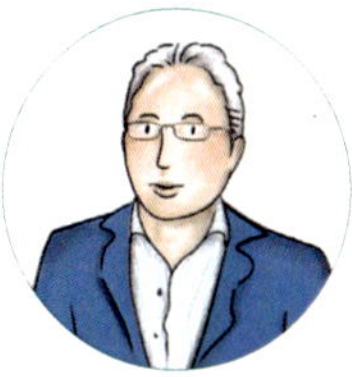

Adding ezetimibe is more than three times as effective as doubling a statin dose and is the obvious next step if maximum statin therapy does not achieve sufficient LDL-C lowering. We often use a moderate or low-dose statin combined with ezetimibe as the first-line therapy – especially for patients who are concerned about statins, have a history of intolerance, or need LDL-C reductions greater than 50 per cent. Using two drugs at lower doses helps minimise side effects while achieving strong lipid-lowering results.

bempedoic acid

Bempedoic acid lowers LDL-C by about 30 per cent. Its main use is for patients who are statin-intolerant.

As an adenosine triphosphate (ATP) citrate lyase inhibitor[1], it works 'upstream' from the statins (HMG-CoA reductase inhibitors) in the cholesterol production process blocking the ATP enzyme. The ATP enzyme plays a crucial role in the production of cholesterol and fatty acids in the liver by converting citrate to acetyl-CoA (acetyl coenzyme A), a key building block for cholesterol and fatty acid synthesis. By inhibiting this ATP enzyme, bempedoic acid **reduces the liver's ability to produce cholesterol,** leading to lower levels of LDL-C by about a 30 per cent.

Bempedoic acid is taken as a prodrug[2] and is converted to an active form only in the liver cells. As the enzyme needed for the conversion is not found in the skeletal muscle, issues with muscle pain should not arise. Bempedoic acid has been used internationally as an adjunct therapy, meaning it is used

---

1 *An ATP citrate lyase inhibitor works by inhibiting the enzyme ATP citrate lyase (ACLY), a key player in cholesterol synthesis.*

2 *A prodrug is a medication or compound that, after administration, is metabolised (converted) within the body into a pharmacologically active drug. Unlike active drugs, prodrugs are initially inactive or have reduced activity and require metabolic transformation to release the active drug, exerting the desired therapeutic effect.*

in addition to ezetimibe and/or statin, especially in individuals who may not tolerate high doses of statins, or need additional LDL-C reduction. It is due to be released in Australia in 2026.

Of note, Dr K.'s Brisbane research centre was one of the first in Australia to assess this therapy in large clinical trials.

bile acid sequestrants

Bile acid sequestrants were versatile team players early in the fight against cholesterol. Although not highly favoured today, they still have their uses.

Bile acids are produced by the liver and play a role in digestion. Bile acid sequestrants (which need to be taken with each meal) bind to these acids in the intestine, forming complexes that cannot be reabsorbed by the intestines. So, they are excreted from the body through faeces, taking with them some of the cholesterol present in the bile and thus reducing the amount of cholesterol circulating in the bloodstream. While their primary effect is to lower LDL-C, they can also modestly increase levels of HDL-C.

They are rarely used today as ezetimibe is more effective, has fewer side effects and, at one tablet a day with or without meals, is much easier to take.

targeting the PCSK9 protein

PCSK9 inhibitors[3] target a key regulatory pathway in LDL-C metabolism. The protein proprotein convertase subtilisin/kexin type 9 (PCSK9) is produced mainly in the liver and plays an important role in controlling the number of LDL receptors (LDLR) on the surface of liver cells. Under normal circumstances, when PCSK9 binds to LDLR, the receptors are directed towards degradation rather than being recycled back to the cell surface. This reduces the liver's capacity to clear LDL particles from the bloodstream. By inhibiting PCSK9, these therapies preserve LDLR recycling, increase LDL uptake from the blood, and produce substantial reductions in circulating LDL-C levels.

---

3 *PCSK9 inhibitor development was made possible by genetic studies in African American families with a naturally mutated non-functioning PCSK9 gene leading to very low LDL-C levels and lowered cardiovascular risk.*

Two newer therapies achieve this: **monoclonal antibody therapy**, which blocks PCSK9 from binding to the LDLR, and **siRNA therapy**, which reduces production of the PCSK9 protein.

evolocumab, monoclonal antibody

The monoclonal antibody[4] PCSK9 inhibitor, evolocumab, is a valuable option for people at very high cardiovascular risk, especially those with familial hypercholesterolaemia (FH) or those who do not reach target LDL-C levels despite optimal oral therapy. It can lower LDL-C levels by as much as 60 per cent. It is usually prescribed as a third-line therapy with statins and ezetimibe.

Its cost and prescribing guidelines currently limit broad use, but for the right people it is highly effective and transformative. For those who do use it, evolocumab is administered by subcutaneous injection (under the skin) fortnightly or monthly.

inclisiran, siRNA therapy

The newest approach to blocking PCSK9 is a developing therapy called small interfering RNA (siRNA) therapy that involves using small RNA (ribonucleic acid) molecules to block the production of very specific proteins. In the case of cholesterol, PCSK9. siRNA stays in the cytosol[5] of the cells, so it does not interact with DNA and, therefore, does not affect a person's genes.

The first drug in this class is **inclisiran**. Given as a simple subcutaneous injection every six months by a health professional, it not only supports excellent adherence but also ensures persistence with therapy.

---

4 *A monoclonal antibody is a laboratory-made antibody designed to recognise and bind to one specific target in the body.*

Normally, the immune system produces many different antibodies, each recognising a different feature of a foreign substance. In contrast, a monoclonal antibody is made from a single cell line, so every antibody molecule is identical and targets the same protein.

In cholesterol treatment, monoclonal antibodies are designed to bind specifically to PCSK9, preventing it from interacting with LDLR. This allows more LDLR to remain active on liver cells, increasing the removal of LDL from the bloodstream.

Two drugs were approved for use in Australia (and elsewhere): evolocumab and alirocumab. The latter was discontinued in Australia in 2024 for commercial reasons.

5 *Cytosol is the liquid portion of the cytoplasm inside a cell, excluding the organelles.*

Inclisiran is generally well tolerated and has shown significant efficacy in lowering LDL-C by about 50 per cent. It is especially helpful for individuals with FH or those who cannot achieve sufficient cholesterol control with statins and ezetimibe. It has been approved for use in many countries.

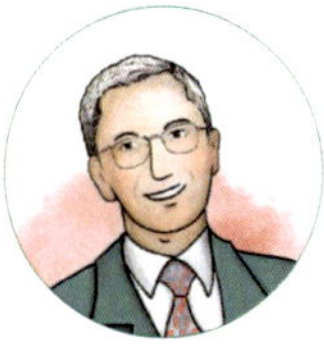

When a PCSK9 inhibitor is prescribed, patients must continue their statin and ezetimibe tablets, as the combination works synergistically to achieve the best cholesterol-lowering effect.

lowering LDL-C independently of LDLR

evinacumab, ANGPTL3 inhibitor (monoclonal antibody)

Another innovative approach for people with severe cholesterol disorders is to block the liver-derived angiopoietin-like 3 (ANGPTL3) protein.

Evinacumab is a monoclonal antibody that targets ANGPTL3, lifting its inhibitory effect on lipid breakdown and lowering LDL-C even when LDLR are defective – a key advantage in homozygous familial hypercholesterolaemia (HoFH), a rare but severe inherited condition causing extremely high LDL-C from birth. (HoFH will be discussed later.)

Evinacumab is given as a once-monthly intravenous infusion and offers a breakthrough option for patients who do not respond adequately to traditional LDL-C-lowering therapies.

lomitapide, MTP inhibitor

Lomitapide – a microsomal triglyceride transfer protein (MTP) inhibitor – is an oral medication used mainly for people with homozygous familial hypercholesterolaemia (HoFH), as mentioned above. Lomitapide blocks MTP in the liver and intestine. MTP is a protein essential for assembling and releasing VLDL and chylomicrons, the lipoproteins responsible for transporting TG and cholesterol from the liver and intestines into the circulation. By inhibiting MTP, lomitapide markedly reduces the production of these precursor lipoproteins and, consequently, the amount of LDL that can be produced and released into the bloodstream.

Because it interferes with normal fat metabolism, it can cause gastrointestinal side effects and fat accumulation in the liver (hepatic steatosis), so careful monitoring is required. It is typically reserved for patients in whom standard therapies are insufficient.

Worldwide, evinacumab and lomitapide are the first drugs approved in their classes. In Australia, they are currently (early 2026) available only for compassionate use. Research is ongoing.

target: triglycerides

omega-3 fatty acids

Omega-3 fatty acids, found in fish oil supplements, are classified as medications when highly purified and specifically prescribed to treat hypertriglyceridaemia (elevated TG). This classification stems from their concentrated form and targeted therapeutic benefits. As fish oil is a popular over-the-counter supplement, we will take a closer look at it soon

fibrates

Fibrates are particularly effective in lowering TG levels and elevating HDL-C. They have only a modest effect on reducing LDL-C. Fibrates have a particular benefit in **mitigating diabetic complications** such as retinopathy and even amputation. They are usually prescribed in conjunction with lifestyle changes, such as a heart-healthy diet and regular exercise. Common fibrates include **fenofibrate** and **gemfibrozil,** although various fibrates are available in different countries. (Also, see next page.)

historical therapies

niacin

Niacin (nicotinic acid), also known as vitamin B3, influences the production and breakdown of fats, including cholesterol. It lowers TG, LDL-C and lipoprotein(a) and increases HDL-C. Yet, it has not shown significant benefits in large clinical trials to date. Niacin can cause side effects. Its role in cholesterol management has diminished due to the availability of other medications with fewer side effects.

A CLOSER LOOK

fenofibrate

Fenofibrate is an example of the fibrate class of drugs. These are medications used primarily to manage and treat **high TG levels** and, to a lesser extent, high cholesterol.

Fenofibrate works by activating the **peroxisome proliferator-activated receptor alpha** (PPARα), which plays a key role in lipid metabolism. PPARα activation increases lipoprotein lipase activity[1], enhancing lipolysis[2] and breaking down TG into free fatty acids (FFA) for energy. PPARα also decreases the expression of ApoC-III (by reducing the production of ApoC-III at the genetic level). This reduction helps lower TG levels in the bloodstream because ApoC-III inhibits the lipoprotein lipase enzyme, which breaks down TG.

Fenofibrate is prescribed with **lifestyle changes,** such as diet, exercise and weight loss, to reduce very high TG levels and to prevent pancreatitis.

The cardiovascular benefits of fenofibrate were tested in the FIELD (Fenofibrate Intervention and Event Lowering in Diabetes) Trial[3]. The Australia-based, double-blind, randomised, placebo-controlled trial assigned participants to receive either 200 mg of fenofibrate daily or a placebo. Researchers looked at nearly 10,000 patients, aged 50 to 75 years, with a wide range of cholesterol and TG levels. Although no significant problems or side effects were experienced with using fenofibrate as a medication, it did not significantly reduce the trial's primary endpoint, coronary events. However, it had a **significant impact** on the microvascular complications (small blood vessel damage caused by high blood sugar levels) of the **diabetics** who were in the trial. They experienced improved kidney function, reduced risk of amputation linked to diabetes, and better outcomes with their eyes.

While the FIELD Trial was technically a negative study for the benefit of fenofibrate in relation to heart issues, practically, it showed **benefit for the diabetic group,** protecting the retina and reducing amputations.

---

1 *Lipoprotein lipase activity refers to the role of the lipoprotein lipase (LPL) enzyme in breaking down TG in the bloodstream, facilitating their uptake and use by cells, and helping maintain healthy blood lipid levels.*

2 *The process by which fats (lipids) are broken down in the body to release fatty acids and glycerol. This process primarily occurs in adipose (fat) tissue and is crucial for providing energy to the body, especially during fasting or exercise.*

3 *The Lancet https://www.thelancet.com/journals/lancet/article/PIIS0140-6736(05)67667-2/abstract*

action of lipid-lowering drugs on the liver

Statins and bempedoic acid (which act in the liver) and ezetimibe (which works in the intestines) all reduce the amount of cholesterol available to the liver. In response, the liver increases the number of LDLR, which remove more LDL-C from the blood. When used in combination, these drugs have a greater effect than when used alone.

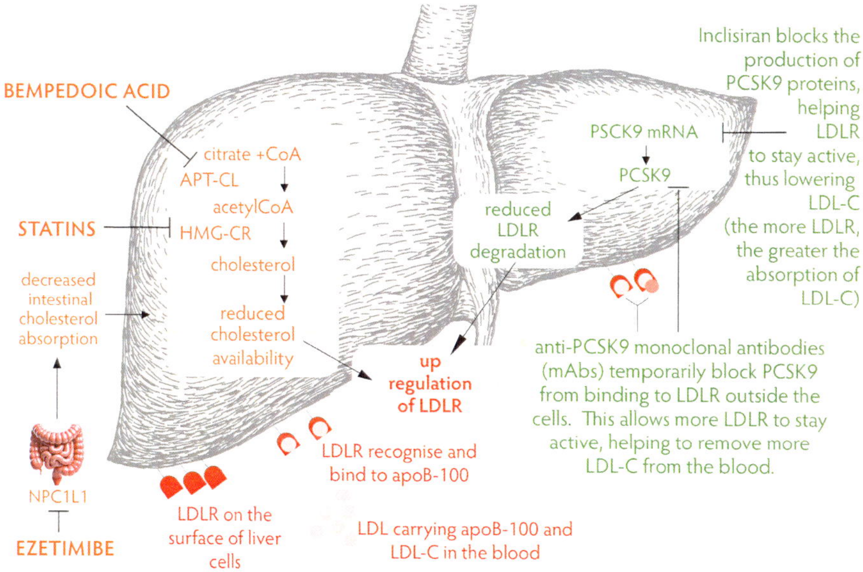

Inclisiran and anti-PCSK9 monoclonal antibodies work through different mechanisms to inhibit PCSK9 activity. This allows more LDLR to remain active on the liver surface, increasing the clearance of LDL particles (and the LDL-C they carry) from the blood.

Recent chapters have focused on cholesterol-lowering medications. Let's not forget lipoprotein(a) – the highly atherogenic particle we encountered earlier. Lp(a) is genetically determined and does not respond to standard cholesterol-lowering therapies. Currently, lipoprotein apheresis, a dialysis-like procedure, is the only treatment available. Promising new drugs are being trialled around the world, including in Australia. Other pioneering therapies are also in development. **See the following pages for details.**

on the horizon: new therapies in development

While current cholesterol-lowering therapies, especially statins, have revolutionised heart disease prevention through their cholesterol-lowering abilities, the search continues for even better and more personalised options.

Several promising drugs and therapies are in late-stage clinical trials, aiming to help people who remain at high risk despite existing treatments.

Lp

As we have noted, current drug therapies do not significantly lower lipoprotein(a) levels. However, several new treatments targeting Lp(a) are being trialled – including trials in Australia. They are showing great promise.

The most advanced include **antisense therapies**[1] such as the agent **pelacarsen,** and **siRNA drugs**[2] such as **olpasiran**, **zerlasiran** and **lepodisiran**. These are **injectable** therapies given either monthly or every six months, and work by directly blocking the production of Lp(a) in the liver.

An **oral** treatment, **muvalaplin**, is a small molecule drug[3] that also inhibits Lp(a) formation, but through a different mechanism to the injectable agents.

It must always be remembered that one of the most important things with elevated Lp(a) is to significantly reduce other risk factors, especially LDL-C, to very low levels.

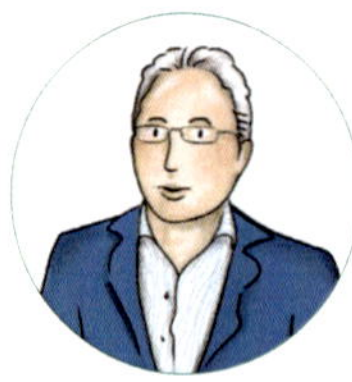

1 *Antisense therapies are an exciting new type of genetic treatment that work by blocking the body's instructions for making a key part of Lp(a), offering a targeted and effective way to lower high Lp(a) levels and reduce cardiovascular risk. (further information, page 12, ftn 2)*

2 *siRNA drugs are a new kind of genetic treatment that work by "silencing" the specific instructions inside cells that make harmful proteins – like the kind involved in high Lp(a). This can also target elevated LDL-C and TG. They help reduce the production of these proteins at the source, offering a powerful and targeted way to lower certain cholesterol levels and reduce heart disease risk.*

3 *A small molecule drug is a low molecular weight compound that can enter cells easily and interact with specific targets inside the body.*

CETP inhibition

Another class of drug targets the **cholesteryl ester transfer protein** (CETP), which helps move cholesterol between HDL and LDL particles. Blocking this protein may raise HDL-C while lowering the number of TG- and LDL-C-rich particles.

Earlier CETP inhibitors failed due to safety concerns or lack of efficacy.

A new agent, **obicetrapib**, is a once-daily oral medication designed for use alongside statins. It is being tested in several Phase III studies – BROOKLYN, BROADWAY, TANDEM, and PREVAIL – which are assessing its lipid-lowering efficacy, safety, and potential cardiovascular benefits in people with established CVD.

Early findings show that obicetrapib raises HDL-C, substantially lowers LDL-C, and moderately lowers TG, all with a favourable safety profile.

Results are expected in 2026.

a cure for life?

CRISPR – clustered regularly interspaced short palindromic repeats – is often called **molecular scissors**. This revolutionary **gene editing tool** allows scientists to cut and modify DNA with remarkable precision.

CRISPR-based therapies are now being developed to target genes such as PCSK9 and ANGPTL3, both of which are involved in cholesterol metabolism. **The goal is simple but bold**: to permanently lower LDL-C – and reduce cardiovascular risk – with a **single** treatment.

The **promise** is extraordinary: a one-time therapy that could offer lifelong protection. Still, the **challenges** are enormous, including how to deliver the treatment safely, ensure lasting effect, and manage the ethical implications of altering human DNA.

The **potential** is nothing short of **a cure for life**.

IMPORTANT POINTS

NON-STATIN THERAPIES

- Medical options beyond statins exist and are highly effective.
- EZETIMIBE reduces the reabsorption of dietary cholesterol.
- BEMPEDOIC ACID, a pro-drug, is generally used in combination with ezetimibe.
- BILE ACID SEQUESTRANTS increase cholesterol excretion.
- PCSK9 INHIBITORS (monoclonal antibodies and siRNA therapy) reduce PCSK9 function and so increase the number of LDLR. This helps remove LDL particles from the blood, thus lowering LDL-C.
- EVINACUMAB blocks ANGPTL3, a protein that normally inhibits lipid breakdown, helping to lower LDL-C even when LDLR are defective.
- LOMITAPIDE inhibits MTP, a protein essential for forming VLDL and chylomicrons, so reducing the production and release of LDL into the bloodstream.
- Medications used for lowering TG include
  - OMEGA-3 FATTY ACIDS (in very high concentration)
  - FIBRATES, which also elevate HDL-C and can lessen diabetic complications.
- New drugs and gene-based therapies in development are opening exciting new horizons for cholesterol lowering and even lifelong cardiovascular risk reduction.

Why cholesterol targets matter, and how low we should go.

chapter 16

CHOLESTEROL TARGETS: WHY AIMING LOW MATTERS

When it comes to managing cholesterol, knowing **where you're headed** is as important as knowing **where you are**. LDL-C targets matter.

Once people are identified as high risk for CVD – whether they've already had a heart attack or stroke, or they have key risk factors like diabetes, familial hypercholesterolaemia, or high-risk plaque on imaging – we don't just hope for improvement. **We aim for it. And we aim low.**

targets

Targets[1] give both patients and clinicians a clear goal. They guide decisions about **which** medications to start, **when** to escalate treatment, and **how** to monitor progress. They also give patients a **reason** to stay the course, especially when there may be multiple tablets, regular blood tests, and little immediate reward.

The idea is simple: the lower the LDL-C, the lower the risk – a principle consistently reinforced by ongoing research.

When the 4S trial (see page 121) was published in the 1990s, it was a turning point. It showed that lowering cholesterol with statins could reduce the risk of heart attack and death. But it was only the beginning. Subsequent studies, including the TNT[2] and PROVE-IT (see page 130) trials, found that

1 *The terms 'target' and 'goal' can be used interchangeably in doctor-patient discussions. In this book, we use goal as an aspirational focus, and target as a measurable specific.*

2 *The TNT trial (Treating to New Targets), published in 2005, was a landmark study that helped redefine how low we should aim when treating cholesterol in patients with existing heart disease. The trial enrolled over 10,000 people with stable coronary disease and assigned them to receive either 10 mg or 80 mg of atorvastatin daily. The group on the lower dose achieved an average LDL-C level of around 2.6 mmol/L, while the high-dose group reached a much lower level of approximately 1.8 mmol/L. The results were clear: those in the high-dose group experienced significantly fewer major cardiovascular events, including heart attacks and strokes. This trial demonstrated that lowering LDL-C well beyond the then-standard targets brought additional benefit, reinforcing the idea that in high-risk*

lowering cholesterol even further brought additional benefit. In high-risk patients, there had been no clear threshold below which LDL-C lowering stopped being useful. This concept – **lower is better** – became a new cornerstone of cardiovascular care.

guidelines

Today, global guidelines reflect this shift. The European Society of Cardiology recommends LDL-C levels of 1.4 mmol/L (55 mg/dL) or lower for very high-risk individuals, and 1.0 mmol/L (40 mg/dL) or less in those with recurrent events. These targets have been adopted worldwide.

While international guidelines offer strong direction, targets must still be **tailored to the individual**. Age, frailty, other medical conditions, and personal choice all shape the decision. For some, a moderate reduction in cholesterol may be appropriate if it aligns better with the person's overall risk, goals, and tolerance of treatment.

Lowering cholesterol often requires more than one medication, particularly when aiming for the most ambitious targets. This can bring added complexity, including side effects, cost, and the need for ongoing blood tests. For patients already managing multiple conditions, it's important to weigh the long-term benefit against the day-to-day burden.

plaque can change

Many patients naturally ask:

"Do I really need all these medications?"

"What's the point of more blood tests?"

The answer is both clinical and visual. Not only does lowering LDL-C reduce the risk of future events, it can **improve** the health of the arteries.

We have already introduced that plaque build-up can be altered for the

---

patients, "lower is better". TNT played a key role in shifting clinical guidelines towards more intensive cholesterol management in secondary prevention.

Treating to New Targets (TNT) trial (2005) LaRosa JC, Grundy SM, Waters DD, et al. Intensive Lipid Lowering with Atorvastatin in Patients with Stable Coronary Disease. N Engl J Med. 2005;352(14):1425-1435.

better. Its significance warrants a brief recap here. Early evidence came from Dean Ornish's 1998 study on intensive lifestyle changes[3], which used invasive coronary angiography to show a small but measurable regression of plaque. This opened the door to asking whether medication alone could do the same.

It could – and it did[4]. Statin therapy was shown to stabilise and even shrink plaque burden, using repeated angiograms. With improved imaging, researchers like Steven Nissen and Stephen Nicholls advanced this work further. They used high-resolution intravascular ultrasound (IVUS) to demonstrate that intensive cholesterol lowering with statins could reduce plaque volume and stabilise the vessel wall (see ASTEROID trial, page 127).

In 2016, Nicholls again broke ground, this time using PCSK9 inhibitors in the GLAGOV trial (see page 129). These powerful agents drove LDL-C levels down to an average of 1.6 mmol/L (about 62 mg/dL), with 60 per cent of patients showing plaque regression. A remarkable outcome,

low, early, and sustained

We now know that aiming low is more than a number. It's a strategy:

- as **low** as possible
- from as **early** as possible
- for as **long** as possible.

While this approach helps reduce cardiovascular events, improve arterial health, and engage patients in long-term care, targets are not meant to be imposed but shared. When patients understand not just the numbers but the reason behind them – when they see that treatment can lead to stronger arteries and fewer events – they are more likely to engage and then persist.

Targets are not just about statistics. They're about **confidence, clarity,** and a **shared plan** between patient and doctor for better outcomes.

---

3 *Ornish D, Scherwitz LW, Billings JH, et al. 1998. Intensive lifestyle changes for reversal of coronary heart disease. JAMA 280:2001–7 [PubMed]*

4 *Blankenhorn DH, Azen SP, Kramsch DM, et al. 1993. Coronary angiographic changes with lovastatin therapy. The Monitored Atherosclerosis Regression Study (MARS). Ann. Intern. Med 119:969–76 [PubMed]*

residual risk

Despite effective LDL-C lowering, high-risk individuals may still experience events. This is known as residual risk and highlights that LDL-C is only part of the complex atherosclerosis picture.

Residual risk may stem from factors like raised TG, prediabetes, chronic inflammation, elevated Lp(a), and other less defined influences such as diet, exercise, medication, difficult relationships, and psychological and emotional stress. Fish oil, discussed next, may help reduce this risk, alongside managing key issues such as blood pressure. Notably, some anti-inflammatory agents have also been shown to lower residual risk.

Understanding residual risk better is driving new areas of research.

IMPORTANT POINTS

CHOLESTEROL TARGETS

- Cholesterol targets guide treatment decisions, helping to determine when to start, adjust, or escalate therapy. They give patients a clear goal to work towards.
- Lower LDL means lower risk especially in high-risk patients.
- Plaque can be stabilised or reduced through intensive LDL-C lowering.
- Targets need to be individualised, tailored to each person's health status, choices, and ability to manage treatment.
- Despite effective LDL-C lowering, high-risk patients can still experience events. This is called residual risk.

Does fish oil deserve its reputation and widespread use?

chapter 17

FISH OIL: BALANCING THE SCALES

Fish oil sits at the intersection of medication, supplementation, and diet.

Apart from being probably the most consumed over-the-counter supplement in the Western world, what is fish oil?

Fish oil, renowned for its numerous health benefits, is derived from marine TG. Interestingly, these potent oils originate from plankton in the cold, deep waters of the ocean, rather than directly from fish. Small fish consume this plankton and are then eaten by larger fish, a process that continues up the food chain until it reaches fish such as salmon, tuna, sardines, and anchovies – all rich sources of these beneficial oils.

When consumed by humans, these marine TG are broken down into the essential fatty acids, **eicosapentaenoic acid** (EPA), ($C_{20}H_{30}O_2$ or 20:5 ω3) and **docosahexaenoic acid** (DHA), ($C_{22}H_{32}O_2$ or 22:6 ω3), which are then absorbed into and utilised by the body.

These essential fatty acids, especially EPA offer several heart-health benefits, such as reduced TG production and enhanced TG clearance from the body.

trials

Extensive trial data[1] exist.

GISSI P (*Gruppo Italiano per lo Studio della Sopravvivenza nell'Infarto Miocardico – Prevenzione*) (Italy)

In this randomised, controlled trial, more than 11,000 people who had recently suffered a heart attack were given 1 g of omega-3 fatty acid/day versus a control group. The trial found a significant reduction for individuals with impaired heart function – a 45 per cent reduction in sudden cardiac

1 *The reference material for all the trials mentioned in this chapter is listed at the end of the chapter.*

A CLOSER LOOK

omega-3 and omega-6 fatty acids

Omega-3 and omega-6 are essential fatty acids that play crucial roles in our diet, but they have distinct functions and come from different sources.

Omega-3 fatty acids are known for their **anti-inflammatory** properties (reduce inflammatory responses) and numerous health benefits. They are found in fatty fish like salmon, mackerel, and sardines, as well as in plant sources such as flaxseeds, chia seeds, walnuts, and hemp seeds. There are three main types of omega-3s: **alpha-linolenic acid** (ALA), **eicosapentaenoic acid** (EPA), and **docosahexaenoic acid** (DHA). ALA is found in plant oils, while EPA and DHA are mainly found in fish oil.

DHA omega-3 is essential for brain function and development and maintaining good eye health. EPA omega-3 is beneficial for heart health, helping to reduce TG, lower blood pressure, and decrease the risk of heart disease.

Omega-6 fatty acids are more common in the typical Western diet than omega-3s. Omega-6 is found in vegetable oils like corn oil, soybean oil, and sunflower oil, as well as in nuts, seeds, and meat. The most common types of omega-6 are **linoleic acid** (LA) and **arachidonic acid** (AA).

As omega-6 fatty acids have **pro-inflammatory** properties, they can promote inflammation. While inflammation is often seen as negative, it is necessary for immune response and healing. Omega-6s are also important for skin and hair growth, bone health, and reproductive system function. They play a role in brain function and development as well.

The **key difference** between omega-3 and omega-6 lies in their **effects on inflammation.**

Both types are necessary for our health, but maintaining a balance is crucial. With the typical Western diet tending to be high in omega-6 and low in omega-3, increased inflammation and various chronic diseases often are the result. To achieve a healthier balance, it is important to increase omega-3 intake by consuming more fish, flaxseeds, and walnuts, and to moderate omega-6 intake from vegetable oils and processed foods.

Striving for a **ratio close to 4:1** of omega-6 to omega-3 can help reduce inflammation and promote overall health. In Western diets, the ratio is often much higher – around 15-20:1. (Also see page 186.)

death (SCD) with a reduction in overall mortality of about 20 per cent in the omega-3 fatty acid group compared with the control group.

The GISSI P trial was one of the first large trials to show the benefits of omega-3 fatty acids in **secondary prevention** of CVD. Unfortunately, not all the following trials were quite as glowing for the use of fish oil.

VITAL (VITamin D and omega-3 TriAL)

This randomised, double-blind, placebo-controlled trial investigated the effects of vitamin D and omega-3 fatty acid supplements on the risk of developing cancer, heart disease, and stroke in more than 25,000 American adults without prior history of the diseases **(primary prevention)**. They were given 1 g of omega-3 fatty acid/day or a placebo. The trial showed a potential benefit for heart attack reduction, but no major overall cardiovascular event reduction in a primary prevention population. This trial tells us that fish oil will probably be beneficial for people who have had a heart attack (secondary prevention), while in the primary prevention arena it is more complicated.

ASCEND (A Study of Cardiovascular Events iN Diabetes)

This randomised, double-blind, placebo-controlled trial involved more than 15,000 patients with **diabetes but no CVD**. Participants were given either 1 g of omega-3 fatty acid/day or a placebo. As there was no significant reduction in serious vascular events, the findings cast doubt on the role of omega-3 supplementation in primary prevention for diabetic patients.

More trials were performed.

OMEMI (Omega-3 Fatty Acids in Elderly Post-Myocardial Infarction Patients)

This randomised, double-blind, placebo-controlled trial involved 1027 elderly patients aged 70 to 82 years, who had recently suffered a heart attack. They were given almost 2 g of omega-3 fatty acid/day or a placebo.

The trial found that the additional treatment did not significantly reduce the rate of cardiovascular events, or all-cause death over a two-year period compared with a placebo. The trial also noted a small, although non-significant, increase in the incidence of new atrial fibrillation in the omega-3 group compared with the placebo group.

The results suggest that omega-3 supplements may not be effective for cardiovascular prevention in this high-risk group of older adults, especially in the context of other recent trials that also reported neutral outcomes.

ORIGIN (Outcome Reduction with an Initial Glargine Intervention

Another randomised, double-blind, placebo-controlled trial, this time involving more than 12,000 people with impaired fasting glucose, impaired glucose tolerance, or early type 2 diabetes who had not had a cardiovascular event. They were given 1 g of omega-3 fatty acid/day or a placebo. Again, there was no significant reduction in cardiovascular outcomes, adding to the evidence questioning the role of omega-3 fatty acids in cardiovascular prevention for diabetic and prediabetic populations. As to whether it was beneficial in terms of cardiovascular prevention, again, the result was borderline.

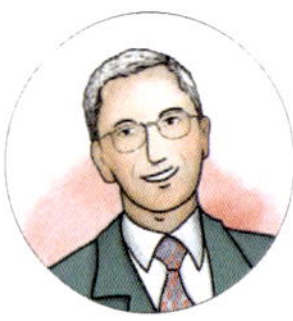

These studies seem to show a positive impact of fish oil only for people who have had an event (secondary prevention) and have a damaged heart. From my perspective, that can be too late.

Some studies then looked at using **EPA** (eicosapentaenoic acid) **only.**

JELIS (Japan EPA Lipid Intervention Study) 2007

JELIS was a large-scale, prospective, randomised, open-label, blinded endpoint (PROBE) trial conducted in Japan. It involved more than 18,000 Japanese participants with hypercholesterolaemia who were on statin therapy. One group received 1.8 g EPA/day in addition to their statin therapy; the second group received statin therapy alone. The study followed participants for an average of almost five years. EPA seemed to be well-tolerated without any significant side effects.

The trial group (EPA and statin) showed a 19 per cent relative reduction in major coronary events compared with the control (statin-only) group. Specifically, the incidence of major coronary events was 2.8 per cent in the EPA group and 3.5 per cent in the control group. The study also found that the benefits of EPA were pronounced in patients with high TG levels and low HDL-C levels.

JELIS concluded that adding EPA to statin therapy could further reduce the risk of major coronary events in hypertriglyceridaemic patients, highlighting the potential benefits of omega-3 fatty acids in CVD prevention.

STRENGTH (Statin Residual Risk Reduction with EpaNova in High Cardiovascular Risk Patients with Hypertriglyceridemia) study (about 2023)

This was a large-scale clinical trial to evaluate the effects of omega-3 carboxylic acids (epanova – a pharmaceutical compound of EPA and DHA) on cardiovascular outcomes in patients with high TG levels and at risk for cardiovascular events. In this double-blind, randomised, placebo-controlled trial, more than 13,000 participants were assigned either omega-3 carboxylic acids or a placebo in addition to their statin therapy.

The study concluded that the omega-3 carboxylic acids did not provide additional cardiovascular benefits beyond the statin therapy alone in these high-risk individuals.

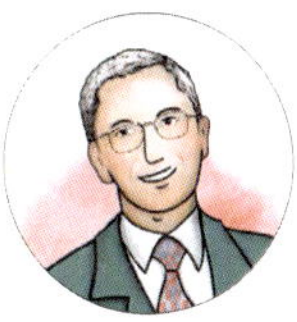

These individuals were considered high risk although they hadn't necessarily had an event. So, a very big study, again, causing more confusion.

In 2019, **REDUCE-IT** (Reduction of Cardiovascular Events with Icosapent Ethyl-Intervention Trial) considered if icosapent ethyl, a highly purified, pharmaceutical-grade form of EPA, could reduce the risk of major adverse cardiovascular events in high-risk patients with elevated TG who were already on statin therapy.

It was a double-blind, randomised, placebo-controlled trial. More than 8000 participants had elevated TG levels (135-499 mg/dL or 1.52 to 5.63 mmol/L) with either established CVD or diabetes as additional risk factors. All participants were on stable statin therapy. Participants received either 4 g of icosapent ethyl/day or a mineral oil placebo.

Icosapent ethyl significantly reduced the risk of the primary endpoint by 25 per cent compared with the placebo. The incidence of the primary composite endpoint was 17.2 per cent in the icosapent ethyl group versus 22 per cent in the placebo group. Secondary endpoints, including individual components of the primary endpoint, also showed significant reductions, notably a 20 per cent lower risk of cardiovascular death, a 31 per cent lower risk of non-fatal heart attacks, and a 28 per cent lower risk of stroke.

REDUCE-IT concluded that icosapent ethyl significantly reduced the risk of major adverse cardiovascular events in high-risk patients with elevated TG who were on statin therapy. This finding supported the use of icosapent ethyl as an additional therapy for risk reduction in this patient population. The trial provided robust evidence for the cardiovascular benefits of icosapent ethyl in specific high-risk patient groups and has led to its approval in many countries, including Australia, as a reimbursable treatment for cardiovascular risk reduction.

The risk reduction in REDUCE-IT using EPA is as good as we have seen with potent medications.

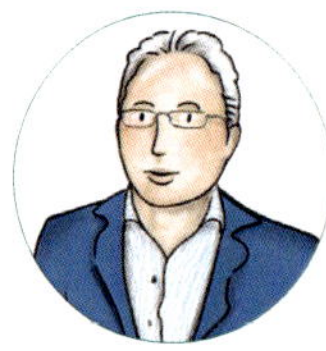

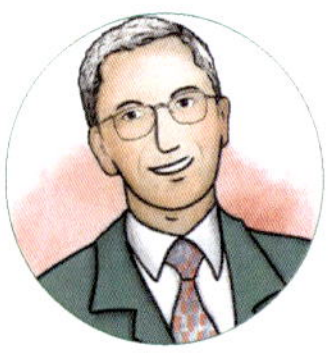

It is also worth noting that the trial used mineral oil as the placebo, raising concerns of possible harm rather than a neutral impact. For some, this remains unresolved.

Omega-3 Index

While the above-mentioned studies show that EPA is particularly good for the heart, **DHA** plays a crucial role in **eye and brain health** where it is a major structural component of these organs. It supports brain development, cognitive function, and communication between brain cells, while also maintaining retinal health and good vision, especially during pregnancy, early childhood, and throughout life.

The **Physicians' Health Study** is a large-scale, long-term, prospective, observational research project involving US physicians investigating the health effects of various supplements and medications.

Regarding omega-3 fatty acids, the study aimed to determine their impact on cardiovascular health and other medical outcomes. Critical to that was the **Omega-3 Index**[2], which measures the percentage of EPA and DHA in red blood cell membranes – a key marker of long-term omega-3 status. Researchers noted that **a higher** Omega-3 Index was beneficial in **reducing** the risk of heart disease and related conditions. Looking at different quartiles (see diagram below), they found a 90 per cent relative risk reduction in the highest quartile of individuals with higher omega-3 levels.

Beyond general cardiovascular benefits, the study found that the **single strongest predictor of sudden cardiac death (SCD) was the Omega-3 Index**[3] – not cholesterol levels, good or bad, nor inflammation markers. Simply put, **the lower your index, the greater your risk of dying suddenly from a heart attack**.

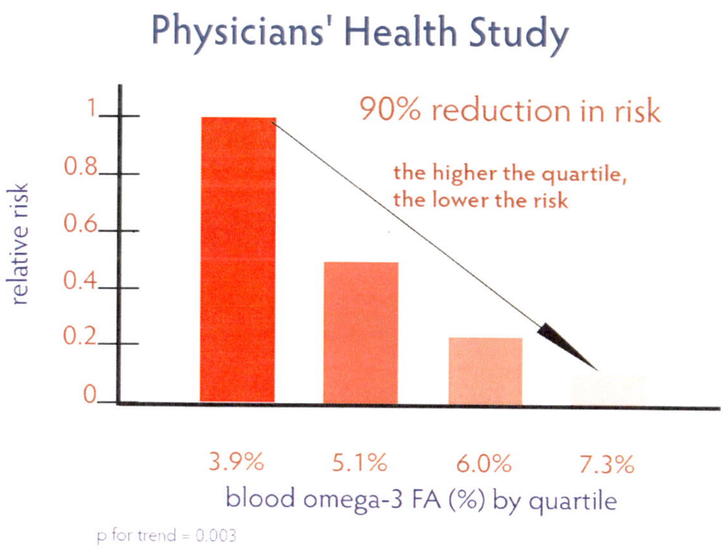

2 *A small (finger prick) blood sample is analysed, and the percentage of EPA and DHA is calculated as a fraction of the total fatty acids in the red blood cell membrane. Less than 4% is high risk for CVD and sudden cardiac death (SCD), 4-8%, intermediate risk, 8% or higher is the optimal range associated with a lower risk of heart disease and SCD.*

3 *The omega-3 level, if measured in free blood, would fluctuate from minute to minute depending on what the person had eaten. Omega-3s in fatty tissue have a very long turnover (the length of time the fatty acids persist and function before they are broken down and replaced by new fatty acid), too long for clinical relevance. However, omega fats accumulate in the membrane of red cells. These last in our body for 90 days which gives a weeks-to-months-long measurement of the person's omega-3 consumption and the body's omega-3 level.*

Another useful measurement is the **omega ratio** that looks at the balance between omega-3s and omega-6s, assessing inflammatory potential. The ideal omega-3 to omega-6 ratio is considered to range from 1:1 to 1:4. Modern Western diets often have ratios of 1:10 to 1:25, which is associated with increased inflammation and higher chronic disease risk. A lower, more balanced ratio is thought to support heart health and reduce inflammation.

The **PREDIMED** (*Prevención con Dieta Mediterránea*) study confirmed that saturated fatty acids that were 12, 14 or 16 carbon molecules long tended to drive worse CVD outcomes. This could be improved if these C12-14- or 16-long saturated fatty acids were replaced with monounsaturated fats or polyunsaturated fats, particularly like fish oil, which are PUFA (polyunsaturated fatty acids).

Interestingly, observation also suggests that the **source** of saturated fatty acids can be important in understanding cardiovascular outcomes.

Saturated fats from sources such pastries and processed foods tend to increase CVD risk, and those from dairy may also contribute. However, saturated fatty acids from fish, vegetables, and nuts can have a protective effect. Similarly, very long-chain saturated fatty acids (VLCFA) - such as C20, C22, and C24 - are associated with a reduced risk of CVD.

several questions

While differences in study design, patient populations, and omega-3 formulations help explain the varied results, questions remain.

Oily fish certainly seems to be a powerful component of a healthy diet. We highly recommend eating fish regularly, particularly oily fish such as sardines or herrings. We haven't touched on the epidemiological data (the study within populations), which also support fish being a regular component of a healthy diet.

When should you take fish oil supplements?

Fish oil supplements are recommended

- if you do not eat oily fish, and
- if you have elevated TG and residual cardiovascular risk.

Even more importantly, **a strong argument exists for knowing your Omega-3 Index**. In Australia, as there is no Medicare rebate for this testing, the out-of-pocket cost is about $100. However, the information received is very informative and we both support patients accessing the test. You now know that you want an index of eight or above to minimise your risk of sudden cardiac death.

Should supplementation use EPA + DHA or EPA alone?

Dr K. says that pharmaceutical-grade EPA (icosapent ethyl), mainly, is the one that has been shown to reduce cardiovascular risk and, can be reimbursed in many countries. However, both EPA and DHA are effective in reducing TG.

Dr W. believes that the cardiac space will follow the path of EPA in isolation. However, for **total well-being** – heart, brain and eyes – a combination of the marine fish oil components seems to be the sensible approach.

issues

Before we move away from fish oils, several significant issues need to be addressed.

quality, purity of supplements

Quality and purity are at the top of the list, as over-the-counter supplements are not prepared under the same strict regulations as pharmacological preparations. Quality and purity are closely linked to efficacy. High-quality, pure supplements are more likely to be effective, safe, and reliable. Labelling is also far more stringent for pharmacological products than supplements.

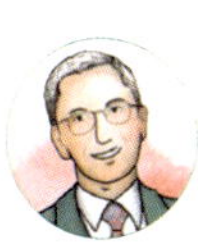

Go for good quality. You generally get what you pay for!

blood thinning

A concern with taking fish oil, particularly without medical supervision, is its blood-thinning effect. The omega-3 fatty acids EPA and DHA reduce the blood's ability to clot.

While this can lower the risk of heart attacks and strokes, it may also increase the risk of bleeding, especially in people taking other blood-thinning medications or those with bleeding disorders. For this reason, anyone in these groups – or anyone facing an upcoming operation – should consult their healthcare team before starting fish oil supplements.

atrial fibrillation

Recent studies using moderate-to-high doses of fish oil supplementation have observed a small but real increased risk in the development of atrial fibrillation. It is noteworthy that dietary omega-3 from fish is associated with a decreased risk.

sustainability

The source of the fish used in fish oil supplements is an important consideration, both for the quality of the product and its environmental impact. Fish harvested from clean, uncontaminated waters are less likely to contain harmful toxins, helping ensure the safety and purity of the oil.

Equally important is the sustainability of that source. Overfishing and destructive harvesting practices can deplete fish populations and damage marine ecosystems, so it's essential to choose products that support responsible fishing.

Reputable fish oil producers adhere to strict sustainability standards and have their products certified by independent organisations that monitor environmental and ecological practices. Choosing fish oil derived from responsibly sourced fish contributes to the long-term health of ocean ecosystems.

Ultimately, these factors – the cleanliness of the water, the methods of harvest, and the sustainability of the source – not only influence the environmental footprint of fish oil production but also affect the overall quality and efficacy of the final product. Consumers looking for fish oil supplements should look for clear labelling that identifies the fish species used, the region from which they were harvested, and the sustainability credentials of the brand.

costs

Supplements can be costly. Dr K. recommends **liquid** fish oil formulations for TG-lowering as they are cost-effective and contain high concentrations of EPA and DHA. In general, it is important to consider the cost-benefit ratio. Individuals need to assess whether the health benefits justify the expense.

---

actions of common lipid therapies in summary

lipid therapy	LDL-C lowering	HDL-C raising	TG lowering	Lp(a) lowering
statins	++++	++	++	0/-
ezetimibe	++	+	+	0
PSCK9 inhibitors	++++	+	+	++
niacin	++	++++	+++	++
fibrates	+/-	+++	++++	0
purified EPA (fish oil)	0/-	+	++++	0

key

++++	strong positive effect
+++	moderate positive effect
++	mild positive effect
+	minimal positive effect
0	no meaningful effect
-	potential adverse effect

references for the trial data

GISSI P Gruppo Italiano per lo Studio della Sopravvivenza nell'Infarto miocardico   Dietary supplementation with n-3 polyunsaturated fatty acids and vitamin E after myocardial infarction: results of the GISSI-Prevenzione trial. The Lancet 1999, 354:447–455. (https://www.thelancet.com/journals/lancet/article/PIIS0140-6736(99)07072-5/fulltext)

VITAL (VITamin D and omega-3 TriAL) Study   Division of Preventive Medicine on the Brigham and Women's Hospital's Division of Preventive Medicine website (https://prevmed.bwh.harvard.edu/vital/)

ASCEND (A Study of Cardiovascular Events iN Diabetes)   homepage managed by the Clinical Trial Service Unit & Epidemiological Studies Unit (CTSU) at the University of Oxford. (https://www.ctsu.ox.ac.uk/research/ascend)

OMEMI (Omega-3 Fatty Acids in Elderly Post-Myocardial Infarction Patients)   Omega-3 fatty acids supplementation and risk of atrial fibrillation: an updated meta-analysis of randomized controlled trials, Marco Lombardi et al, European Heart Journal - Cardiovascular Pharmacotherapy, Volume 7, Issue 4, July 2021, Pages e69–e70, https://doi.org/10.1093/ehjcvp/pvab008 (https://academic.oup.com/ehjcvp/article/7/4/e69/6255232)

ORIGIN (Outcome Reduction with an Initial Glargine Intervention)   Basal Insulin and Cardiovascular and Other Outcomes in Dysglycemia; the ORIGIN Trial Investigators, published July 26, 2012, N Engl J Med 2012;367:319-328 DOI: 10.1056/NEJMoa1203858

VOL. 367 NO. 4 (https://www.nejm.org/doi/full/10.1056/NEJMoa1203858) Effect of Basal Insulin Glargine on First and Recurrent Episodes of Heart Failure

Hospitalization: The ORIGIN Trial (Outcome Reduction With Initial Glargine Intervention) Circulation Volume 137, Number 1 (https://doi.org/10.1161/CIRCULATIONAHA.117.030924)

JELIS (Japan EPA Lipid Intervention Study)   Effects of eicosapentaenoic acid on major coronary events in hypercholesterolaemic patients, Yokoyama et al, The Lancet, volume 369, issue 9567, p1090-1098, March 31 (https://www.thelancet.com/journals/lancet/article/PIIS0140-6736(07)60527-3/abstract)

Japan EPA Lipid Intervention Study - JELIS   (https://www.acc.org/Latest-in-Cardiology/Clinical-Trials/2010/02/23/19/10/JELIS#references-for-article)

STRENGTH (Statin Residual Risk Reduction with EpaNova in High Cardiovascular Risk Patients with Hypertriglyceridemia)   The Effect of High-Dose Omega-3 Fatty Acids vs Corn Oil on Major Adverse Cardiovascular Events in Patients at High Cardiovascular Risk

STRENGTH Randomized Clinical Trial   Stephen J. Nicholls et al JAMA. 2020;324(22):2268-2280. doi:10.1001/jama.2020.22258 Published Online: November 15, 2020. doi:10.1001/jama.2020.22258 Correction: This article was corrected on December 18, 2020, to fix the units of measure for EPA and DHA in Table 4. (https://jamanetwork.com/journals/jama/fullarticle/2773120)

REDUCE-IT (Reduction of Cardiovascular Events with Icosapent Ethyl-Intervention Trial) Cardiovascular Risk Reduction with Icosapent Ethyl for Hypertriglyceridemia   Published November 10, 2018 N Engl J Med 2019;380:11-22 DOI: 10.1056/NEJMoa1812792 VOL. 380

NO. 1 PHYSICIANS' HEALTH STUDY   the Division of Preventive Medicine at Brigham and Women's Hospital. https://prevmed.bwh.harvard.edu/physicians-health-study/ and https://phs.bwh.harvard.edu/

PREDIMED (Prevención con Dieta Mediterránea) Primary Prevention of Cardiovascular Disease with a Mediterranean Diet Supplemented with Extra-Virgin Olive Oil or Nuts N Engl J Med. DOI: 10.1056/NEJMoa1800389

IMPORTANT POINTS

FISH OIL

- Fish oil is renowned for its health benefits. Derived from marine TG, the potent oils originate in plankton and are passed along the food chain until consumed by the fish from which we obtain it.
- When eaten by us, the marine TG are broken down into fatty acids, especially eicosapentaenoic acid (EPA), and docosahexaenoic acid (DHA), which are then absorbed and utilised by the body.
- The primary observed effects of fish oil are that it decreases TG production and increases the body's ability to rid itself of TG. There is very little effect on LDL-C.
- Many fish oil trials have produced mixed cardio results.
- Knowing your omega-3 Index is significant.
- Pharmaceutical-grade EPA (icosapent ethyl) is available and reimbursable under certain conditions.
- If using fish oil, consider
  - taking EPA alone (heart) or with DHA (brain and eyes)
  - the product's quality and the sustainability of its source
  - that it can reduce the blood's ability to clot, so please take only under medical advice
  - the cost-benefit to you personally.

Healthy habits not only improve heart well-being, they also enhance the effectiveness of cholesterol-lowering medications.

cholesterol curiosities

fish oil does not contain cholesterol

Fish oil supplements provide omega-3 fatty acids, not cholesterol. Any cholesterol in fish comes from the flesh, not the oil.

fish oil lowers TG, not cholesterol production

Omega-3 fats primarily reduce triglycerides and do not directly suppress cholesterol synthesis.

a polar bear would alarm a cardiologist

With an almost entirely fat-based diet and extremely high LDL cholesterol, a polar bear would appear high-risk by human standards – yet its arteries remain free of atherosclerosis due to profoundly different lipoprotein biology, inflammatory responses, and arterial wall behaviour.

dolphins have high LDL-C, too, but little plaque

Despite a high-fat, fish-based diet, dolphins develop minimal arterial plaque, again highlighting important species differences in lipid handling.

high LDL-C alone does not tell the whole story

Whether plaque develops is complex and depends not just on cholesterol levels, but on inflammation, particle behaviour, arterial responses, and more (as you are learning as you read this book).

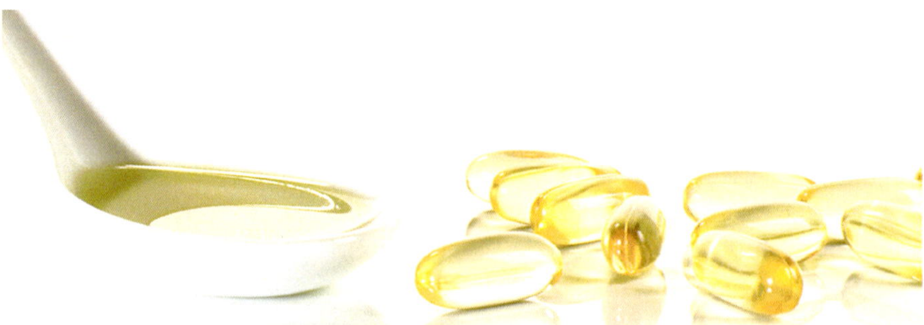

Although fish oil is among the most commonly consumed over-the-counter supplements in the Western world, individuals with heart-related conditions should take it under medical supervision.

chapter 18

LIFESTYLE CHANGES: HEALTHIER HABITS MAKE A DIFFERENCE

Lifestyle changes lay the foundation for a healthier, more fulfilling life – and they're essential for preventing CVD. The four key areas that make the biggest difference are diet, weight control, exercise, and quitting smoking. While these changes may have only a **modest** direct effect on cholesterol levels, **they significantly reduce overall cardiovascular risk** and **enhance the benefits of cholesterol-lowering medications**. They're powerful, proven, and far too important to ignore.

Doctors and patients often consider risk factors in isolation. While each one is an independent predictor of disease – meaning it increases risk on its own – risks also have a **cumulative effect**. The more risk factors present, the higher the overall risk. That's why lifestyle changes matter so much: they help reduce multiple modifiable risk factors. It's **never too late to start**, but the earlier you act, the better your long-term health prospects.

> *The Australian Institute of Health and Welfare estimates that high cholesterol is responsible for more than a third of all the years of healthy life lost to heart disease in Australia. As one important risk factor for heart disease, among others, cholesterol should always be considered within the context of an individual's global risk of CVD.*[1]

In the previous Bishop-Kostner collaboration, *10 Commandments of Heart Health Explained* (2024), knowing your cholesterol level and acting on it is one of the '10 commandments'. Among the others are:

- *eat well, maintain a healthy weight,*
- *exercise regularly for your physical and mental health,* and
- *don't smoke.*

---

1 *a paraphrased summary of information from the Australian Institute of Health and Welfare (AIHW). According to the AIHW's Australian Burden of Disease Study 2018, high cholesterol contributed to 2.7% of the total disease burden in Australia and accounted for 37% of the burden from coronary heart disease.*

Sound familiar? These practices are crucial for overall heart health and, implemented in association with cholesterol-lowering medications, provide a **dual advantage**.

frustrations

Two key frustrations often arise when trying to change cholesterol levels through lifestyle changes alone: genetic coding and homeostasis.

Genetics: You can thank your parents! Your genes play a major role in cholesterol metabolism and significantly influence your blood lipid levels.

Homeostasis: The body strives to maintain a stable internal environment. Homeostasis governs factors such as temperature – heating up triggers perspiration, while getting cold triggers shivering – helping to **maintain the status quo despite changes** in the external environment. **Homeostasis regulates cholesterol.** If you **increase** your cholesterol consumption, your body will make less, and your cholesterol levels **will not move much**. If you eat **less** cholesterol-rich food, your body will sense that and make more, so your cholesterol levels **will not move much.** Homeostasis causes much of the frustration people experience as they try to alter their cholesterol levels through diet alone. And that point is set by – you guessed it – your parents!

Because the body adjusts its cholesterol production in response to our food intake, decreasing your consumption of cholesterol-rich foods such as eggs, milk, prawns, or liver rarely makes much difference. The exception is the approximately 20 per cent of people who are hyper-absorbers of dietary cholesterol.

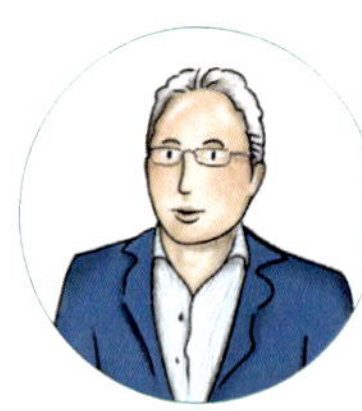

Even when we accept that lifestyle changes are essential, it can be overwhelming. The good news? **Small, sustainable changes** can make a real difference.

For the remainder of this chapter, we'll look more closely at foods that help or hinder cholesterol, diet, and weight control along with the roles of exercise and a smoke-free life.

food and fats

We know we should make healthy food choices (no question), but there's often confusion about how best to approach it. Keeping it simple helps:

- eat whole, unprocessed foods – fruit, vegetables, whole grains and healthy proteins and fats;
- avoid packaged foods – packets with barcodes and food that won't spoil when exposed to air;
- limit saturated fats and processed foods – meats, such as salami and bacon, which are high in saturated fats and preservatives, and
- keep refined sugars – soft drink, lollies, cake – as occasional treats.

Beyond these general guidelines, people follow a specific diet for one of three main reasons:

- to **lower cholesterol** (the Portfolio Diet is one of the very few that can achieve this);
- for **heart-healthy eating** (e.g., the Mediterranean Diet), or
- to **lose weight** (e.g., the Keto Diet or calorie restriction).

cholesterol

So, where does cholesterol fit into the equation? How much cholesterol is there in the food we consume?

cholesterol in foods	cholesterol
butter (1 tsp, about 5 g)	11 mg
egg (1, about 60 g)	203 mg
milk (whole, 1 cup, 250 mL)	35 mg
salmon, raw (100 g)	60 mg
crab, raw (100 g)	49 mg
beef (lean mince, 100 g)	75 mg
veal (top, round, 100 g)	127 mg
chicken liver (100 g)	631 mg
tofu, firm (0.5 cup)	0 mg

The total cholesterol in the average, healthy human body is 35 g.
(sources: FSANZ Australian Food Composition Database [Release 1.1, 2019], and UCSF Cholesterol Content of Foods.)

The amounts of cholesterol in our food are **relatively small**. For example, a 30 g serving of cheddar cheese contains about 30 mg of cholesterol and 100 g of a pork chop contains roughly 80-90 mg. A 100 g of raw prawns contains roughly 130-160 mg and a 100 g of squid contains around 230-270 mg.

Remember, cholesterol is found only in animal products. Fruits, vegetables, grains and other plant foods contain none.

So what happens after we eat cholesterol-containing foods?

Let's recall our lipoprotein transporters – particularly **chylomicrons**.

After digestion, dietary fats are packaged into chylomicrons in the small intestine. Chylomicrons move through the lymphatic system to reach the bloodstream. Once in the circulation, chylomicrons deliver TG and some cholesterol to peripheral tissues such as muscle and adipose tissue.

After offloading most of their TG, the chylomicron remnants are taken up by the liver, where they are broken down. Their remaining components – now mostly cholesterol – are either used by the liver or repackaged into VLDL and sent back into the bloodstream.

A CLOSER LOOK

eggs

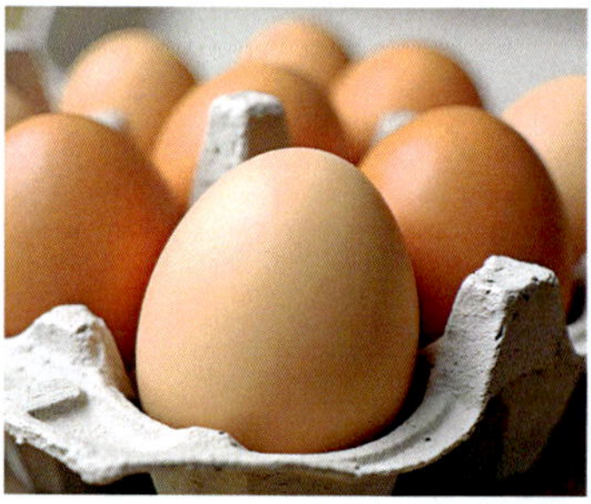

According to the Australian Eggs website[1], the latest Heart Foundation recommendations[2] put no limit on how many eggs **healthy people** can eat each week. The Heart Foundation says that eggs have a **minimal effect** on blood cholesterol levels. Additionally, eggs are **low in saturated fat** (3.4g per serving), which has a greater impact on cholesterol levels than dietary cholesterol intake.

Eggs also contain 13 essential vitamins and nutrients[3], including quality protein, antioxidants and healthy fats: vitamin D, vitamin B12, choline, iron, lutein and zeaxanthin (antioxidants), riboflavin (vitamin B2), pantothenic acid (vitamin B5), vitamin A, vitamin E, phosphorus, folate, iodine, selenium.

The Heart Foundation encourages the consumption of eggs as part of a heart-healthy eating pattern with a reminder to be mindful of what you choose to eat with them!

video: unscrambling eggs and heart disease (QR code, left, or) visit: https://Dr Warrickbishop/post/unscrambling-eggs-and-heart-disease

1 *Australian Eggs – https://bit.ly/eggs-cholesterol*

2 *National Heart Foundation (of Australia) – https://bit.ly/eggs-heart-cholesterol*

3 *Australian Eggs – https://bit.ly/eggs-nutrients*

know your fats

Now it is time to have a closer look at fats. Does eating saturated fats increase the body's cholesterol levels?

As we learned earlier, there are two main types of fat found in food:

- **saturated**, which can **increase LDL-C** and
- **unsaturated**, which can help **decrease LDL-C,** while
  - a third form of fat, **trans fats**, although technically unsaturated, behaves differently by **increasing LDL-C** and **decreasing HDL-C**, contributing to cardiovascular risk.

Research shows that replacing unhealthy fats with healthy ones can improve a person's cholesterol profile, thus reducing heart disease risk.

Saturated fats, which are solid at room temperature, are found in acids such as palmitic (meats, dairy products, vegetable oils), stearic (animal fats, cocoa butter, some plant oils) and lauric (coconut and palm oils). These fats act on the same homeostatic protein as cholesterol, **increasing** the body's cholesterol production. More significantly, they **interfere** with the liver's ability to clear LDL by reducing LDLR activity, a key mechanism driving higher LDL-C levels.

While dietary cholesterol is often blamed, **saturated fats are far more influential** in raising LDL-C. **Processed meats** (such as bacon and sausages), **oils** (like coconut and palm oil), **baked goods**, and **deep-fried** foods are **major contributors**. These foods create a perfect storm for high cholesterol and heart disease risk. Eating just 50 grams of processed meat per day - about one to two slices of deli meat or a single sausage - has been linked to a 42 per cent higher risk of heart disease[2]. By contrast, fibre-rich foods such as oats, legumes, and vegetables can help remove cholesterol by binding it in the intestines.

---

2 *Micha, R., Wallace, S. K., & Mozaffarian, D. (2010). Red and Processed Meat Consumption and Risk of Incident Coronary Heart Disease, Stroke, and Diabetes Mellitus: A Systematic Review and Meta-Analysis. Circulation, 121(21), 2271–2283. https://doi.org/10.1161/CIRCULATIONAHA.109.924977 see also Harvard Gazette+6Europe PMC+6ScienceDaily+6 This meta-analysis, published in Circulation, reviewed data from over 1.2 million participants across 20 studies. It found that each daily 50-gram serving of processed meat –approximately one to two slices of deli meat or one hot dog – was linked to a 42% increased risk of coronary heart disease and a 19% higher risk of type 2 diabetes.*

However, not all sources of saturated fat have the same impact. According to Sydney's Victor Chang Cardiac Research Institute[3], classifying all saturated fats uniformly may be misleading. The health effects depend on the overall food matrix, which includes a wide range of nutrients and compounds that interact in complex ways.

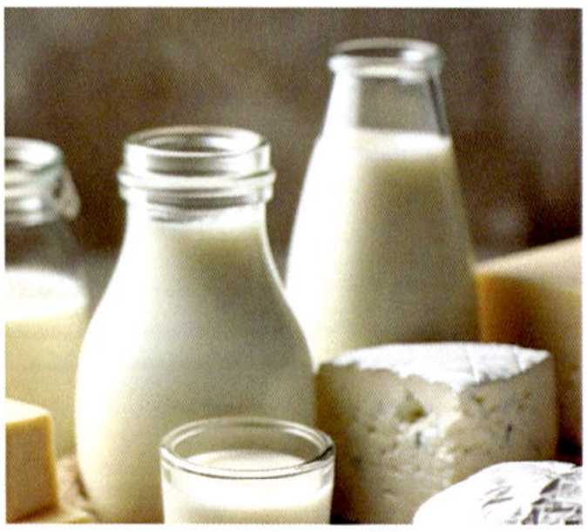

Take full-fat dairy foods such as milk, cheese, and yoghurt. While they contain saturated fat, they also provide **beneficial nutrients** like calcium, protein, vitamin K2, and probiotics. Consumed in **moderation**, these dairy products are **not associated** with increased cardiovascular risk. That said, they do not **reduce** risk in the same way as plant-based foods like olive oil, fruits, vegetables, legumes, and nuts.

Unsaturated fats have two main types – **poly**unsaturated and **mono**unsaturated fats, and **both** should be included in the **daily** diet.

Plant-based oils, including sunflower and grapeseed oils, as well as some nuts, seeds, and fatty fish contain **polyunsaturated fatty acids (PUFA)**. There are two main types:

- **omega-6**, such as linoleic acid found mainly in plant-based oils, and
- **omega-3**, such as alpha-linolenic acid, found in flaxseeds, chia seeds, and walnuts, and the marine-derived EPA and DHA found in oily fish and fish oil.

Omega-3 PUFA, particularly EPA (best recognised as fish oil) are known for **reducing TG levels**[4]. Omega-3 oils can also directly reduce TG production by inhibiting various enzymes involved in its synthesis. So, omega-3 PUFA can lower TG levels **without** significantly affecting cholesterol levels.

---

3 *the Victor Chang Cardiac Research Institute (https://www.victorchang.edu.au/heart-disease/high-cholesterol/saturated-fat-and-heart-disease)*

4 *Lowering TG levels is achieved through multiple mechanisms, including inhibiting TG-producing enzymes and modulating particle synthesis involved in VLDL-C and ApoB-100. Omega-3 PUFA also interact with the peroxisome proliferator-activated receptor alpha (PPAR alpha), which is implicated in diabetes, further reducing TG production.*

Oleic acid, found in olive oil, is a prime example of **monounsaturated fatty acids (MUFA)**. Foods such as avocado and almonds and their oils, and egg yolks also contain oleic acid. Palmitoleic acid (in macadamia nuts, and some animal fats) and nervonic acid, which is synthesised in the body from other fatty acids, are types of MUFA. While MUFA do not affect cholesterol levels significantly, they can **reduce TG levels** through effects on apolipoproteins (such as ApoE and ApoC-III) involved in lipoprotein metabolism.

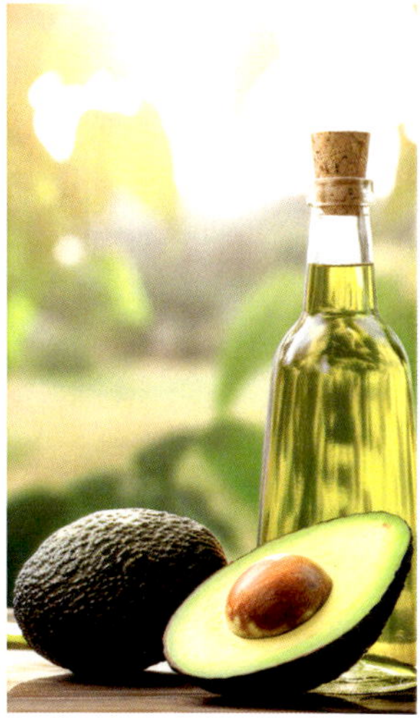

nutritional interventions

Plant sterols, fibre, and soy are 'top-of-the-pops' for lowering LDL-C with the help of nature.

Plant sterols (phytosterols) can lower LDL-C because they actively compete with cholesterol for absorption in the gut. They are found naturally in plant-based foods but only in small amounts, making it difficult to achieve the recommended two to three grams per day without using enriched foods.

It is worth mentioning here that plant sterols also reduce the level of carotenoids (beneficial antioxidants) in your blood. Hence, it is important to eat at least two fruits and five vegetables every day, especially yellow and orange ones, to ensure plenty of antioxidants are in your diet.

Soluble fibre is found in plant foods. Because it is not absorbed in the intestine, soluble fibre can bind cholesterol in the intestine and remove it from the body. It is found in fruits, vegetables, grains, and legumes. Importantly, as you eat more fibrous foods, drink plenty of water to prevent constipation.

Soy is a nutraceutical rich in isoflavones, which may help lower LDL-C by mimicking oestrogen and supporting cardiovascular health. Its plant-based protein and fibre content also contribute to improved cholesterol management.

For more detail on nutraceuticals, see chapter 19.

but what do I eat?

How does all this information come together in our daily eating?

As we have already said, three eating styles are worth mentioning:

- the **Portfolio Diet** or plant-based diets to help reduce LDL-C,
- a **Mediterranean-style diet** to support heart health and help lower overall cardiovascular risk, and
- **calorie-restriction** and **low carbohydrate** eating for weight loss.

for LDL-C reduction – Portfolio Diet

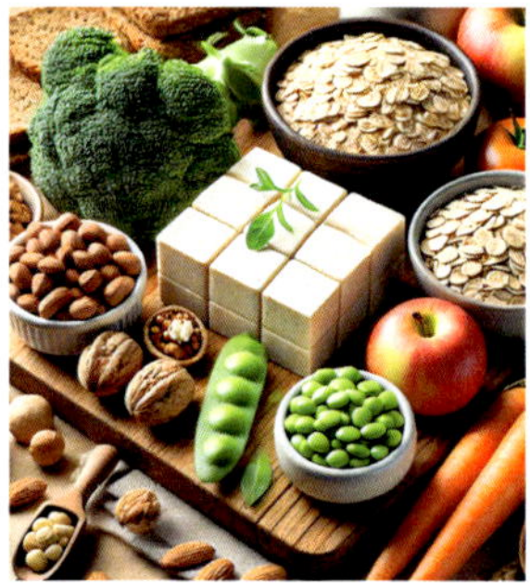

The **Portfolio Diet** is based on combining cholesterol-lowering foods to maximise their impact on reducing LDL-C levels.

Key ingredients include soy protein (found in tofu, tempeh, edamame), plant sterols (naturally occurring in nuts, seeds, whole grains, fruits, vegetables), tree nuts (such as almonds, walnuts, and other nuts that are rich in unsaturated fats), and soluble fibre (from oats, barley, legumes, fruits, vegetables), all of which have been shown to reduce LDL-C.

This way of eating encourages incorporating these cholesterol-lowering foods instead of foods high in saturated fat such as meat, processed foods, sweets, and refined foods. It offers a way to lower cholesterol levels while promoting overall health. Discussing this diet with your primary care provider or cardiologist as part of a therapeutic approach is essential. While solid evidence supports the cholesterol-lowering effects of the Portfolio Diet, its impact on reducing cardiovascular events is not yet established. Nonetheless, it is a valuable dietary option for lowering plasma cholesterol.

plant-based diets

Dean Ornish was one of the initial advocates for plant-based diets in association with improved cardiovascular health. Plant-based diets include vegan (no animal products), vegetarian (includes dairy and eggs but no meat or fish), and flexitarian (mostly plant-based with occasional meat or fish), making them similar to the Mediterranean Diet without animal products. Because they are rich in fruits, vegetables, whole grains, legumes, nuts, and seeds, such diets are abundant in fibre, vitamins, and minerals. They help lower blood pressure and LDL-C, reduce the risk of diabetes, and help maintain a healthy weight – all of which can help lower the risk of developing CVD, including heart attack and stroke.

It's important to note that plant-based diets are not automatically healthy. Focusing on whole, minimally processed plant foods is crucial, as some vegetarian or vegan diets can include high amounts of refined grains and sugars, which do not confer the same cardiovascular benefits.

for heart health – Mediterranean Diet

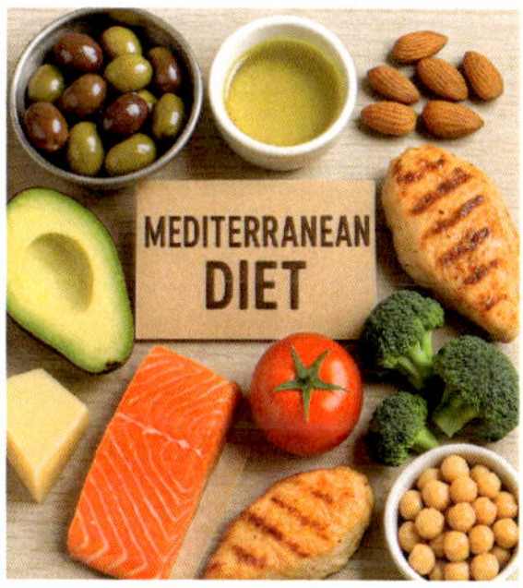

A **Mediterranean eating style**, inspired by the traditional diets of countries bordering the Mediterranean Sea, focuses on whole, minimally-processed foods such as fruits, vegetables, whole grains, lean proteins, and healthy fats.

Olive oil, an essential fat source containing monounsaturated fats and antioxidants, is a cornerstone of the Mediterranean diet. Fish – especially fatty fish rich in omega-3 – poultry, legumes, and moderate amounts of dairy provide lean protein, while red meat and processed foods are limited.

Several influential studies point to Mediterranean-style eating as a means of healthy eating for the heart and overall well-being.

The **PREDIMED** study (Spain) showed that, in people at high cardiovascular risk, a Mediterranean diet supplemented with olive oil or nuts reduced major cardiovascular events by about 30 per cent compared with a low-fat diet.

The **Lyon Diet Heart Study** (France) found that patients who had already suffered a heart attack and adopted a Mediterranean-style diet had a 72 per cent reduction in cardiac death and recurrent heart attacks and a 56 per cent reduction in overall mortality.

The **DART** trial (Wales) highlighted the benefits of omega-3 rich fatty fish, showing a 30 per cent reduction in all-cause mortality among men post-heart attack who increased their fish intake.

The **Heart Institute of Spokane Diet Intervention and Evaluation Trial** study (USA) demonstrated that both a low-fat and a Mediterranean-style diet lowered cardiovascular risk by around 30 per cent compared with usual care after a heart attack.

Most recently, the **CORDIOPREV** trial (Spain) confirmed that a Mediterranean diet was superior to a low-fat diet in preventing major cardiovascular events in people with established heart disease, providing strong contemporary evidence of its benefit in secondary prevention.

The message is consistent across decades and countries: Mediterranean-style eating protects the heart.

If you would like to delve further into the details of these studies, please refer to *a closer look: studies support the Mediterranean diet* beginning on page 205.

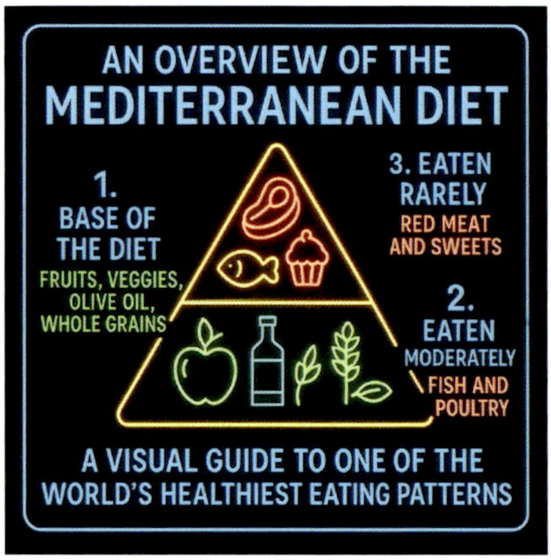

weight loss – Ketogenic Diet

The **Ketogenic (keto) Diet** (including the Carnivore Diet, see next page) is high in fats, moderate in protein, and very low in carbohydrates. It aims to put the body into a state of ketosis so that **fat** is burned for energy instead of **carbohydrates**. This diet can be effective for weight loss and reducing blood sugar levels. However, some adherents can develop very high LDL-C levels. This is not necessarily a short-term problem, but if the diet is used longer-term, it can elevate cardiovascular risk.

DR KOSTNER:

> *Some people experience a sharp rise in LDL-C after switching to a low-carb, high-fat diet. These individuals are often referred to as*

***hyper-responders** – defined by a 50 per cent or greater increase in LDL-C (typically due to an increase in saturated fat intake). At the same time, HDL-C usually rises and TG fall, which is common with low-carb eating.*

*A subgroup known as **lean mass hyper-responders** (LMHRs) takes this to another level. As the name suggests, LMHRs are usually lean and/or athletic, and follow a very low-carb diet. Some are ultra-endurance athletes who thrive on this way of eating – but may also develop extremely high LDL-C levels. This paradox continues to raise questions about long-term cardiovascular risks, especially in those who appear otherwise metabolically healthy.*

I have seen increases in LDL-C of more than 500 per cent in some individuals on keto diets! While this may not increase cardiovascular risk over the short term, I believe it does over longer periods, especially if other risk factors are present.

An April 2025 research paper[5] by the Budoff group showed that for individuals following a keto diet who started with healthy arteries, there was no relationship between ApoB exposure and plaque development over a one-year period. However, those who had plaque from the onset showed significant plaque progression. This highlights the complexity of the early stages of atherosclerosis, where LDL-C may not be the primary driver, but rather one of several contributors to the environment that supports plaque formation and progression.

Several other well-known weight-loss diets and patterns of eating help with weight loss.

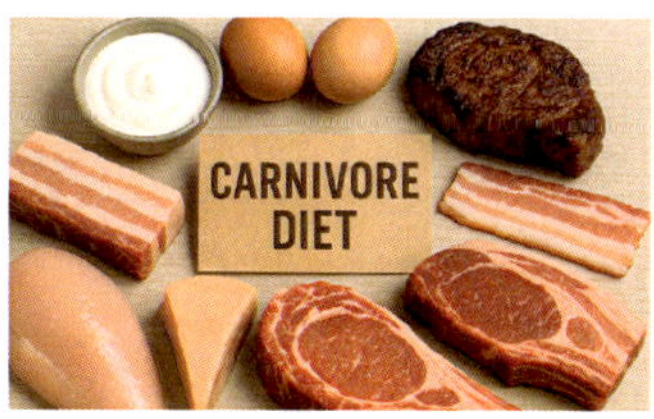

The **Carnivore Diet** is a controversial eating plan that consists entirely of animal-based foods. Eliminating all plant-based foods, it focuses solely on meat, fish, eggs, and animal fats with some variations allowing for limited dairy products.

5 *Soto-Mota A, Manubolu VS, Kinninger A, Norwitz NG, Feldman D, Wood TR, Fialkow J, Cury R, Feldman T, Nasir K, Budoff MJ. Plaque begets plaque, ApoB does not: longitudinal data from the KETO-CTA trial. JACC Adv. 2025 Apr 7;4(7):100365. doi:10.1016/j.jacadv.2025.100365.*

The idea is that by avoiding carbohydrates and plant-based foods, the body becomes more efficient at burning fat for fuel, potentially leading to weight loss and other health benefits. **Advocates** claim that the carnivore diet can help with weight loss, inflammation, and autoimmune conditions. **Critics** raise concerns about its lack of essential nutrients such as fibre, vitamins, and antioxidants found in plant-based foods. **Recent studies** have shown that the **long-term effects** of the carnivore diet are **raised** LDL-C and **increased** cardiovascular event rates.

The **Paleo Diet** focuses on eating foods that our ancestors might have eaten, such as meat, seafood, fruits, vegetables, nuts, and seeds, while avoiding processed foods, grains, and dairy.

Intermittent fasting involves cycling between periods of eating and fasting. Common methods include 16–8 (16 hours fasting, eight hours eating) and 5–2 (eating as usual for five days and drastically reducing calories for two days in the week).

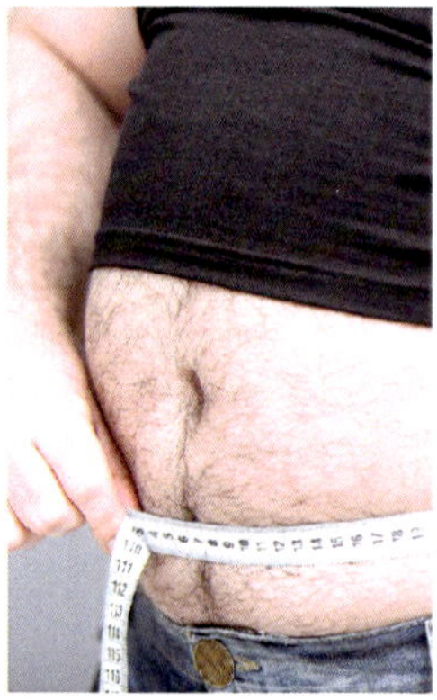

Calorie-restricted eating involves consuming fewer calories than the body needs to maintain its current weight.

weight

Maintaining a healthy weight is crucial to good heart health. Its significance in the cholesterol story is its effect on TG and HDL-C levels. Weight loss typically **lowers TG** and **increases HDL-C**. *Good!*

Sustainable weight management requires timely action, supportive strategies, and an understanding of each person's broader social and psychological context.

beyond the plate, page 208

scan for Dr Bishop's weight loss program
or
https://drwarrickbishop.com/s/tfbsg

A CLOSER LOOK

studies support the Mediterranean diet

Looking closely at the major trials supporting the Mediterranean diet shows how their outcomes, designs, and patient groups built its reputation in both primary and secondary prevention.

primary prevention

The **PREDIMED study**[1] (*Prevención con Dieta Mediterránea*, or Prevention with Mediterranean Diet) (conducted in Spain, published in 2013 and re-released several years later) was a large primary prevention trial of more than 7000 mainly Spanish men and women at high cardiovascular risk but without established disease. Over nearly five years of follow-up, it showed that a Mediterranean diet supplemented with either extra virgin olive oil or nuts significantly reduced the risk of major cardiovascular events – by about 30 per cent – compared with a low-fat diet.

Notably, although cholesterol levels were slightly higher in the Mediterranean diet group, rates of CAD and cardiovascular events were lower, underscoring the importance of fat quality over fat quantity in prevention.

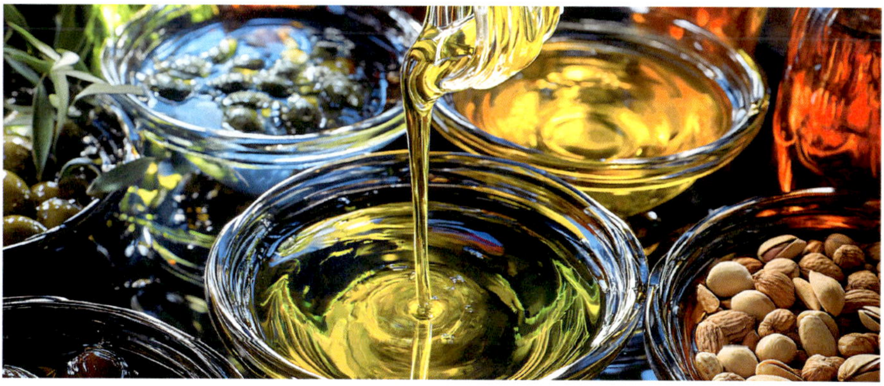

1 *Prevención con Dieta Mediterránea – PREDIMED Anthony A. Bavry Trial Sponsor: Spanish government's Instituto de Salud Carlos III. Food donated by Hojiblanca and Patrimonio Comunal Olivarero, California Walnut Commission, Borges, La Morella Nuts. Date Published: 01/01/2013 Date Updated: 02/25/2013 Original Posted Date: 02/25/2013 American College of Cardiology https://www acc.org/latest-in-cardiology/ clinical-trials/2014/08/08/15/35/predimed see also*

PREDIMED trial of the Mediterranean diet: retracted, republished, BMJ 2019; 364 doi: https://doi.org/10.1136/bmj.l341 (Published 07 February 2019) BMJ 2019;364:l341 https://www.bmj.com/content/364/bmj.l341

secondary prevention

The **Lyon Diet Heart Study**[2] (conducted in France in the 1990s) was a trial of 605 patients who had previously suffered a heart attack.

Participants were randomly assigned to either a Mediterranean-style diet – emphasising fruits, vegetables, legumes, whole grains, olive oil, fish, and omega-3 fatty acids – or the standard Western diet then recommended for heart disease prevention – typically, a low-fat, high-carbohydrate diet with limited saturated fat and cholesterol.

Over a median follow-up of just 27 months, the Mediterranean diet group experienced a 72 per cent reduction in cardiac death and recurrent heart attacks and a 56 per cent reduction in overall mortality, prompting the trial to be **stopped early** because the **benefits were so pronounced**.

It offered foundational evidence by showing that comprehensive dietary change could rival or even surpass the pharmacological therapies of the time, thus establishing an enduring reputation as one of the most compelling demonstrations of diet's role in secondary prevention.

The **Diet and Reinfarction Trial** (DART)[3] (conducted in Wales and published in 1989) was a trial of more than 2000 men who had survived a heart attack.

Participants were randomised to one of three diets: a low-fat diet with more polyunsaturated than saturated fat, an omega-3-enriched diet through increased fatty fish consumption, or a high-fibre cereal-based diet.

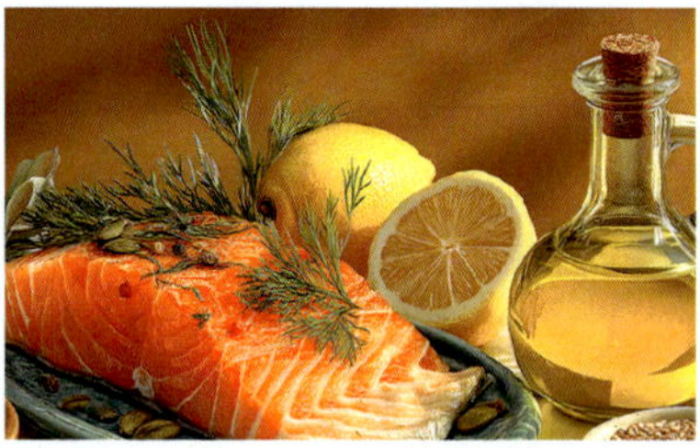

After two years of follow-up, the fatty fish group showed a 30 per cent reduction in all-cause mortality, although this was not matched by a reduction in reinfarction (another heart attack) rates.

As the first randomised trial to demonstrate a mortality benefit from dietary advice in post–heart attack patients, DART is regarded as historically significant and highlights the value of omega-3 fatty acids in secondary prevention.

---

2 *Lyon Diet Heart Study; de Lorgeril M, Salen P, Martin JL, Monjaud I, Delaye J, Mamelle N. Mediterranean diet, traditional risk factors, and the rate of cardiovascular complications after myocardial infarction: final report of the Lyon Diet Heart Study. Circulation. 1999;99(6):779-785*

3 *Diet and reinfarction trial (DART): design, recruitment, and compliance; M.L. Burr et al, European Heart Journal, Volume 10, Issue 6, June 1989, Pages 558–567, https://doi.org/10.1093/oxfordjournals.eurheartj.a059528 Published: 1 June 1989*

Heart Institute of Spokane Diet Intervention and Evaluation Trial (HIS-DIET)[4] (conducted in the United States late in the 1990s) was a trial of about 100 patients who had recently suffered a heart attack. Participants were randomised to usual care, a low-fat diet, or a Mediterranean-style diet that reduced saturated fat and increased omega-3 intake.

After follow-up, both dietary intervention groups showed about a 30 per cent relative risk reduction in cardiovascular outcomes compared with usual care, reinforcing that even modest dietary changes after a heart attack can meaningfully reduce risk.

The **CORDIOPREV trial** (Long-term Secondary Prevention of Cardiovascular Disease with a Mediterranean Diet and a Low-Fat Diet)[5] was conducted at Reina Sofía University Hospital in Córdoba, Spain, and published in 2022.

This trial was a single-centre randomised study of 1002 patients with established CAD, aged 20 to 75 years. Participants were assigned to either a Mediterranean diet or a low-fat diet and followed for seven years, with interventions delivered by dietitians.

The primary outcome was a composite of major cardiovascular events including heart attack, revascularisation, stroke, peripheral artery disease, and cardiovascular death. The Mediterranean diet group experienced significantly fewer events than the low-fat group, confirming the superiority of the Mediterranean diet for long-term secondary prevention.

CORDIOPREV is the largest and longest trial of its kind to date and provides strong, contemporary evidence that Mediterranean dietary patterns remain central to cardiovascular risk reduction.

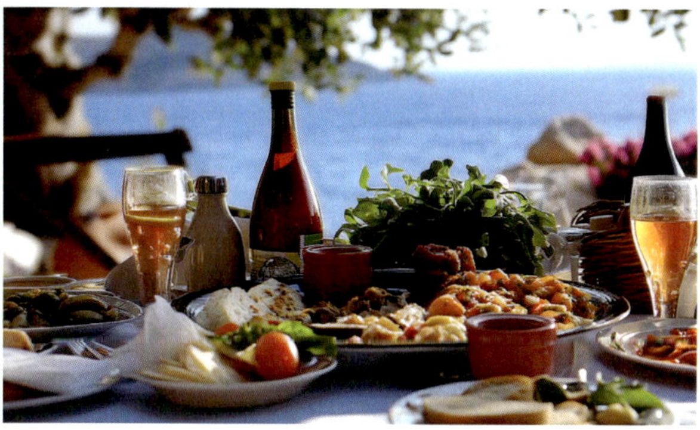

4 *Heart Institute of Spokane Diet Intervention and Evaluation Trial; Tuttle KR, Shuler LA, Packard DP, Milton JE, Daratha KB, Bibus DM, et al. "Comparison of low-fat versus Mediterranean-style dietary intervention after first myocardial infarction." Am J Cardiol. 2008;101(11):1523-30. https://www.ajconline.org/article/S0002-9149(08)00236-1/fulltext see also (SPOKANE) https://clinicaltrials.gov/ct2/show/NCT00269425*

5 *Long-term secondary prevention of cardiovascular disease with a Mediterranean diet and a low-fat diet (CORDIOPREV): a randomised controlled trial. Delgado-Lista, JavierAlcala-Diaz, Juan F et al. The Lancet, Volume 399, Issue 10338, 1876 - 1885*

beyond the plate

Now, we shift our focus beyond dietary choices to examine the interconnected effects of exercise and smoke-free living on cholesterol levels. These complementary lifestyle habits enhance the benefits of a healthy diet, paving the way for a stronger and more resilient cardiovascular system.

physical exercise

Physical activity plays **a crucial role in lifestyle adjustments** targeting multiple risk factors. While exercise alone does not significantly lower cholesterol, it improves blood pressure, weight, glucose control, and overall fitness – all of which reduce the risk of heart problems. Exercise **raises HDL-C**, a beneficial outcome, as HDL-C helps remove cholesterol from the arteries. Moderately intense exercise, where you're slightly short of breath but can still talk, can **increase HDL-C** by 5-15 per cent, performing as well as more intense workouts. Exercise also improves muscle metabolism, shifting energy use from glucose to lipids, which can lower blood fats and sugars.

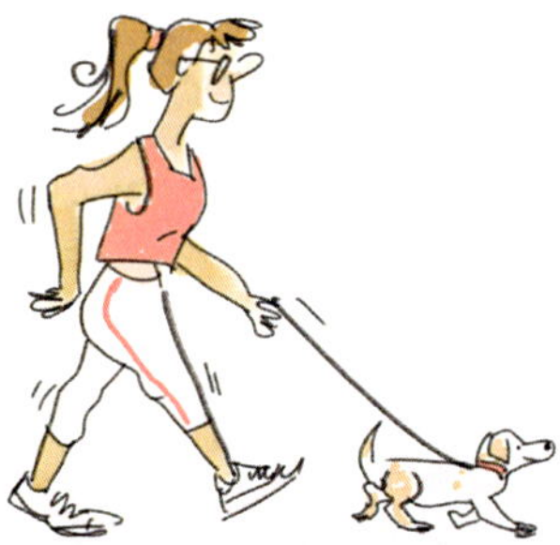

The impact of exercise on **LDL-C is less clear**, with some studies showing a slight decrease. However, exercise effectively **lowers TG** levels, improving metabolic health by aiding weight loss, better sugar utilisation, and insulin sensitivity. Elevated TG, linked to heart disease and stroke, can be reduced through exercise, diet, and, if needed, medication.

Aim for **at least five 30-minute sessions of moderate exercise**, such as brisk walking, each week. A daily goal of 8000–10,000 steps is beneficial.

And it's not just cardio that helps. **Resistance training** – using weights, resistance bands, or your body weight – has also been shown to improve LDL-C and TG levels. It reduces visceral fat, a key driver of inflammation and cardiovascular risk. Including **two to three sessions of strength training each week**,

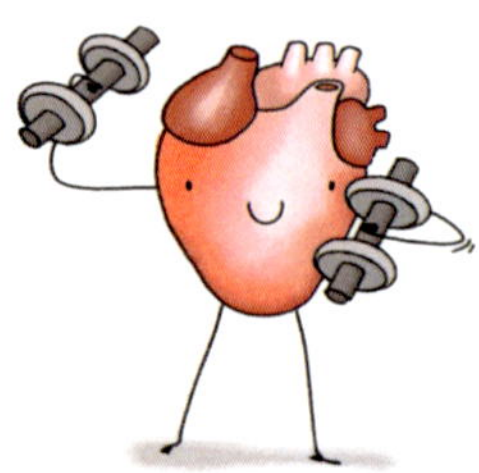

alongside aerobic activity, enhances both metabolic and lipid health, especially in middle-aged and older adults.

To make exercise a lasting habit, choose activities you **enjoy**. Regular exercise supports physical health and boosts mental well-being by reducing stress, anxiety, and depression, and improving self-esteem and cognition.

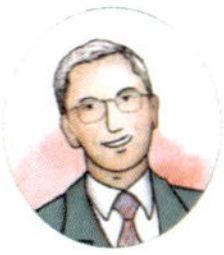

For a 5–15 per cent increase in HDL-C, a possible 5–7 per cent reduction in LDL-C, a 10–15 per cent reduction in TG, and a 5–7 mmHg reduction in blood pressure, exercise delivers an impressive 30–40 per cent reduction in CVD risk. This makes it a cornerstone intervention for better health – even before considering its benefits for endothelial function, reduced inflammation, improved insulin sensitivity, enhanced autonomic balance, and, crucially, a better mood.

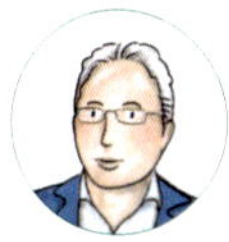

smoking/vaping

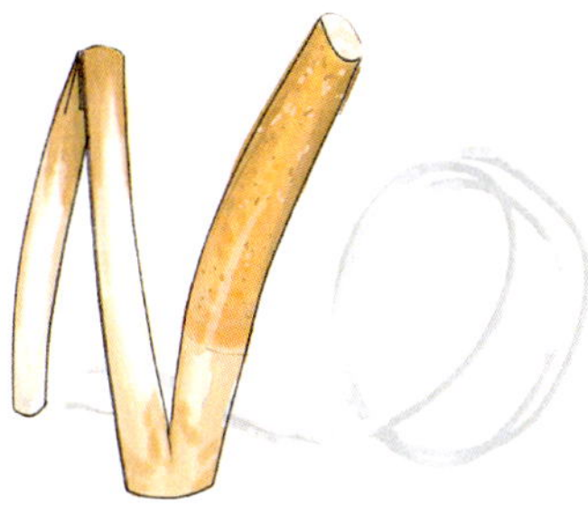

Don't – **please!**

Smokers face elevated risks of heart attacks, strokes, and angina at a younger age, with a four-fold increase in heart disease mortality compared with non-smokers. In Australia, lives are claimed daily by CVD linked to smoking. **Female smokers** are particularly susceptible to heart attacks. Smoking is a major **preventable** cause of mortality and morbidity globally. It not only impacts the heart but also affects lung function, raises cancer risks, and contributes to peripheral vascular disease, thin bones, and skin problems.

From a cholesterol perspective, smoking **increases** inflammation and **negatively** affects lipid metabolism, leading to **higher TG levels**. Even a few cigarettes a day increases health risks.

Cutting back may slow lung damage, but **only quitting** can significantly lower cardiovascular risk. It takes planning and persistence, but the benefits are huge – **within two years** of quitting, your cardiovascular risk is **almost the same** as that of a **non-smoker** of the same age and sex.

Quitting also protects others from **second-hand smoke**, which can harm the health of unborn children, children, and adults. While less studied, **e-cigarettes** and **vaping** appear to carry similar risks as smoking.

coordinated approach

It is exceedingly challenging to shift cholesterol levels more than about 15 per cent through lifestyle changes alone – and sustaining such changes requires **dedication** that can be hard to maintain in everyday life. That said, **eating well, managing weight, staying active and not smoking offer powerful benefits beyond cholesterol**. They improve metabolic health, reduce inflammation, lower blood pressure, and support vascular function – all vital for long-term cardiovascular well-being.

Lifestyle and **medication** work best **together.** Each enhances the other, especially for those at higher risk, making long-term success more likely.

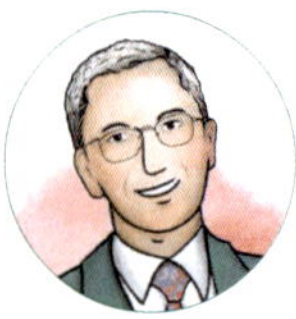

We, as doctors, are like mechanics, ensuring everything under the bonnet runs smoothly. But if the driver ignores speed limits, doesn't wear a seatbelt, is inattentive – then, the journey's safety is more at risk.

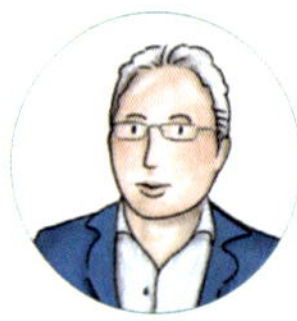

IMPORTANT POINTS

LIFESTYLE CHANGES

- Adopting healthy habits – including a balanced, whole food diet, regular exercise, maintaining a healthy weight, avoiding/quitting smoking – works harmoniously with medications to lower cholesterol, improve cardiovascular health, and enhance overall well-being.

Central to everything discussed in this book is the belief that **education is pivotal to meaningful change.** Alongside your GP and cardiologist, consider help from professionals such as an accredited practising dietitian, exercise physiologist, physiotherapist, and/or psychologist.

More detailed information on the heart health '10 commandments' is available in the Bishop-Kostner collaboration, *10 Commandments for Heart Health Explained*.

Dr Bishop has a weight loss program https://Dr Warrickbishop.com/s/tfbsg

Because of its focus on prevention, the Bishop-Begg collaboration, *Cardiac Rehabilitation Explained,* is also an excellent resource.

10 Commandments of Heart Health Explained

weight loss

Cardiac Rehabilitation Explained

While medications are essential for lowering LDL-C levels, natural adjuncts can help enhance their effectiveness.

cholesterol curiosities

coffee, cafestol, and cholesterol

Coffee contains a natural compound called cafestol, found in coffee oils. Cafestol is one of the most potent dietary substances known to raise LDL cholesterol.

The effect depends largely on how coffee is prepared.

Unfiltered coffee methods – such as French press (plunger), Turkish or Greek coffee, and boiled coffee – allow cafestol to pass into the cup. Regular consumption can lead to a measurable rise in LDL-C.

Paper-filtered coffee removes most cafestol and has little impact on cholesterol levels. Espresso contains some cafestol, but the small serving size limits its overall effect.

For people managing cholesterol or cardiovascular risk, paper-filtered coffee is the preferred choice.

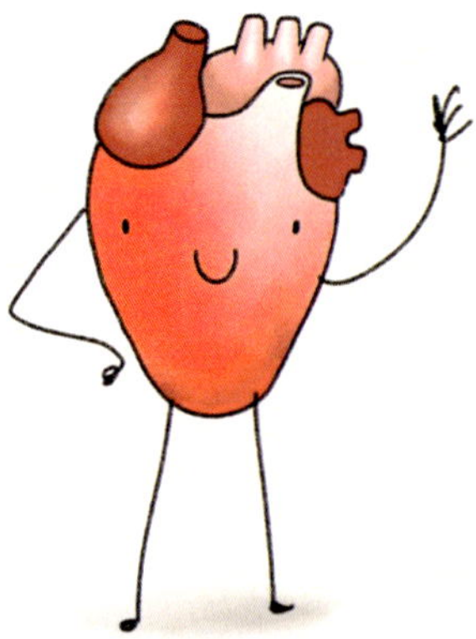

change is possible

- with the help of education
- through seeking medical advice and using medications when needed, supported by lifestyle adjustments and consideration of nutraceuticals
- asking for the support and encouragement of others

chapter 19

COMPLEMENTARY STRATEGIES: BROADER LIPID MANAGEMENT

Medication prescriptions are often accompanied by a recommendation to make healthy lifestyle changes (as discussed in the previous chapter), and the possible use of nutraceuticals. These can offer valuable reinforcement, amplifying the effects of medications for improved outcomes.

nutraceuticals

Nutraceuticals are not drugs in the traditional sense. The term combines *nutrition* and *pharmaceutical* and refers to foods or food-derived products that provide health benefits beyond basic nutrition. They often contain bioactive compounds believed to support specific bodily functions or help prevent disease. Unlike pharmaceutical drugs, nutraceuticals are usually derived from natural sources and are not subject to the same rigorous testing or regulation. Common examples include dietary supplements, functional foods and herbal products.

In the context of cardiovascular health, nutraceuticals are natural components of plants, legumes and vegetables that may help improve key risk factors such as cholesterol levels.

While nutraceuticals can modestly lower LDL-C, they are generally **not potent enough** to achieve the levels required to significantly reduce the risk of heart attacks and strokes. Their strength lies in serving as an **additional** measure for people already receiving appropriate, guideline-based therapy, particularly those motivated to do more to support their heart health.

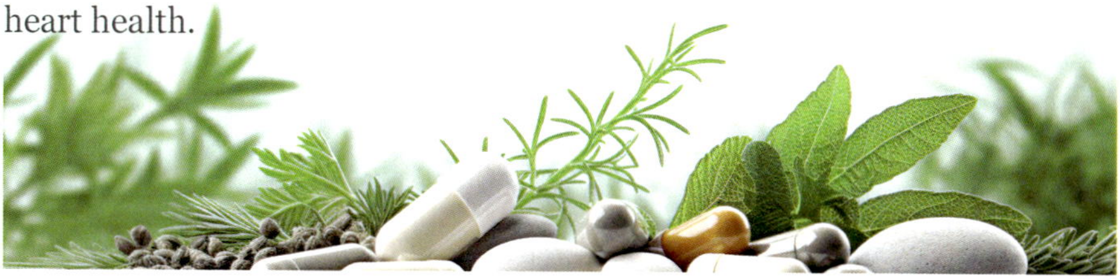

As we know, cholesterol in our body comes from two sources, **production** (primarily the liver, although most cells in our body produce their own cholesterol) and **absorption** (from the food we eat).

People who are very good **producers** of cholesterol and whose liver cannot get rid of cholesterol sufficiently often have inherited this ability. No matter how good their diets are, they will have lifelong high cholesterol levels, and if there is plaque in their arteries, they will have an increased risk of heart disease unless treated with medication. People who **absorb** more cholesterol from their diet than others respond better to a reduction in saturated fat-containing foods such as butter, red meat, cheese, and cream.

cholesterol absorption inhibitors

One of the most effective natural ways to lower cholesterol is by inhibiting cholesterol absorption. Plant sterols and fibre are the most important nutraceuticals to help with this.

Plant sterols and **stanols** occur naturally in vegetables and fruit. However, a person with high cholesterol would need to consume very large amounts of food to ingest enough to make a difference. Plant sterols block cholesterol absorption and work in a similar way to ezetimibe. They can be taken as supplements (capsules) and are also available in a variety of enriched foods, including 'proactive' margarine, yoghurt and cereal, that can be sourced in any supermarket.

dose: 3 g of plant sterols or stanols a day reduces LDL-C by up to 10–15 per cent

Fibre – such as psyllium, oats, beta-glucan and pectin – causes increased gastric emptying time, decreased cholesterol production and increased faecal excretion of cholesterol. Usually, fibre can be consumed as a drink with water and juices or as a powder and added to cereals.

dose: 10–20 g per day can reduce cholesterol by 5–10 per cent

cholesterol synthesis inhibitors

Red yeast rice, bergamot, artichoke and garlic are nutraceuticals that can reduce cholesterol production within the body.

Red yeast rice is extracted from fermented rice and is structurally **similar to lovastatin**, one of the first statins. It, too, works by inhibiting one of the key enzymes of cholesterol production, HMG-CoA reductase. It can have similar side effects to statins and is **not safe** to take during breastfeeding and pregnancy.

dose: 1–5 g per day can reduce LDL-C by 10-20 per cent

Bergamot (*citrus bergamia*) is derived from a citrus fruit and is rich in flavonoids and flavones that can reduce LDL-C by inhibiting cholesterol synthesis (the body's biological process in which cells produce cholesterol).

dose: 500–1000 mg of bergamot extract daily (for at least 30 days) can lead to a reduction in LDL-C levels for some people by between 8-15 per cent

Garlic and its active ingredient, allicin, inhibits cholesterol production similar to statins by blocking the enzyme HMG-CoA reductase.

dose: usually, 1200 mg of garlic powder per day is recommended, leading to LDL-C reductions of five per cent

Artichoke and its leaf extract contain flavonoids and acids such as caffeic acid that inhibit HMG-CoA reductase. They are said to protect the liver, too.

dose: 300 mg per day can reduce LDL-C by 5–10 per cent

cholesterol excretion enhancers

Soy protein, green tea and berberine increase cholesterol excretion into the bile and faeces.

Soy proteins contain bioactive peptides and isoflavones which can reduce cholesterol biosynthesis and increase the faecal excretion of bile salts, which then prevents reabsorption of cholesterol.

dose: up to 30 g per day can reduce LDL-C by five per cent

Green tea and its extracts are rich in polyphenols (potent antioxidants) which prevent lipid peroxidation[1], which in turn prevents LDL from entering

1 *Lipid peroxidation occurs when free radicals oxidise unsaturated fatty acids in cell membranes, causing damage linked to ageing, inflammation, CVD, neurodegeneration, and cancer. Antioxidants help protect by neutralising free radicals and stabilising membranes.*

plaques. They can also inhibit HMG-CoA reductase and increase the biliary excretion of cholesterol.

dose: 3–5 cups a day may lead to an LDL-C reduction of 5–10 per cent

Berberine is an alkaloid that inhibits the protein PCSK9. This compound is found in different plants such as berberis (known for their distinctive, often spiny stems and clusters of bright, colourful berries), coptis (particularly the rhizomes of *coptis chinensis*), and hydrastis (particularly the roots of *hydrastis canadensis*, or goldenseal). Inhibiting PCSK9 increases the clearance of LDL-C via receptors on the liver. Berberine can also reduce LDL absorption in the intestine. Although it can have some mild gastrointestinal side effects such as constipation and diarrhoea, it also has a positive effect on blood pressure and glucose levels. It may interact with some medications.

dose: 900–1500 mg a day might reduce LDL-C by up to 20 per cent

worth noting

Before we conclude this discussion on the benefits of nutraceuticals as aids to lowering LDL-C, we need a few words on vitamin K, coenzyme Q10 (CoQ10), and magnesium. Vitamin K (in its K1 and K2 forms) and CoQ10 are naturally occurring compounds, while magnesium is a naturally occurring mineral. Each can be consumed through diet or as supplements.

They are often promoted as improving health outcomes. **Vitamin K1** is important for clotting and **K2** in calcium regulation, while **CoQ10** is crucial for cellular energy production. **Magnesium** plays a role in lipid metabolism and cardiovascular health, with potential benefits for improving endothelial function and reducing inflammation. However, you should be aware of several things.

Vitamin K2 is essential for bone health, ensuring calcium is deposited in the bones, not in soft tissues such as blood vessels and cartilage. It activates proteins like osteocalcin (crucial for bone mineralisation – making bones hard and strong), and matrix Gla protein (MGP), which inhibits calcium build-up in the wrong places like arteries or the aortic valve.

DR BISHOP:

I share with my patients that by inhibiting HMG-CoA reductase, statins may reduce the production of vitamin K2. Additionally, ezetimibe, another lipid-lowering agent, affects not only the reabsorption of cholesterol but potentially vitamin K in the intestines. This dual mechanism could, theoretically, lead to a vitamin K deficiency, causing less calcium to be deposited in bones and more in places where it shouldn't be. This scenario could contribute to conditions such as osteoporosis and aortic stenosis.

While there is no conclusive clinical evidence linking statin use with an increased risk of bone or heart valve issues, biological mechanisms support the theory.

For patients on lipid-lowering therapies, it might be worth considering – in consultation with your medical team – if vitamin K supplementation could help mitigate potential calcium mismanagement. This is an evolving area of research, and more studies are needed to understand the full implications.

Coenzyme Q10 (CoQ10), also known as ubiquinone, is a vital compound involved in energy production within cells, particularly in the mitochondria (cell structures that produce energy and regulate cell functions). Statins, in blocking the HMG-CoA reductase pathway, may reduce CoQ10 levels, potentially leading to muscle-related side effects, such as aches and pains.

The study, A Randomised Trial of Coenzyme Q10 in Patients with Confirmed Statin Myopathy[2], assessed CoQ10 levels in individuals with statin-related muscle symptoms. While it found no clear link between CoQ10 levels and symptoms or significant changes with supplementation, it remains a point of interest. For patients with statin-related muscle aches, trying CoQ10 might be worthwhile. Alternatively, bempedoic acid, a newer lipid-lowering drug targeting the liver higher up the cholesterol pathway, may be an option for statin-sensitive patients without affecting CoQ10 levels in the muscles, as it is active only in the liver.

---

2 *Taylor, B. A., Lorson, L., White, C. M., & Thompson, P. D. (2015). A randomized trial of coenzyme Q10 in patients with confirmed statin myopathy. Atherosclerosis, 238(2), 329–335. https://doi.org/10.1016/j.atherosclerosis.2014.12.016*

Magnesium is important for heart health and is generally safe to take. It helps keep the heart beating steadily, supports healthy blood flow, and relaxes muscles, which may also ease cramps and soreness. Anecdotally, magnesium orotate is considered a good choice because the body absorbs it well, and it may also help with sleep.

IMPORTANT POINTS

COMPLEMENTARY STRATEGIES

- Patients have the option to discuss with their doctors the use of nutraceuticals as a safe way to optimise outcomes.
- While nutraceuticals have a small effect on their own, they are used in conjunction with pharmaceutical medications. Their value lies in being an adjunct to appropriate medical (pharmacological) care.
- Nutraceuticals help to
  - inhibit cholesterol absorption
  - reduce cholesterol production
  - increase excretion.
- Nutraceuticals must be used in consultation with your doctor / specialist.
- Although current research does not strongly support using vitamin K, CoQ10, or magnesium supplementation to counteract deficiencies potentially caused by lipid-lowering medications, these supplements are gaining interest and may benefit some individuals.

Some patients face an even greater inherited burden than most high-risk sufferers and require a distinct approach to treatment and management.

chapter 20

GENETIC RISKS: FAMILIAL HYPERCHOLESTEROLAEMIA, Lp(a)

Some people face an unavoidably high risk of CVD because of their genetics, a prior event, or particular life circumstances. In these vulnerable groups, the link between cholesterol and disease is not in question.

After briefly reiterating the importance of treatment for secondary prevention patients, this and the next chapter will focus on **primary prevention** in specific high-risk groups.

This chapter will look at the impact of familial hypercholesterolaemia (FH) and elevated lipoprotein(a) [Lp(a)]. *Chapter 20* will discuss groups with distinct risk profiles: people concerned about the risk of developing dementia, older adults, women (and specifically pregnant women), people whose ethnicity has an impact, and individuals with kidney or liver disease. For all these people, **early and tailored** cholesterol management is also **essential**. The risks are real; the stakes are high. Timely and personalised treatments matter.

secondary prevention

Our secondary prevention patients are high-risk patients. They are being treated after a major cardiovascular event, such as a heart attack, stroke, peripheral vascular disease, or revascularisation (stent implantation or bypass surgery). There isn't a guideline document in the world that does not recommend cholesterol-lowering therapy for these patients.

The **message is unambiguous**,
the **data is undeniabl**e, and the **science is solid**:
this group of patients **will benefit** from cholesterol-lowering
'for life' treatment.

Even the cholesterol non-believers and the anti-statin voices concede that there is a **clear benefit** for these high-risk individuals when it comes to lowering cholesterol.

primary prevention

The other patients to be considered are those for whom we want to prevent the first event – our primary prevention group. These patients are **yet to define themselves as high-risk by having an event**. They can be **'hiding'** anywhere in low-risk or intermediate-risk groups. Of the clues, **cholesterol** is the most significant. Remember our discussion about association and causation? These individuals have **associations** that **suggest** the risk group they **may** be in but it does **not** determine if they will have an event or not. *Tricky!* And yet there are a couple of instances where this is not the case.

familial hypercholesterolaemia

In this **primary prevention** setting, familial hypercholesterolaemia (FH), which affects about 1 in 250 people, provides **clear evidence of treatment benefit**.

Familial hypercholesterolaemia is a relatively common **genetic** condition characterised by **high LDL-C from birth** and **early** cardiovascular events. FH affects **how** the body clears cholesterol from the blood because inherited gene variants impair this process. These variants most often involve LDL receptors (LDLR), apolipoprotein B (ApoB), or PCSK9 genes.

- **LDLR** sit on the surface of liver cells and are responsible for 'grabbing' LDL particles from the bloodstream and 'pulling' them into the liver for processing. If LDLR are faulty or missing, LDL particles can't be cleared efficiently so the LDL-C level rises.
- **ApoB** is the protein on the surface of LDL particles that the LDLR recognise and to which they bind. If ApoB is abnormal, the receptors can't properly identify or bind the LDL particles, again leading to reduced clearance of cholesterol from the blood.
- **PCSK9** regulates the number of LDLR available. If PCSK9 activity is too high, LDLR are broken down more quickly, reducing the number available to clear LDL from the blood and so increase the LDL-C level.

forms

FH presents in three main forms: heterozygous (HeFH), compound heterozygous (cHeFH), and homozygous (HoFH).

Heterozygous familial hypercholesterolaemia **(HeFH)**, the most common form of FH (1:250-300 patients), occurs when a person inherits **one** copy of a faulty gene from **one** parent[1]. If one parent has HeFH, there is a 50 per cent chance of passing it on to each child.

Without treatment, LDL-C is typically twice the normal level by early adulthood. Because the arteries are exposed to high cholesterol for many years, people with HeFH have a higher risk of early heart disease, especially if the condition goes untreated.

Most people with HeFH **feel** healthy, and the condition is often only discovered through a blood test or after a heart event in the family. As is the case in each form, **family history** is crucial in detecting the condition early.

Compound heterozygous familial hypercholesterolaemia **(cHeFH)** is **very rare.** It occurs when a person inherits **two *different*** faulty FH-related genes – **one from each parent.** The two inherited variant genes are not identical (as in HoFH), yet both disrupt the body's ability to remove LDL from the blood and so lower LDL-C. This leads to **extremely high** LDL-C from birth and **significantly increases** the risk of **early** and **aggressive** heart disease. cHeFH sufferers require strong, early, and comprehensive treatment to manage their cholesterol levels and protect their heart health.

Homozygous familial hypercholesterolaemia **(HoFH)** is very rare and the **most serious** form of FH, causing the **very highest** of cholesterol levels (even higher than cHeFH) from birth. It occurs when a person inherits the **same** faulty FH gene from **each** parent.

With HoFH, LDL-C levels can be four to six times higher than normal, even in childhood. This massive cholesterol build-up leads to the early development of plaque in the arteries, often starting in childhood or adolescence.

---

1 *Most genes come in pairs – one copy from each parent. These two copies may be the same or slightly different. Sometimes, a change (variant) in one or both copies can affect how the gene works.*

A CLOSER LOOK

rare familial hypercholesterolaemia – homozygous (HoFH) and compound heterozygous (cHeFH)

Homozygous familial hypercholesterolaemia (HoFH) and compound heterozygous familial hypercholesterolaemia (cHeFH) are **rare** forms of FH, affecting about **one in a million Australians**.

They are characterised by **extreme** elevations in LDL-C (above 10 mmol/L), resulting in aggressive and early-onset CAD, even without other risk factors.

Affected individuals have inherited the FH gene from both parents and face a very high risk of heart attacks, stent placements, and even bypass surgery before the age of 20, with survival beyond 30 years being difficult.

They can also have cholesterol infiltration and calcification of the aortic valve and root, causing valve narrowing. Heart surgery to replace the aortic valve is often needed at an early age.

All options are on the table for treating HoFH and cHeFH patients, including all agents that can be taken to lower cholesterol and some new agents such as the microsomal transfer protein (MTP) inhibitor, lomitapide[1], and the angiopoietin-like 3 (ANGPTL3) inhibitor, evinacumab[2].

These patients are also considered for LDL apheresis, a process not unlike dialysis. The patient is hooked up to a machine that removes the LDL particles from the blood.

In certain cases, HoFH patients progress to a liver transplant when all other treatment options fail.

---

1 *Microsomal transfer protein (MTP) inhibitors block the action of microsomal TG transfer protein , which is essential for assembling and secreting apoB-containing lipoproteins such as VLDL and chylomicrons. Lomitapide is the only MTP inhibitor approved for clinical use. Currently (2026), it is available in Australia for compassionate use only.* *(Please see page 168 for further information.)*

2 *Evinacumab is a fully human monoclonal antibody that targets angiopoietin-like 3 (ANGPTL3), a protein involved in lipid metabolism. By inhibiting ANGPTL3, evinacumab promotes the clearance of LDL-C and TG independently of the LDLR pathway. Evinacumab, administered by monthly intravenous infusion, remains the only approved ANGPTL3 inhibitor for the treatment of HoFH. Currently (2026), it is available in Australia for compassionate use only.* *(Please see page 168 for further information.)*

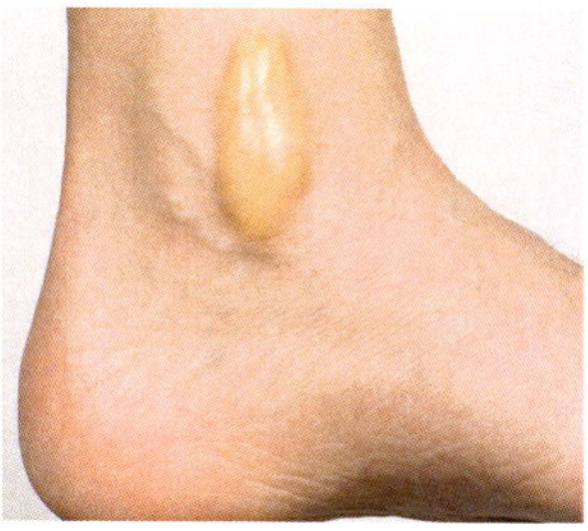

xanthomas

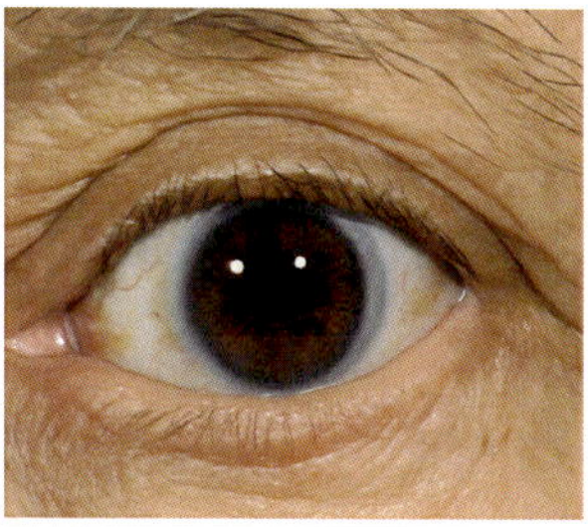

corneal arcus

Without treatment, individuals with HoFH are at **very high risk** of heart attack or other serious cardiovascular problems **at a young age**. Children or teens with HoFH often develop xanthomas (yellow cholesterol deposits in the skin or tendons) or corneal arcus (a grey-white ring in the eye). Both conditions are diagnostic tools for FH.

Standard therapies such as statins are not enough. Combinations of drugs and specialised treatments may be needed to bring cholesterol levels down. Because the condition is so aggressive, **early** identification and strong, **lifelong** treatment are essential to prevent serious cardiovascular complications.

evidence

The evidence is clear. Like the secondary prevention group, individuals with FH benefit from cholesterol-lowering therapy. For them, it's not a question of 'if' coronary problems will develop, but 'when'.

Despite clear diagnostic criteria and effective treatments that can greatly reduce this risk, FH remains **underdiagnosed.** With early detection and appropriate management, individuals with FH can lead full, healthy lives.

testing

the Dutch Lipid Clinical Network Score (DLCNS) online calculator

In modern clinical practice, **genetic** testing is often used to confirm an FH diagnosis by identifying variants in the LDLR, ApoB, or PCSK9 genes (for the LDLR, ApoB protein and PCSK9 protein, respectively). Before genetic tests, diagnosis was based on clinical characteristics and probability scoring. The **Dutch Lipid Clinical Network Score** (DLCNS) remains the most widely used tool for this. DLCNS is a validated set of criteria to determine the likelihood of an adult having FH. It is based on factors such as the patient's family history of premature CVD in first-degree relatives, their own CVD history, untreated lipid levels, and physical signs, for example, the presence of tendon xanthomata (see previous page). The scoring system helps guide decisions about genetic testing and lipid-lowering treatment.

history is important

Early identification of FH depends on eliciting a **thorough** history that reveals **patterns** of inherited risk. A detailed pedigree allows clinicians to trace patterns such as

- elevated LDL-C,
- premature CVD,
- early statin use, or
- sudden cardiac death (SCD).

family pedigree for heterozygous FH

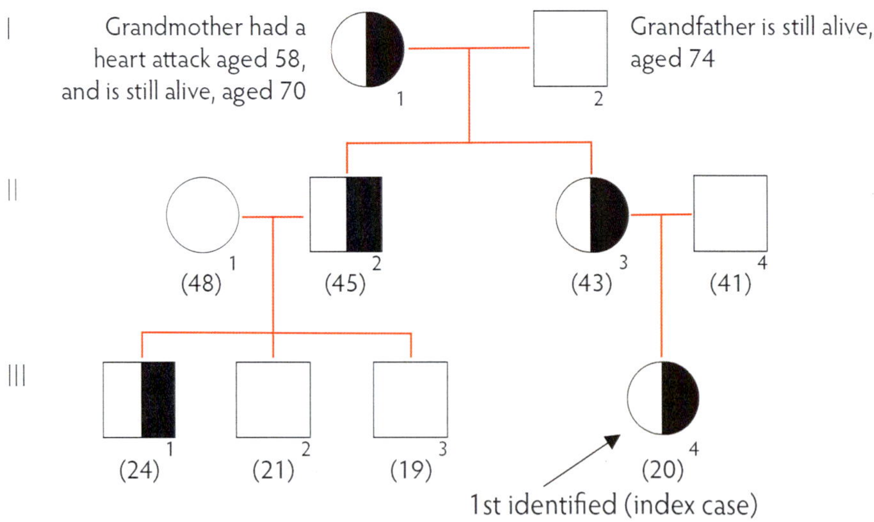

This family pedigree shows a typical pattern of HeFH inheritance. The 20-year-old female (III-4, bottom right) was the first to be diagnosed. She inherited FH from her mother (II-3), who had inherited it from her mother (I-1). After the diagnosis, other family members were tested, using a process known as cascade testing. This led to the diagnosis of her uncle (II-2) and one of his children (III-1).

This history then

- guides clinical suspicion,
- prompts genetic testing, and
- triggers cascade screening of relatives.

Despite its significance, family history is too often **overlooked or poorly detailed** in routine clinical practice – a gap that continues to delay diagnosis and intervention. Family history should be an important focus for treating GPs (primary care providers), cardiologists, and specialist nurse practitioners.

children

As FH is present from birth, lowering cholesterol in children helps prevent complications later, improves both lifespan and quality of life, and **should begin as early as possible** (from the age of **eight years**, depending on the child's additional risk factors) **with the target for cholesterol levels as low as possible.**

Statins are very **safe** for children, and side effects are **rare**. In contrast, ezetimibe and PCSK9 inhibitors have not been extensively studied in children and are usually introduced in the **young adult** years. Another important aspect of managing children with significant hypercholesterolaemia is to begin **early conversations about healthy lifestyle habits** such as not smoking, maintaining a balanced diet, and staying active.

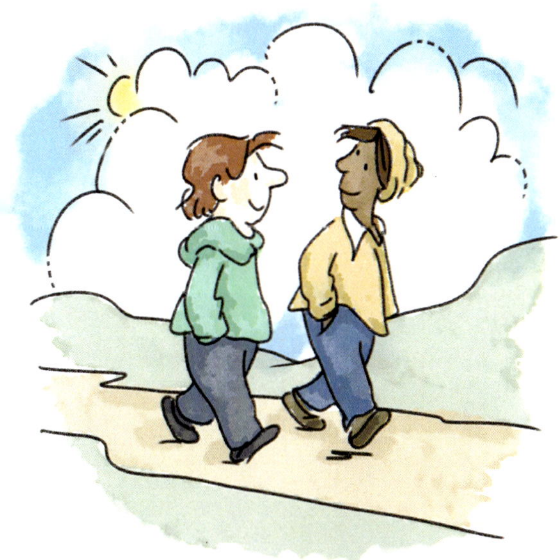

Screening is also vital. If a parent has a history of early CVD, it is common practice to screen their children for hypercholesterolaemia and elevated Lp(a), even if they appear otherwise healthy.

case study ANGELA

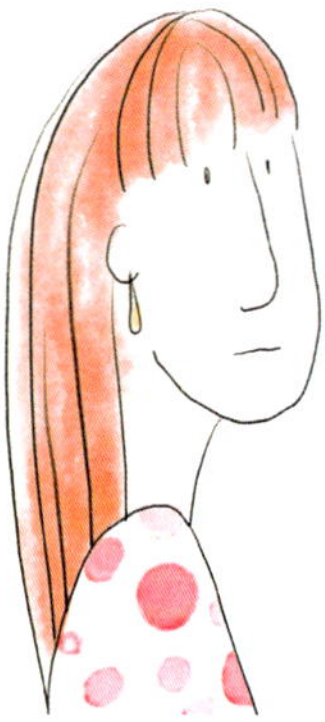

Angela was a 22-year-old woman who was referred to me, Dr K., for a second opinion through her GP as her mother was concerned about her cardiovascular risk.

Unfortunately, her dad had died from a massive heart attack at age 36 when Angela's mum was pregnant with Angela.

Angela's grandad had also died from a heart attack, aged 41.

Angela was a healthy young woman who did not smoke, consumed a healthy diet, had normal blood pressure, and exercised regularly without problems. Her only risk factor was moderately elevated LDL-C at 3.9 mmol/L.

She had seen another specialist who had ordered a genetic test for familial hypercholesterolaemia. However, this did not show any of the common gene variants responsible for FH. That plan was to continue with a healthy lifestyle and assess her arteries with a CT scan in her mid 30s.

When I saw her, a routine physical exam and electrocardiogram (ECG)[1] showed no clinical signs of FH. However, I sent Angela for more blood tests including lipoprotein(a) because this is often elevated in patients with a family history of premature heart disease.

Angela's Lp(a) came back at 390 nmol/L, which is very high (normal is < 75 nmol/L) and explains her family's increased cardiovascular risk.

I started her on atorvastatin and ezetimibe to reduce her LDL-C to very low levels.

I was also able to tell her that I am trialling several therapies for elevated Lp(a) and that they should be available in a couple of years.

---

1 *An electrocardiogram is a test that records the electrical activity of the heart over time. It's used to diagnose heart conditions like arrhythmias, heart attacks, and other cardiovascular issues.*

public health perspective

DR KOSTNER

Despite its prevalence and effective treatments, FH remains ***severely underdiagnosed and undertreated****. The World Health Organization identified it as a global health priority in 1998, and a Global Call to Action followed in 2020. Yet more than* ***90 per cent of cases remain undetected*** *worldwide. In Australia, a Medicare rebate has covered genetic testing since 2020 – $1300 for the first diagnosed person in a family (the proband or the index case) and $200 for cascade testing of relatives. Shockingly, genetic testing has been used just over 300 times, despite more than 100,000 Australians being affected. Addressing this gap demands* ***better screening****,* ***stronger implementation****, and* ***greater clinical vigilance****, beginning with a thorough family history.*

A CLOSER LOOK

the lower, the sooner, the better

A compelling concept for anyone – and particularly those with FH – is the idea of **lifelong exposure** to LDL-C associated with a **theoretical threshold** for the development of CAD. The concept suggests thresholds of **15 years** for HoFH patients, **40 years** for HeFH patients, and **65 years** for people with less severe cholesterol elevation. A valuable aspect of this concept is that it helps visualise the impact of therapy: the **earlier** LDL-C is reduced, the **greater** the lifelong benefit. As we've observed, the principle 'the lower, the better' holds true, with the added emphasis, 'the sooner, the better.'

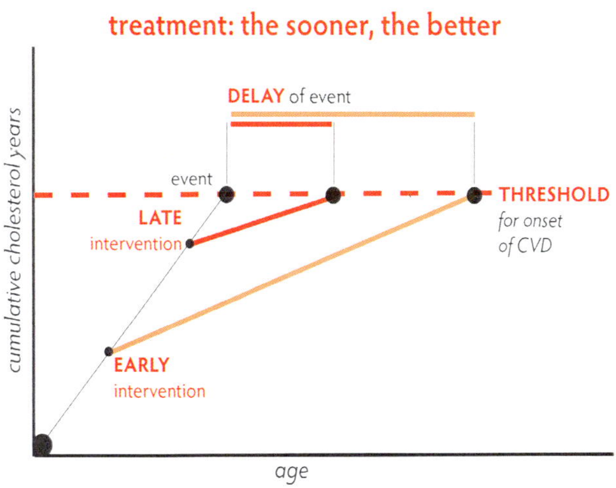

lipoprotein(a) and FH

As part of this discussion, it is also important to consider another distinct and often overlooked contributor to cardiovascular risk: lipoprotein(a) [Lp(a)]. As we have already seen, elevated Lp(a) levels can significantly increase CVD risk.

We know that Lp(a) is a genetically determined lipoprotein that behaves like LDL but includes an additional protein, apo(a), making it **more atherogenic** and **more likely** to contribute to **clotting** and **inflammation**. It's a known, independent risk factor for CVD. Diet, exercise, and traditional cholesterol-lowering therapies do not significantly influence its levels. Nor does its level change much during a person's life, except for several specific health events, of which pregnancy, menopause, and chronic kidney disease are the most significant. In patients with FH, elevated Lp(a) can **compound** an already high lifetime risk, even if LDL-C is well managed. Importantly, many FH patients have significantly elevated Lp(a) levels.

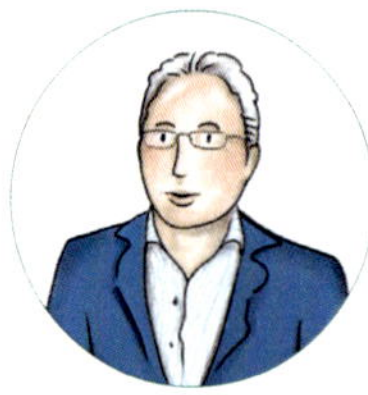

We consider Lp(a) levels to be elevated if they are above 50 mg per decilitre or above 125 nanomoles per litre. Lp(a) can be measured in either milligrams per decilitre or nanomoles per litre, depending on the laboratory that undertakes the testing. So, it's important to check which unit of measurement is used.

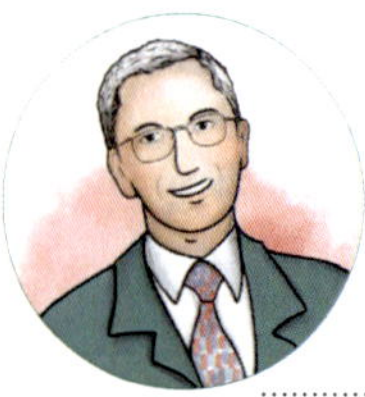

lowering Lp(a)

No widely available medications specifically lower Lp(a) to target (2026).

Niacin lowers Lp(a) by up to 30 per cent.

PCSK9 inhibitors, a therapy we have already discussed for elevated LDL-C, can also lower Lp(a) by up to 25 per cent. However, while they are not indicated solely for lowering Lp(a), high-risk patients with high LDL-C who qualify for PCSK9 inhibitors and also have high Lp(a) levels will benefit dually from this therapy.

Lipoprotein apheresis, a dialysis-like procedure, is the only Lp(a) treatment available. It can be performed weekly or biweekly on patients who have very high Lp(a) levels and who have not responded adequately to medication and lifestyle changes, and who also are at a high risk of CVD. While this treatment can be **effective**, it is **expensive, invasive**, and **not widely used** in many countries due to its **high cost** and **complexity.**

Several **promising therapies** specifically targeting Lp(a) are now in late-stage clinical trials, including injectable antisense and siRNA drugs, and an oral agent called muvalaplin.

(see page 172 for details)

Dr K. is conducting several trials with new therapies for elevated lipids. If the trials show benefits, these agents will be for patients with elevated Lp(a) or TG, and will likely be available in Australia in a couple of years.

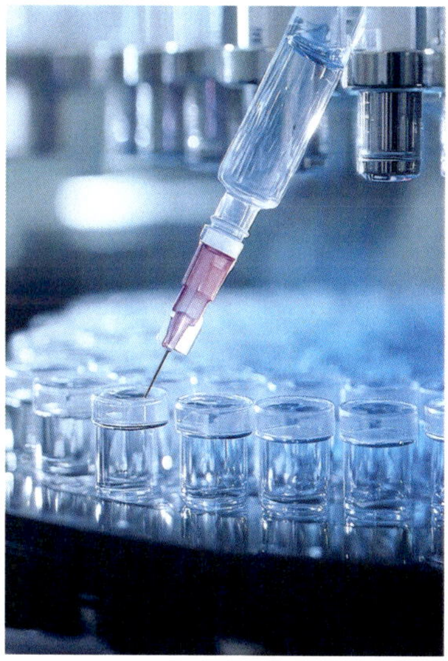

DR KOSTNER:

Individuals with high Lp(a) and LDL-C require aggressive LDL-lowering – ideally to the lowest possible level – because we can't yet directly manage Lp(a). We also need to manage all other modifiable risk factors, such as smoking, blood pressure, and diabetes, carefully. Even though they don't lower Lp(a), statins remain essential because they reduce overall cardiovascular risk.

IMPORTANT POINTS

GENETIC RISKS

- FH is a common lifelong, genetics-driven, high-risk condition that significantly increases the risk of premature CVD.
- Early and aggressive treatment of FH is essential (ideally from childhood) to reduce long-term CVD.
- Statins are safe and effective for treating FH children from the age of eight years. The other, newer cholesterol-lowering drugs have not been studied in children and are introduced in young adult years.
- Lipoprotein(a) adds extra CVD risk for many patients and requires careful management. While it is not responsive to current treatments, new therapies are in late-stage clinical trials.
- Drugs under development to lower Lp(a) are showing great promise and could be available in a couple of years (before the turn of the decade).

Certain other groups also require specialised cholesterol management.

chapter 21

VULNERABLE GROUPS: RISKS BEYOND GENETICS

This chapter continues our focus on vulnerable populations, shifting from the genetic conditions of FH and elevated Lp(a) to large, yet often under-recognised, groups: people concerned by the risk of developing dementia, older adults, women, women who are pregnant, people from different ethnic backgrounds, and those suffering liver failure or kidney disease. Although their risk factors and treatment considerations differ, one message is consistent – **thoughtful, individualised, sooner rather than later** cholesterol management remains **essential** for cholesterol control, CVD risk mitigation and quality of life.

dementia

The relationship between cholesterol-lowering therapy and dementia has sparked both interest and concern. While early reports raised fears about memory loss with the use of statins, extensive recent research has since shown that these medications – and other lipid-lowering strategies – are not only safe but may help prevent dementia, particularly vascular dementia. Rather than causing cognitive decline, they are increasingly recognised as part of a broader strategy to **protect brain health**, especially in those at high cardiovascular risk.

The latest trial (relative to the release of this book) was published online in the *Journal of Neurology, Neurosurgery and Psychiatry* on 1 April 2025. The Low-Density Lipoprotein Cholesterol Levels and Risk of Incident Dementia: a Distributed Network Analysis Using Common Data Models trial[1] demonstrated that aggressively lowering LDL-C was associated with a reduced risk of developing dementia in high-risk individuals.

1 *Low-density lipoprotein cholesterol levels and risk of incident dementia: a distributed network analysis using common data models. Lee M, Lee KJ, Kim J, et al. Journal of Neurology, Neurosurgery & Psychiatry published online first: 1 April 2025. doi: 10.1136/jnnp-2024-334708*

The study found that having **an *LDL-C level below 70 mg/dL* (1.8 mmol/L) was linked to a *26 per cent lower risk of all-cause dementia* and a *28 per cent lower risk of Alzheimer's disease-related dementia* (ADRD), with statin use offering additional benefit.**

While earlier studies hinted at a protective effect from lower LDL-C, these findings highlight a specific target that could guide clinical practice.

"These findings emphasize the importance of targeted LDL-C management as part of dementia prevention strategies, with potential integration into clinical guidelines," lead investigator Yerim Kim, MD, PhD, Department of Neurology, Kangdong Sacred Heart Hospital, Hallym University College of Medicine, Seoul, South Korea, and colleagues wrote[2]. "The results support the use of statin therapy within specific LDL-C ranges for both cardiovascular and cognitive health benefits."

The article, *Lower LDL of 'critical importance' in reducing dementia risk,*[3] reports that

> Balancing LDL-C for cardiovascular benefits while being cognizant of potential neurocognitive impacts is "something we deal with constantly in clinical practice", Shaheen Lakhan, MD, PhD, a neurologist and researcher based in Miami, Florida, said.
>
> "Until now, it's been hard to say what level is 'safe' or even beneficial for the brain," said Lakhan, who was not part of the new research.
>
> "The study's identification of <70 mg/dL as a target that significantly reduces risk of both all-cause and Alzheimer's-related dementia is incredibly helpful. It gives us a concrete, evidence-based benchmark we can share with patients – especially those at high vascular and cognitive risk."
>
> For Lakhan, the evidence that statins have neuroprotective effects and that those benefits extend beyond lowering cholesterol are the most important findings for clinical care.

---

2 *quoted in a Medscape Medical News article by Jeff Craven published on 2 April 2025*

3 *ibid*

"It gives clinicians a strong rationale to continue statins in older adults and those at risk for dementia, not just for their hearts, but for their brains as well." Lakhan said the study's "size, consistency, and methodologic rigor make this a valuable contribution that should absolutely inform clinical decision-making and future guidelines".

In earlier trials ...

A trial, the Pravastatin in Elderly Individuals at Risk of Vascular Disease (PROSPER)[4], a randomised, controlled trial, used pravastatin (one of the older cholesterol agents) at 40 mg with nearly 6000 patients, with nine-monthly cognitive testing over about three and a half years. Because it was an elderly group, as expected, the cognitive function across the group declined. However, there was no difference between the treatment and non-treatment groups, confirming that statins do not cause measurable cognitive decline in the elderly.

Another study, The Heart Protection Study[5], using simvastatin at 40 mg, followed a large number of patients for between three and five years for follow-up and found no significant difference in cognitive outcome between treatment and non-treatment groups.

The Justification for the Use of Statin in Prevention: an Intervention Trial Evaluating Rosuvastatin (JUPITER)[6] rationale and prespecified analysis, although not explicitly set up for testing brain function, did include cognitive testing. JUPITER, which involved nearly 20,000 people (more men than women), found no change in cognitive decline. However, persistent concerns about statin-related confusion led the US Food and Drug Administration (FDA) to list "potential impact on thought processes" as a possible side effect of rosuvastatin. This warning was based on anecdotal reports, and subsequent trials have not confirmed consistent cognitive effect.

---

4 *Shepherd J, Blauw GJ, Murphy MB, et al. Pravastatin in elderly individuals at risk of vascular disease (PROSPER): a randomised controlled trial. Lancet. 2002;360(9346):1623–1630. DOI: 10.1016/S0140-6736(02)11600-X*

5 *Heart Protection Study Collaborative Group. MRC/BHF Heart Protection Study of cholesterol-lowering with simvastatin in 20,536 high-risk individuals: a randomised placebo-controlled trial. Lancet. 2002;360(9326):7–22. DOI: 10.1016/S0140-6736(02)09327-3*

6 *Ridker PM, Danielson E, Fonseca FAH, et al. Rosuvastatin to prevent vascular events in men and women with elevated C-reactive protein. N Engl J Med. 2008;359(21):2195–2207. DOI: 10.1056/NEJMoa0807646*

Another 12 small trials have specifically looked at the question of cognitive function for people on cholesterol-lowering statin therapy:

- nine trials showed no difference
- one suggested a decline in function, and
- two suggested a benefit.

no clear evidence

While there is no certainty that taking a statin to lower cholesterol can cause cognitive problems, there is more scientifically-supported evidence to say that it does not. However, certain individuals can respond differently to the 'crowd'. For example, some people say their thinking is clouded if they drink coffee, others if they have too much sugary food. Some people report mental clouding on taking medication – including cholesterol agents. Medication side effects and concerns should be addressed on an **individual** patient basis.

another option

DR BISHOP:

Should a patient raise a concern, the option exists to try cholesterol tablets that are less likely to be absorbed into the brain's fatty tissue. As we have already seen, some cholesterol tablets are ***lipophilic*** *(absorbed into fat), and some are* ***lipophobic*** *(not absorbed into fat). As atorvastatin is lipophilic, it is potentially more likely to impact the brain. Rosuvastatin, being lipophobic and remaining in the aqueous bloodstream, is, theoretically, less likely to affect brain tissue and could be preferred. It's crucial to discuss any concerns about, or experienced changes in, cognitive function with your cardiologist.*

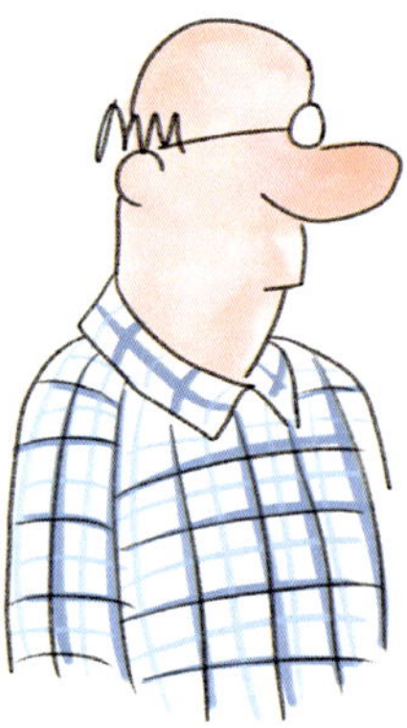

the elderly

Older age is another critical factor that shapes risk.

Those who are living well and enjoying a good quality of life should be considered for proactive treatment. As cardiovascular risk rises with age, the potential benefit from cholesterol-lowering therapy should support continued health and independence. At the same time, treatment considerations such as overall health, life expectancy, and personal preferences are especially important for the more frail, older patients whose quality of life has already significantly declined.

These are important patient-doctor conversations.

women

Women's cardiovascular risk is often **underestimated** because their symptoms can differ from the typical chest pain seen in men. They may not present with classic angina, making diagnosis more challenging. Before menopause, higher oestrogen levels offer some cardiac risk protection. However, **after menopause**, oestrogen levels drop and the protective effect fades. Further, cholesterol levels generally **rise** – significantly increasing cardiovascular risk. For many women, **hormone replacement therapy** (HRT) can help offset this risk, but **timing** is crucial. HRT seems most beneficial when initiated within 10 years of the onset of menopause or before age 60. Later initiation offers less benefit and may even carry some risk. Other female-specific conditions that increase CVD risk include early menopause, gestational hypertension (high blood pressure after 20 weeks of pregnancy), preeclampsia (high blood pressure and organ damage after 20 weeks), and polycystic ovary syndrome.

pregnancy

Most cholesterol-lowering medications have not been tested in clinical trials involving pregnancy and are not considered safe for use during pregnancy or breastfeeding. **Statins** and **PCSK9 inhibitors**, in particular, should be **stopped** as soon as pregnancy is confirmed. While these medications don't affect fertility, they must be paused during pregnancy and only restarted after breastfeeding has been completed. This can mean up to 30 months off therapy for high-risk women – and must be considered in the decision-making.

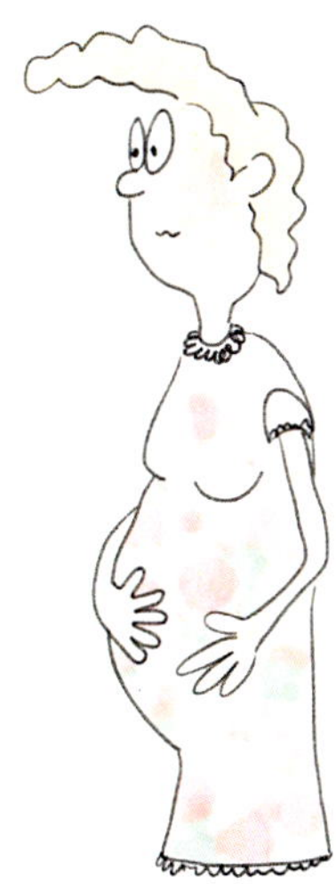

Cholesterol, TG, and Lp(a) levels naturally rise during pregnancy. This is a normal physiological response. However, in a woman with **genetic dyslipidaemia** such as FH, it is important to begin treatment early. That way, when medications need to be paused during one or more pregnancies, the woman has already benefited from cholesterol-lowering therapy and has protection in place.

ethnicity

Different ethnic groups show **genetic differences** that influence cholesterol metabolism – affecting both absorption and synthesis – and these can impact cardiovascular risk. As a result, levels of HDL-C, TG, Lp(a), and comorbidities such as hypertension often vary significantly between populations.

These genetic variations also influence responses to lipid-lowering therapy. For example, individuals of East Asian descent typically have higher blood concentrations of statins at standard doses. They achieve similar LDL-C reductions but may have a greater risk of adverse effects, particularly statin-induced myopathy.

In such cases, it is not only appropriate – but often essential – to start with lower statin doses and combine them with other lipid-lowering agents where needed, rather than relying on higher statin doses alone.

This approach helps **minimise intolerance** and adverse reactions while **supporting target achievement**. It also explains why lower statin doses are commonly used in many Asian countries compared with Western nations.

liver failure

Fatty liver disease – both non-alcoholic and alcoholic – is commonly seen in people with high cholesterol because both conditions often stem from the same underlying issues: insulin resistance, obesity, and poor dietary habits. The liver plays a central role in processing fats and cholesterol, and when there's an excess of these circulating in the blood, the liver begins to store the surplus as fat.

Over time, this can lead to fatty liver disease in which fat accumulates in the liver cells. It's particularly associated with high LDL-C, elevated TG, low HDL-C, and metabolic syndrome.

The same factors that drive high cholesterol also contribute to fat build-up in the liver and are often worsened by lipid disorders and high cholesterol. Fortunately, the cholesterol-lowering strategies discussed in this book can also help improve liver function and reduce fat accumulation in the liver.

Liver function tests may sometimes show **mildly elevated** results in people taking statins. This can cause **unnecessary concern**. We know that the liver is one of the main organs responsible for producing cholesterol, and statins work by blocking an enzyme involved in that process. As a result, the liver may become more active in response, leading to small changes in liver enzymes seen on blood tests.

These changes do not mean the liver is damaged. In fact, serious liver problems from statins are **extremely rare**, and we almost never need to stop statin therapy because of abnormal liver function tests. In most cases, all that is needed is continued monitoring, perhaps with dose adjustment, along with reassurance.

kidney disease

People with impaired renal function – including those on dialysis – are at significantly increased risk of CVD. These patients benefit from lipid-lowering therapy as part of a broader cardiovascular risk reduction strategy.

Renal guidelines, such as the KHA-CARI guidelines[7], recommend the use of statins and other lipid-lowering therapies discussed in this book for patients with chronic kidney disease.

---

7 *The KHA-CARI Guidelines (Kidney Health Australia–Caring for Australasians with Renal Impairment) provide evidence-based recommendations to improve the quality of care and outcomes for patients with kidney disease in Australia and New Zealand. They cover various aspects of kidney disease management, including chronic kidney disease, dialysis, transplantation, and related conditions. These guidelines are developed to assist healthcare professionals in delivering consistent and effective care to individuals with kidney impairment. [www.cariguidelines.org]*

IMPORTANT POINTS

VULNERABLE GROUPS

- Rather than causing cognitive decline, cholesterol-lowering therapies are being increasingly recognised as part of a broader strategy to protect brain health – especially in people at high cardiovascular risk.
- Cholesterol levels in women often rise after menopause, increasing cardiovascular risk.
- Most lipid-lowering medications are **not safe** during pregnancy and breastfeeding.
- HDL-C, TG, and Lp(a) levels can vary significantly between ethnic populations.
- Fatty liver often coexists with high cholesterol. Cholesterol treatment improves liver health and lowers cardiovascular risk.
- People with chronic kidney disease, including those on dialysis, have high CVD risk and benefit from lipid-lowering therapy.
- In all these groups, the message is clear: the benefits of lowering cholesterol are real, and timing matters – for heart health, brain health, and long-term well-being.

Cholesterol management needs to be personalised, considering individual risk factors, genetics, and treatment responses for optimal outcomes.

chapter 22

SHARED CARE: WORKING TOGETHER FOR THE BEST OUTCOME

Each patient is different. Often, we cannot 'buy a suit off the rack' because it might not fit. Dr Bishop recounts two striking examples of this.

Sue

I met Sue in 2018. She was a 60-year-old woman who was focused on investing in her health. She exercised regularly, went to the gym, did weights, cycled, and walked.

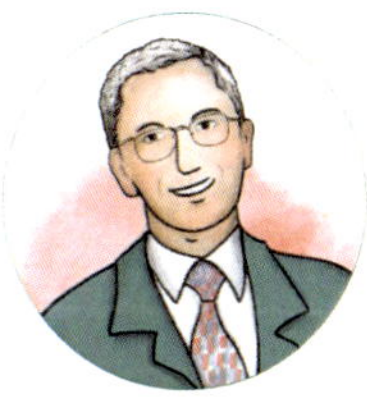

Remember, whatever 'good work' or effort you do today is not for your health now; it's an outlay for your future health. What you do today will count in five or 10 years, especially if your health unravels. You can't rewind time. Please don't ever say, I wish I'd done something sooner.

Sue's husband had come to see me previously and had a heart scan. She wanted to do the same thing, which was appropriate as there was a family history of heart problems and Sue had raised cholesterol. Her total cholesterol was 6.8 (ideally less than 5.0 mmol/L), and her LDL-C was 3.9 (ideally less than 2.5). So, I took the opportunity to undertake a '60,000 km check' for Sue.

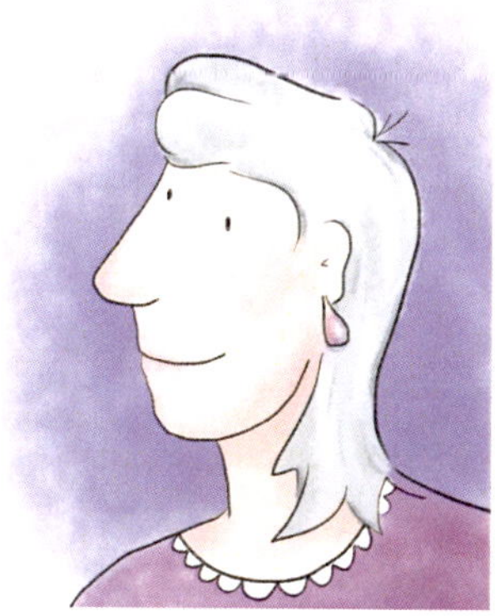

An ultrasound of her heart showed the chambers were functionally and structurally normal. There were no valve problems. The heart, however, was a little stiff. This was in keeping with her elevated blood pressure.

Since then, Sue has been on dual blood pressure therapy to manage the BP, achieving beautiful control. Dual therapy allows use of a low or intermediate dose of two agents harmoniously, rather than driving hard with a single agent. Combining drugs maximises their efficacy and minimises side effects.

Controlling blood pressure is all about reducing the risk – of heart attack, stroke, renal failure, atrial fibrillation, cardiac failure, and dementia. It is a super important component of long-term health management, is straightforward to treat, and excellent medications are available.

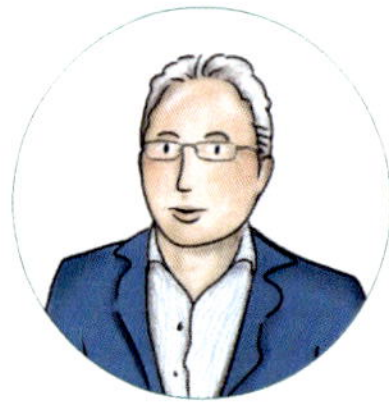

cardiac CT image

We then investigated further with cardiac CT imaging. At 60 years of age, with some family history, elevated cholesterol and a history of elevated blood pressure, Sue was a perfect candidate for this.

Her coronary artery calcium (CAC) score was in the order of 30. While this was not exceptionally high, when we looked at that score compared with other women her age, she sat somewhere between the 75th and 80th percentile. This reading means that if we took 100 women the same age as Sue off the street and arranged them from position one (lowest score) to position 100 (highest score), Sue would be between position 75 and 80 (75-100 is the highest quartile).

This placement told me that she had a significantly **greater propensity** to develop plaque in her arteries than most other women her age. She was in the highest quartile, meaning a three, four, or even five times increased **lifetime** risk of cardiovascular events. This finding ties in with her cholesterol level and family history. Her originally high blood pressure did not help.

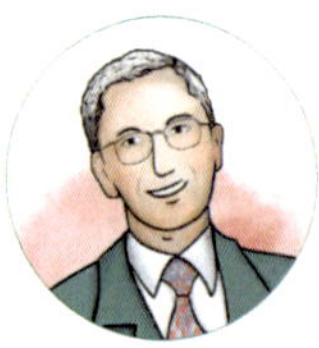

I believe that a CAC scan should be a rite of passage for all men 45 to 50 and all women 55 to 60, even sooner if there is a family history or raised cholesterol.

engaged and eager

Sue was motivated, engaged, and eager to find the best solution for her health journey.

The use of a statin was the first line of therapy to lower her cholesterol levels. I prescribed 20 mg of atorvastatin. I expected a 40 to 50 per cent reduction in LDL-C, which would bring her levels very close to our target of 2 mmol/L, which was in keeping with the current Australian primary prevention recommendations.

Unfortunately, Sue had trouble with the statin as it caused pain in her leg muscles. Because she felt so fit and well, she stopped taking it. So, when I saw her a year or so later for a review, she was off the statin, and her cholesterol levels were back to where they had been previously. This situation was not ideal. We had controlled the blood pressure, and Sue continued her exercise, which was great. However, the cholesterol was too high, especially as her body had a greater tendency than the average woman of her age to develop plaque in her arteries.

So, we revisited that cholesterol-lowering regime. Instead of reintroducing atorvastatin (the most used statin), I recommended the newer rosuvastatin. It is prescribed extensively and used safely, and it has a slightly different chemical structure from atorvastatin. Rosuvastatin is lipophobic (repelled by fat and less likely to enter muscle), while atorvastatin is lipophilic (attracted to fat and therefore more likely to cause muscle-related side effects). Sue tried rosuvastatin at a small dose of five milligrams (when the maximum dose is 40 mg), but she came back reporting symptoms.

It became apparent while speaking with Sue, that the medication took several days to accumulate in her bloodstream before causing side effects. When we talked about her previous atorvastatin experience, the same pattern emerged. So, as an experiment, we retried the atorvastatin – and there it was again. The drug took several days to cause problems.

So, what could we do?

I suggested to Sue that she could try low doses on alternative days.

Success! She tolerated this without problems and they did the job for her. However, when I saw Sue again in April 2024, her LDL-C had crept up to a fraction over 2 mmol/L. I suggested adding 10 mg of a completely different agent, ezetimibe, daily. These drugs, working synergistically, will easily and without side effects, bring LDL-C down to under two millimoles/litre.

Why is this target important?

At under two millimoles/litre, there's an excellent chance we will slow down and possibly even arrest further plaque formation.

For a woman in her 60s with a 'bad heart' family history, raised cholesterol, and high blood pressure now treated, there's every chance that we have mitigated her future risk of a heart attack. And that is important. *The goal!*

Many people forget – or don't know – that women are affected by heart attacks as much as men. Men have heart attacks earlier in life, from about 50 years of age, when they reach that intermediate to high-risk category. Women often follow a decade later.

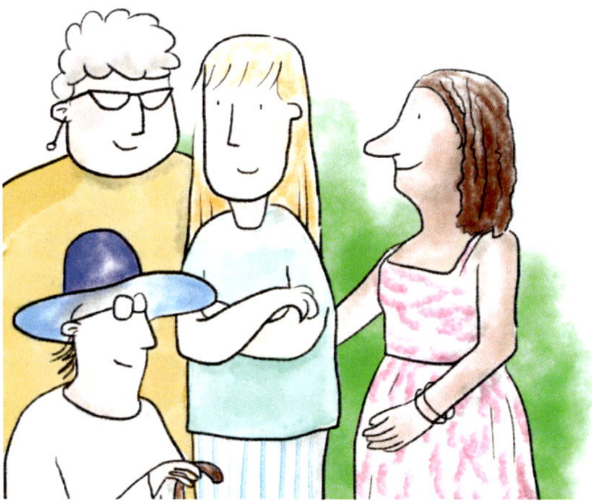

Heart attack is the leading cause of death among the female population in the Western world.

All forms of cancer added together have a similar mortality rate, but **no single disease impacts as many women as CAD**. While the community gives more attention to breast cancer recognition, skin cancer awareness, pap smears and other female issues, none is as prevalent as CAD.

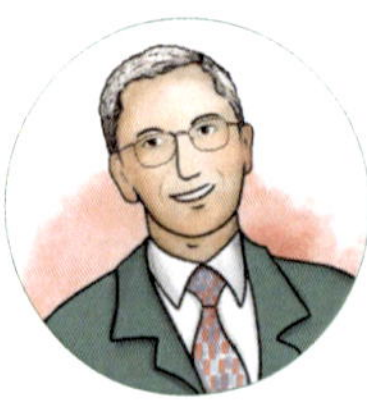

Women, PLEASE have your heart checked!

Phil

I met Phil in April 2024. Phil – a nurse in his late 30s – approached me at an event after a presentation I gave on cholesterol, diets, and heart disease. Phil had a terrible family heart history and raised cholesterol. About five years earlier, he had been seriously overweight – we are not talking five or 10 kilos overweight but more like 50 to 60 kg overweight. Then, he was also prediabetic. Having done his own research, he concluded that he had to drop that weight. *(No question!)* So, he tried a ketogenic diet.

A ketogenic diet cuts out carbohydrates altogether. When you eat carbohydrates, your body preferentially burns sugar, not fat. However, if you do not eat carbohydrates, your body burns ketones as no sugar is available. In a ketogenic state, your body burns fat from its reserves. Phil had dropped 50 or so kilos and returned to a healthy weight.

The consequences were twofold:

- he had become attached to the ketogenic diet because he felt so well, but
- it had raised his high cholesterol levels even higher.

A ketogenic diet, by virtue of the foods being eaten, is enriched with saturated fatty acids, essentially fat found in animal fats such as meats, cheese, butter, and cream. These saturated fats alter the body's production of cholesterol and can drive up cholesterol levels.

Now comes the interesting part.

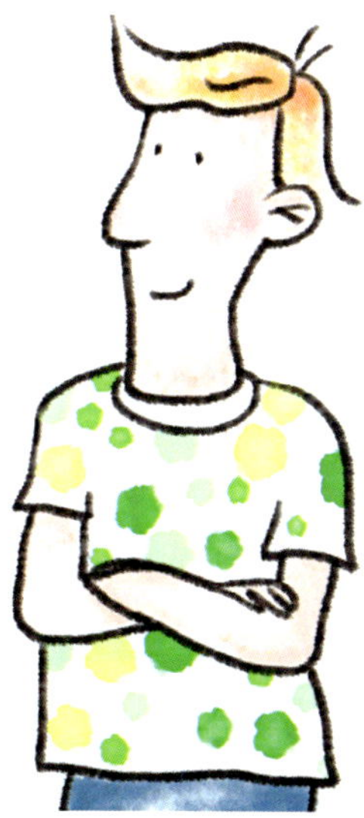

Phil, aware of his family history and rising cholesterol levels, visited his doctor to organise a CAC scan. His CAC score was about 30. To put the absolute numbers into context, zero is a low-risk feature, 100 is an intermediate-risk feature, 300 is a high-risk feature, and 1000 is a very high-risk feature.

red flag

A score in the 30s should not raise immediate alarm bells until it is put through the filter of comparing it to other men his age. Then, the score was over the 90th percentile, meaning that, for his age, there would be a lot of plaque in his arteries compared with his age-matched cohort. This was a red flag for me and drove me to engage with him further, talking about **lifetime risk**, not just the next few years.

Phil's general practitioner had already referred Phil to a cardiologist, who wanted him to immediately stop his keto diet and go on statins. There was a problem. Phil wanted to stay on the keto diet. They were poles apart!

When we met, Phil had visited several cardiologists and was waiting to see another. During this time, he had tried multiple statin therapies at different doses, all with side effects. I don't think he had been on ezetimibe, and I'm not sure that intermittent dosing of the statin had been tried. Regardless, his cholesterol levels were too high – yet Phil was particularly attached to remaining on his ketogenic diet, so we had to find a personalised solution. Could we make it work?

I suggested the possibility of undertaking a CT coronary angiogram of his arteries. While this is not considered a guideline, nor is it generally suggested as a strategy, the scan would provide us with extra information, specifically, the quality of plaque in his arteries. Was it calcified plaque, or did his arteries contain the more concerning non-calcified (or cholesterol-dominant) plaque? Cholesterol-dominant (cholesterol-rich) plaque presents a far greater risk than calcified plaque because that is where inflammation is found and where plaque rupture can occur more easily.

When we look at elevated cholesterol in people's arteries, there are often two situations: people with high cholesterol and clogged arteries or people with high cholesterol and, amazingly, clear arteries. The latter was not Phil's situation.

exactly what was there

The CT coronary angiography would show precisely what type of plaque was in his arteries and its position. If it were to show high-risk plaque, then he would need to review the ketogenic diet and revisit LDL-C lowering therapy. The good thing is he has options such as using ezetimibe, intermittent statin dosing, and possibly the PCSK9 inhibitors – depending on how high that cholesterol is. (Depending on stringent criteria, PCSK9 inhibitors can be subsidised under Australia's Pharmaceutical Benefits Scheme.) The CT coronary angiogram could show that he has dominant calcified plaque, which is more stable, and a feature we might see in people who exercise regularly. The future could include close monitoring to ensure his TG remain down, his HDL-C was maximised (this often happens with ketogenic diets), and a repeat surveillance CT scan to ensure that the atheroma burden in the artery wasn't changing.

I also told Phil that in his situation, in which he wanted to consider holding off on lipid-lowering therapy, I would also check his carotid arteries to ensure any unbeknown plaque was not developing in the neck. There is no point in avoiding a heart attack only to have a stroke!

Phil's story shows us that situations can be complicated, as patients have different responses to therapies and diverse objectives and goals. The ketogenic diet is fantastic for helping people lower weight and avert diabetes. Many people feel very well when on it, like Phil. However, because of the saturated fats, the diet will increase LDL-C levels and recent studies confirm an increase in cardiovascular events.

Although I did not see Phil formally as a patient, the conversation I had with him reflects the importance of the doctor and patient working together to find the very best solution based on cholesterol levels, plaque burden, the type of plaque, the patient's well-being and ability to take medications, together with philosophical beliefs. This is not something that can be solved in a six-minute consultation. This is building a trusted working relationship between doctor and patient to navigate to the best patient outcome.

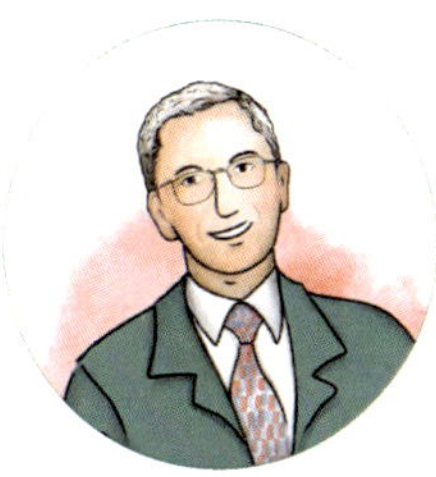

In a previous chapter, we heard about the 2025-published study by the Budoff group that showed plaque can beget plaque. In Phil's case, with a CAC score of 30 that places him in the 90th percentile for his age and sex, the research tells us that a keto diet would accelerate the progression of plaque in his arteries.

IMPORTANT POINTS

SHARED CARE

- As one size does not fit all, it is valuable for doctors and patients to discuss, and experiment with, different treatment options. In medical circles we call working together 'shared decision-making', which is embodied in a quote from the Vienna Declaration on Health (1998), *nothing about me without me*[1]. Ensure you are at the helm of your health journey.

---

1 *The phrase 'nothing about me without me' emphasises the importance of involving individuals in decisions that directly affect their lives. Originating in the disability rights movement, it has since become a guiding principle in healthcare and other fields. It advocates for person-centred approaches in which individuals are front and centre in shaping decisions about their well-being, care, and support. Its significance was reaffirmed in the 1998 Vienna Declaration on Health Promotion, which helped cement this approach in global health policy and reinforced the shift toward shared decision-making and patient empowerment.*

World Health Organization (WHO) Regional Office for Europe. 4th European Conference on Health Promotion: The Vienna Declaration on Health Promotion – Making a Difference. Vienna, 1998. Available at: https://www.euro.who.int/__data/assets/pdf_file/0006/88575/E59546.pdf

We now venture into the maze where the straightforward blends with the baffling and where perpetual mysteries challenge experts and patients alike!

CHOLESTEROL IS NOT THE ENEMY

controversies
myths
mysteries

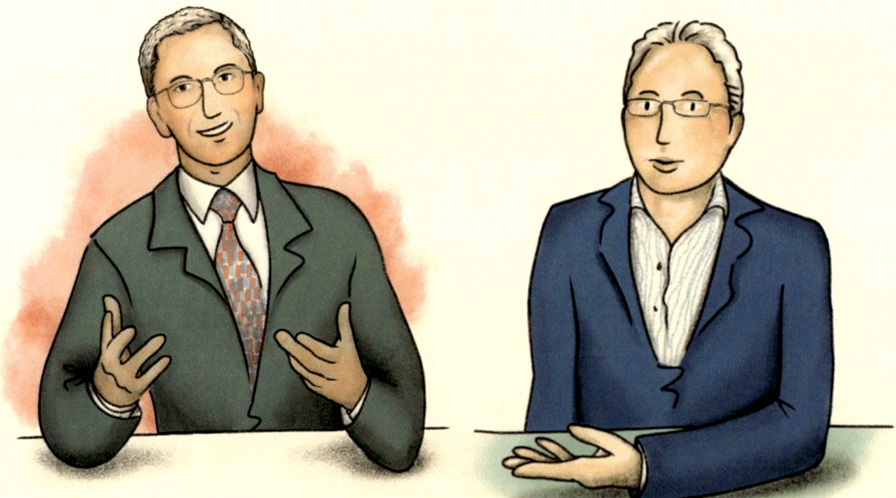

chapter 23

CHOLESTEROL CONTROVERSIES: CLOSING THE DEBATE

By now, you'll have a clear understanding of cholesterol's role in health and heart disease. These final chapters won't alter that foundation, but they will complete the picture by looking at the disputes that have fuelled so much confusion.

Some of these are genuine controversies, where evidence is interpreted differently and research continues to refine our understanding. Others are myths – outdated beliefs that persist despite strong contrary evidence. This chapter focuses on the controversies: the debates in science and medicine that have shaped both confusion and progress.

overview

For decades, cholesterol has been at the centre of clashes between scientists, clinicians, the food industry, pharmaceutical companies, the media, and, more recently, online voices. The result is a swirl of information and misinformation that has shaped public opinion and medical practice.

At the heart of the clashes lie many questions such as:

- Are statins over-prescribed, particularly for people at lower risk?
- Is saturated fat really the main culprit, or should sugar and refined carbs take more of the blame?
- Do cholesterol levels cause heart disease directly, or are they one factor among many?

Conflicting trial interpretations, concerns over side effects, selective reporting, and the influence of social media have all contributed to deepening the divide. For some, the debates have fostered fear or scepticism about proven therapies; for others, they have opened new lines of inquiry into genetics, inflammation, and personalised care.

Our aim here is not to reignite arguments but to set them in context and highlight what the best evidence in 2026 shows.

As we enter the realm of controversies, myths, and mysteries, it is essential to be clear about several distinctions we have already made.

prevention

The first distinction is between primary and secondary prevention. Preventing a first event is **primary** prevention; preventing another event after one has already occurred is **secondary** prevention. Once someone has had a heart attack, stroke, bypass, stent, or imaging has detected high-risk plaque, the evidence is overwhelming: **lowering cholesterol (usually with statins) reduces future risk. No debate**. Most confusion arises in primary prevention – people without established disease but with risk factors. This is where online debates and soundbites thrive.

association or causation

An **association increases risk**, but does not directly cause an event. **Causation is a direct link**. Distinguishing between the two is critical when interpreting cholesterol studies.

individual or population

Risk differs for individuals and populations. A risk calculator might show you have a five per cent chance of an event in 10 years. For a **group** of 100 people like you, five will have an event; 95 will not. For the **individual**, the outcome is either zero or 100 per cent. This **gap** between population risk and personal experience often **drives misunderstanding.**

polarisation

Conversations about cholesterol often reduce to 'absolute' versus 'contributory' or 'single factor' versus 'multifactorial'. **Cardiovascular disease is multi-factorial.** Yet the cholesterol debate has become polarised into 'good or bad', 'right or wrong', ignoring the more useful measures of 'relative risk' and 'benefit'. When distracted by absolutes, we lose sight of subtlety, variation, and personal uniqueness.

Our
understanding
is based on

associations focused on the individual.

Our conversations are
not about 'good' or 'bad'
'right' or 'wrong' but

contributory and multi-factorial.

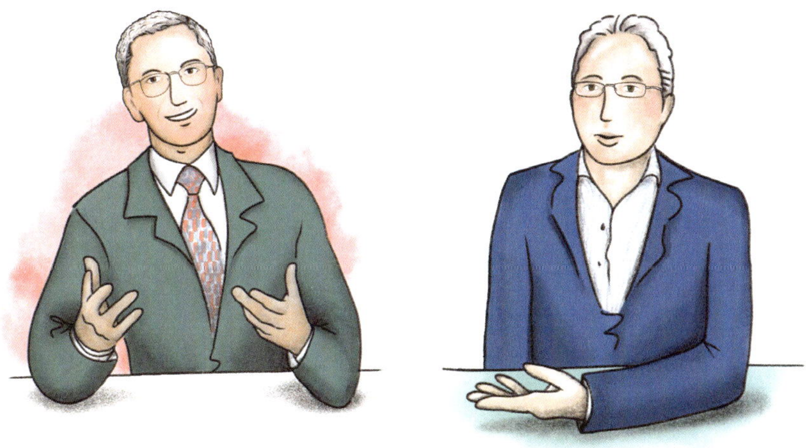

THE controversies

So, to the controversies. These revolve around the extent to which cholesterol itself is a problem, and, if it is, what the best treatments are, from the role of medications to side effects, vested interests, and changing guidelines.

We know plaque formation in the arteries is complicated, with many factors at play, and, in 2026, there's still more to uncover. Against that backdrop, one of the biggest points of contention remains statins.

statins

Few medications have generated as much debate. **Supporters** argue that statins are highly effective in lowering cholesterol and reducing cardiovascular events, pointing to decades of trials confirming their benefits. **Critics**, however, question the balance of risks and benefits. While most people tolerate statins well, some experience muscle pain, weakness, or fatigue, and, in rare cases, rises in blood sugar or liver concerns. These reports, especially when drawn from real-world experience, have fuelled doubt about whether the risks are under-recognised.

This raises a key question: Are statins **overprescribed**? For people at high risk – those with prior heart attack, stroke, bypass surgery, or significant plaque – the benefits are clear and proven. The debate lies in primary prevention, where individuals may have only a moderate risk. Some argue prescribing here is unnecessary; others point to strong evidence that even modest LDL reductions lower future risk. At the centre of the controversy is the question of how much prevention is enough, and for whom.

A further sticking point is the **frequency of side effects**. Clinical trials suggest they are uncommon, yet patient reports often differ. Critics argue that adverse effects are minimised, while defenders note that many symptoms may be explained by the 'nocebo effect' – patients expect them and so experience them. Sorting perception from reality remains one of the most persistent debates.

Another important issue is **adherence**. Even when statins are prescribed, many people stop taking them – sometimes because of side effects, sometimes through fear of harm, or simply from misinformation. Non-adherence is common and can significantly undermine the benefits demonstrated in clinical trials. For doctors, this creates the challenge of supporting patients in continuing their treatment when needed, while also listening carefully to their individual concerns.

Vested interests also play a role in the debate. Statins are among the most prescribed – and most profitable – medicines in the world. This has led to suspicion that pharmaceutical companies have influenced research, marketing, and even clinical guidelines. Critics argue that commercial interests may have promoted wider prescribing than necessary. On the other hand, it is important to note that many independent studies, funded by governments and not-for-profit bodies, also confirm the benefits of statins.

Finally, **guidelines** themselves have evolved. Over the years, thresholds for starting statins have shifted, sometimes broadening the number of people eligible. For some, this represents appropriate recognition of cardiovascular risk across populations; for others, it feeds the perception of 'medicalising' healthy individuals. These changing boundaries have become part of the ongoing controversy.

OUR POSITION

Statins remain one of the most effective and well-studied tools for reducing LDL-C and lowering cardiovascular risk. For people at high risk, the benefits are clear and outweigh the potential harms. In primary prevention, decisions should be individualised, balancing absolute risk reduction, side effect profile, and patient preference. Side effects are usually uncommon but should be taken seriously when they occur. Concerns about vested interests and evolving guidelines are valid, but the core evidence supporting statins is strong and consistent. The priority should be careful, personalised prescribing rather than dismissing statins outright or using them unquestioningly.

is cholesterol really a problem?

A recurring controversy is whether cholesterol is truly a culprit in heart disease, or simply a marker of other processes.

Some argue that atherosclerosis is driven more by inflammation, oxidative stress, or metabolic dysfunction, with cholesterol playing only a supporting role. Others claim that high cholesterol is harmless unless combined with other risk factors.

Decades of research, however, consistently show that LDL-C is **causally** linked to atherosclerosis. Genetic studies of FH, clinical trials of statins and newer therapies, and population data all point in the same direction: lowering LDL reduces risk, across different treatments and patient groups. Still, confusion persists, fuelled by sceptical voices online and by the understandable frustration of patients facing mixed messages.

OUR POSITION

Cholesterol is not the only factor in heart disease, but it is a ***key driver****. High LDL-C increases the likelihood of plaque formation, and lowering LDL reduces that risk, regardless of the method used. At the same time, cholesterol interacts with other pathways – genetics, inflammation, lifestyle – which is why CVD is* ***multi-factorial****.*

The most accurate position is that cholesterol is a major contributor, not the sole cause, of heart disease.

the diet–heart hypothesis

The diet–heart hypothesis – the idea that reducing saturated fat lowers cholesterol and thereby reduces heart disease – has shaped nutrition advice for more than half a century. Early ecological and observational studies gave it traction, and it became the basis for public health campaigns throughout the Western world.

Yet, evidence has not always been straightforward. Some trials showed benefits from reducing saturated fat, especially when it was replaced with unsaturated fats like those found in fish, nuts, and olive oil. Others found little effect when saturated fat was replaced with refined carbohydrates, which is a common unintended consequence of 'low-fat' diets. Critics argue that this weakened the credibility of the hypothesis and over-simplified the role of diet in heart health.

Today, the debate continues, complicated by differing study designs, variable food sources, and the influence of the food industry. Public trust has been eroded by changing advice, with some now dismissing the diet–heart hypothesis altogether.

OUR POSITION

The diet–heart hypothesis remains valid but incomplete. Replacing saturated fat with healthy unsaturated fats reduces LDL-C and improves cardiovascular outcomes. Replacing it with refined carbohydrates does not. The strongest evidence supports dietary patterns rich in vegetables, wholegrains, legumes, nuts, fish, and extra virgin olive oil – the Mediterranean Diet being the most consistent example. The issue is not whether diet matters, but which dietary choices matter most.

fat vs sugar

Is saturated fat really the main culprit, or should sugar and refined carbs take more of the blame?

For many decades, dietary advice had centred on saturated fat as the villain in heart disease. Reducing butter, fatty meats, and full-cream dairy was the cornerstone of prevention campaigns from the 1970s onward. This view was supported by early observational studies and reinforced by the diet–heart hypothesis linking saturated fat, cholesterol, and atherosclerosis.

In recent years, however, attention has shifted. Critics argue that saturated fat has been unfairly singled out, while sugar and refined carbohydrates – abundant in modern diets – are more strongly linked with obesity, insulin resistance, type 2 diabetes, and metabolic syndrome, all of which drive cardiovascular risk. Some point to cultural patterns, noting that populations consuming relatively high amounts of natural saturated fats but low levels of processed foods often show lower heart disease rates.

The debate has been inflamed by selective interpretations of trial data and by the food industry, which has at times promoted low-fat but high-sugar products as 'healthy'. This has led to confusion in both public health messaging and individual decision-making.

OUR POSITION

Both saturated fat and refined carbohydrates matter – but in different ways. High intakes of saturated fat can raise LDL-C and should be moderated, particularly in people at elevated risk. At the same time, diets high in sugar and refined carbohydrates clearly worsen metabolic health and promote weight gain, compounding cardiovascular risk.

The best evidence supports dietary patterns such as the Mediterranean Diet, which emphasises vegetables, fruits, whole grains, legumes, nuts, fish, and extra virgin olive oil, while limiting both saturated fats and processed sugars. The focus should be less on demonising a single nutrient and more on the overall quality of the diet.

cholesterol testing and targets

Two of the more persistent controversies centre on how cholesterol should be measured and what low levels should be considered. For decades, LDL-C has been the standard target, but, in recent years, non-HDL-C, ApoB, and particle numbers have entered the discussion.

Critics argue that shifting markers and 'lower is better' messaging create confusion and medicalise otherwise healthy people. Others point to strong genetic and clinical trial evidence showing that lower ApoB levels consistently reduce risk, with benefits seen even at very low thresholds.

Guidelines have also evolved, sometimes lowering treatment cut-offs and broadening the population eligible for therapy. While this has raised concerns about over-treatment, it has also reflected growing recognition of lifetime risk and the role of cholesterol exposure over time.

OUR POSITION

LDL-C remains the core clinical measure, but non-HDL-C and ApoB provide valuable additional information. For high-risk patients, the evidence supports aggressive targets, while for lower-risk individuals, decisions should be personalised. What matters most is not chasing targets for their own sake but reducing overall cardiovascular risk using the best available evidence.

A CLOSER LOOK

fierce scientific debate

In 2013, two papers in the *British Medical Journal* sparked fierce debate.

John Abramson, an American physician then based at Harvard University, argued that people at low risk of heart disease should not routinely take statins, while **Aseem Malhotra,** a British cardiologist and researcher then based at Croydon University, South London, questioned whether saturated fat had been unfairly blamed for CAD.

Abramson (and several colleagues) suggested in the paper, *Should people at low risk of CVD take a statin?*[1] that people at low risk of heart disease – individuals with less than a 10 per cent risk over 10 years – probably should not take cholesterol tablets routinely as the cost-effectiveness and quality of life impacts meant it was not worthwhile. Essentially, he said not to treat the 100 to help the 10. Abramson's paper was controversial because it questioned whether statins should be prescribed to low-risk people at all, challenging widespread medical practice and sparking a heated debate over benefits, risks, and data transparency.

Dr Bishop:

> *Using imaging, I want to know the plaque burden of the 100 to find the 10 so I can be more targeted in my approach and more precise for the individual patient.*

The paper by Malhotra, *Saturated fat is not the major issue*[2], questioned the landmark Ancel Keys' *Seven Countries Study*[3], launched in 1958. Malhotra suggested that cutting fat often led to increased sugar consumption, since sugar is cheap and widely used in processed foods. This shift raised insulin, promoted fat storage, and contributed to obesity, a problem as harmful as the fats it replaced. He pointed to the PREDIMED study[4], where a Mediterranean diet rich in olive oil or nuts outperformed a low-fat diet in preventing heart disease, despite higher cholesterol levels.

The debate widened when Oxford's **Rory Collins** – representing the Cholesterol

---

1 *Should people at low risk of cardiovascular disease take a statin? BMJ 2013;347:f6123 (correction: 15 May 2014) https://www.bmj.com/content/347/bmj.f6123.full*

2 *Saturated fat is not the major issue BMJ 2013;347:f6340 (correction: 15 May 2014) https://www.bmj.com/content/347/bmj.f6340*

3 *Seven Countries Study, Ancel Keys; https://www.sevencountriesstudy.com/about-the-study/investigators/ancel-keys/*

4 *Prevención con Dieta Mediterránea – PREDIMED (see page 186 and page 205).*

Treatment Trialists' Collaboration[5], a group of trialists interested in cholesterol management and reducing cholesterol to prevent CAD – disagreed with some aspects of Abramson's and Malhotra's papers. The resultant back-and-forth communication led to the request for exposure and openness regarding the data which formed the basis of the CTT Collaboration positions.

Dr Bishop

> *As far as I can follow, the conversation became waylaid in the detail of trying to gather this information which was scattered and difficult to track down. The discussion moved into the space of conspiracy. For me, it's a sub-issue. I prefer to take the controversy away and stay with the facts rather than the to-ing and fro-ing around the accusatory, defensive remarks from Collins, Abramson and Malhotra.*

Later, in 2016, **Christopher Ramsden** revisited the Minnesota Coronary Experiment (1968–73)[6], which had tested replacing saturated fat with corn-oil–based linoleic acid. While cholesterol fell, heart disease outcomes did not improve, suggesting not all fats are equal.

Dr Bishop

> *I am not sure how we can interpret that on its own and apply it to what we would do daily. I think it tells us that using a polyunsaturated fat derived from corn in large amounts to replace saturated fats doesn't really affect the outcome in terms of CVD and in people who may be at higher risk for other reasons, as they are living in institutions. What it doesn't help us with is the replacement of saturated fat with extra virgin olive oil, or nuts,*

Drs Bishop and Kostner

> *We prefer to highlight what the evidence consistently supports: the Mediterranean Diet.*

---

5 *Cholesterol Treatment Trialists' (CTT) Collaboration was established in 1994, with its initial protocol (https://pubmed.ncbi.nlm.nih.gov/?term=ctt+protocol+1995) being published in 1995. It was set up after it was recognised that no single lipid intervention trial would be likely to have a sufficient number of trial participants (and hence statistical power) to reliably assess mortality outcomes or look at events in particular types of patient. Its aim is to conduct periodic meta-analyses of large-scale (≥1000 participants), long-term (≥2 years scheduled treatment duration) unconfounded, randomized controlled trials of lipid intervention therapies. https://www.cttcollaboration.org/*

6 *Re-evaluation of the traditional diet-heart hypothesis: analysis of recovered data from Minnesota Coronary Experiment (1968-73) BMJ 2016;353:i1246 https://www.bmj.com/content/353/bmj.i1246*

other controversies in brief

inflammation, insulin resistance and cholesterol

Critics say inflammation and insulin resistance cause atherosclerosis and LDL-C is just an innocent bystander.

Inflammation and insulin resistance do matter. We know lowering inflammation reduces future cardiac events, and high insulin levels – often tied to weight gain, high TG, and low HDL – do drive inflammation and affect LDL particle size. But to say cholesterol doesn't matter ignores overwhelming data: in high-risk patients, lowering LDL-C by 1 mmol/L reduces cardiovascular risk by about 20 per cent.

OUR POSITION: *Inflammation and insulin resistance are important drivers of heart disease, but LDL-C is central and fuels plaque. All three matter. Reducing LDL-C remains a proven way to cut risk.*

small dense vs large buoyant LDL particle size

It has been suggested that small, dense LDL particles slip more easily through the endothelium, while larger 'fluffy' particles are less harmful. It is true that small, dense LDL are more atherogenic, and insulin resistance tends to increase their number. Low-carbohydrate diets may shift particles toward a larger pattern. But large LDL particles can still form plaque.

OUR POSITION: *Particle size adds nuance, but it does not replace LDL-C as a key risk factor. Total LDL burden remains central.*

lifestyle vs medication

Some claim cholesterol-lowering medication isn't needed if you follow a healthy lifestyle. Lifestyle interventions – such as the Mediterranean Diet, regular exercise, good sleep, stress reduction, and weight management – are powerful and essential. The evidence is clear: lifestyle changes **and** medication are both needed to achieve secondary prevention targets that are known to be beneficial, including saving lives.

OUR POSITION: *We love lifestyle interventions, but* ***medications are needed,*** *especially for high-risk patients. The best results are achieved when they work together.*

brain and sex hormones and low cholesterol

Some people worry that lowering cholesterol harms brain function or sex hormone production. The key here is the difference between cellular cholesterol (the cholesterol the cell itself produces) and cholesterol in the blood (the cholesterol that can form plaque). The brain makes its own cholesterol behind the blood-brain barrier. Blood cholesterol does not limit or affect this process. Large studies show no cognitive harm or dementia from cholesterol-lowering therapy, and some even suggest protection. Similarly, sex hormone production also relies on cellular cholesterol.

OUR POSITION: *The brain and hormones are self-sufficient. Lowering blood LDL-C does not impair their function.*

HDL: good, bad, or irrelevant?

HDL-C lost its shine after drugs that raised it failed to reduce events.

OUR POSITION: *HDL-C level alone isn't protective. Function (how well HDL particles clear cholesterol) matters more. Raising the HDL-C level with drugs has not shown improved cardiovascular outcomes.*

triglycerides: passenger or driver?

Long dismissed as secondary, TG are now recognised as being linked to remnant cholesterol and metabolic risk.

OUR POSITION: *Elevated TG signal risk, especially in metabolic syndrome, but LDL-C remains the primary target.*

imaging vs blood tests

Should coronary calcium scoring or plaque imaging matter more than cholesterol numbers?

OUR POSITION: *Imaging adds precision and powerful risk information, complementing, not replacing, cholesterol testing.*

plant sterols and supplements

While these are often promoted as natural methods for lowering cholesterol, the evidence is mixed.

OUR POSITION: *They modestly reduce LDL but lack outcome data; best used as an adjunct, not a substitute for proven therapy.*

red yeast rice

Is this a natural alternative or is it a 'statin in disguise'?

OUR POSITION: *Red yeast rice contains lovastatin and acts like a low-dose statin, with the same side effects and safety concerns.*

personalised medicine

Should genetics and biomarkers replace one-size-fits-all guidelines?

OUR POSITION: *Personalisation is promising, but core strategies remain effective for the majority of patients.*

very low cholesterol: how low is too low?

Modern drugs achieve extremely low LDL levels, but is that safe?

OUR POSITION: *Current evidence shows risk reduction without signs of harm. Long-term monitoring continues.*

pharma and food industry messaging

Conflicting messages – drugs vs 'eat what you like' marketing – add to public distrust.

OUR POSITION: *Both industries have influence; trust should rest with your caring medical advisers and independent, peer-reviewed evidence.*

in the end ...

Controversies about cholesterol will no doubt continue, but they need not distract from what the evidence makes clear: cholesterol plays a central role in heart disease, and lowering it saves lives. Informed patients show how much they care about their health, and that is always welcome. Cholesterol science is complex, yet the essentials are simple: in secondary prevention, lowering cholesterol is vital, and in primary prevention, imaging, risk scoring, and modern therapies can help prevent heart events. The challenge – and the opportunity – is to apply knowledge wisely and personally.

from a media article

The deadly propaganda of the statin deniers: The drugs DO protect you from heart attacks but as this devastating investigation reveals thousands are refusing them

by Barney Calman, Health Editor, *The Mail On Sunday*[1]

- Millions of middle-aged people who would benefit from taking statins, don't.
- Research suggests many who refuse the pills have already had a heart attack.
- This could be because they've been led to believe that the drugs don't work.

Professor Sir Nilesh Samani, cardiologist and Medical Director of the British Heart Foundation:

> "The stories contain a grain of truth, mixed with speculation and opinion. It makes it very difficult for the public to know what the facts are, or whom to trust.
>
> "Of course we should debate the evidence, but all they have done is confuse people about the benefits of statins, which means those who really need them might stop taking them."

In January (2019), the editors-in-chief of all 30 major heart-health medical journals – each a leading cardiologist – signed a joint open letter, warning:

> "Lives are at stake [due to the] wanton spread of medical misinformation. It is high time that this stopped."

Professor Colin Baigent, an epidemiologist at the University of Oxford, who is also involved in major statins trials, explains that it is misleading to claim observational studies on statins refute what has been proven in clinical trials.

....

No one will force you to take the pills. Whether you take their advice is up to you. But if you do, it might just save your life.[2]

---

1 *The Mail on Sunday, published: 09:05 AEDT, 3 March 2019 | Updated: 12:16 AEDT, 3 March 2019 https://www.dailymail.co.uk/health/article-6764117/Devastating-investigation-reveals-impact-deadly-statin-denier-propaganda.html*

2 *ibid (end of another article on the same page)*

from a media article

There is a special place in hell for the doctors who claim statins don't work

by Barney Calman, Health Editor, *The Mail On Sunday*[1]

... I met 49-year-old Colin Worthing as he recovered in his hospital bed following a heart attack in the early hours of Tuesday. He had been prescribed cholesterol-lowering tablets ten years ago but quit them – without any medical advice – having "heard they don't really work".

Colin suffered his first heart attack in 2009, with little warning. "It was a shock as I'd felt well otherwise," he said. "Later I was told I had high blood pressure and high cholesterol. My mother has heart problems, so I think it runs in my family."

He was prescribed statins and blood pressure-lowering medication. "I took them to start with, but I felt lethargic. I was always hearing on the radio that statins didn't really work, and drug companies were just trying to make money by getting us all on tablets. You do start to think there's no smoke without fire."

In 2013 he decided to stop all medication... Over the next five years he felt well, "although I suppose I was stressed with work, and I did put on quite a bit of weight".

And then, about 1 am on Tuesday, he woke feeling clammy, with a familiar tightness in his chest... Colin was rushed to hospital where he had surgery to insert a stent which will keep blood flowing through his cardiac arteries while he awaits a full heart bypass operation.

His consultant at Hammersmith Hospital, London, Dr Rasha Al-Lamee, said: "We regularly see patients who, like Colin, have stopped taking statins because they believe the myth that they don't do any good. In fact, he's one of the lucky ones. He's alive. There will be numerous reasons his heart disease progressed so far, but one of the factors will be because he stopped taking statins."

Colin added: "I was a fool to stop taking the medication ... If I had carried on taking them, I might not be where I am now."

---

1 *ibid (another article on the same page)*

IMPORTANT POINTS

CHOLESTEROL CONTROVERSIES

- **Statins:** Statins are effective and well-studied, with benefits outweighing problems when prescribed carefully and individually.
- **Is cholesterol really a problem?** LDL-C is a major causal factor in heart disease and lowering it consistently reduces risk.
- **The diet-heart hypothesis:** Replacing saturated fat with unsaturated fat improves outcomes. A Mediterranean-style diet is recommended.
- **Fat vs sugar:** Both saturated fat and refined carbohydrates matter, but overall dietary quality is what protects heart health.
- **Cholesterol testing and targets:** LDL remains central, with non-HDL and ApoB adding value; goals should be personalised to overall risk.
- **Inflammation, insulin resistance, and cholesterol:** Inflammation and insulin resistance matter, but LDL-C remains central and lowering it reduces risk.
- **Small dense vs large buoyant LDL:** Particle size adds nuance, but total LDL burden is what drives risk.
- **Lifestyle vs medication:** Lifestyle and medication work together for everyone, but especially for high-risk patients.
- **Brain and sex hormones:** The brain and hormones make their own cholesterol; lowering blood LDL-C does not impair them.
- **HDL:** HDL level alone does not ensure protection; function matters, and raising HDL with drugs has not helped.

IMPORTANT POINTS

- **Triglycerides:** High TG is an independent risk factor but LCL-C remains the treatment target.
- **Imaging vs blood tests:** Imaging adds valuable risk insight. It complements rather than replaces blood tests.
- **Plant sterols and supplements:** They modestly lower LDL but lack outcome data and are best used as adjuncts.
- **Red yeast rice:** It acts like the statin, lovastatin, with the same effects and risks.
- **Personalised medicine:** Personalisation is promising, but standard strategies still benefit most people.
- **Very low cholesterol:** Evidence shows very low LDL levels bring added benefit without signs of harm.
- **Pharma and food industry messaging:** Industry influence exists, but guidance should rest on independent, scientific evidence.

We (Dr Bishop and Dr Kostner) are closely associated with numerous leading researchers in Australia and globally (Dr K. is one of them), and know that their ethics are beyond reproach. Following their guidance, we prescribe therapies for patients based on the individual's specific needs.

For an even clearer and more accurate understanding of cholesterol, let's clear away some of its most common half-truths and misconceptions.

cholesterol curiosities

statins are one of the most studied drug classes in history

Statins have been studied in hundreds of randomised trials and large outcome investigations over the past four to five decades, involving many millions of participants. Very few areas of medicine have undergone such scrutiny.

statins make up only a tiny fraction of all medications

Despite how often they are discussed, statins make up well under one per cent of all prescription medicines worldwide – yet they draw a disproportionate amount of public discussion.

statins have extensive long-term outcome data

There are more long-term randomised outcome trials for statins than for many commonly used medicines that people take without hesitation, including widely used pain relief.

the first statin came from fungi

The earliest statins were discovered after researchers observed that certain fungi could inhibit cholesterol synthesis – a reminder that some of our most effective medicines originate in nature.

concern about statins often precedes experience

Population studies consistently show that many people who express strong concern about statin side effects have never taken one. For many, apprehension stems from second-hand stories rather than personal experience.

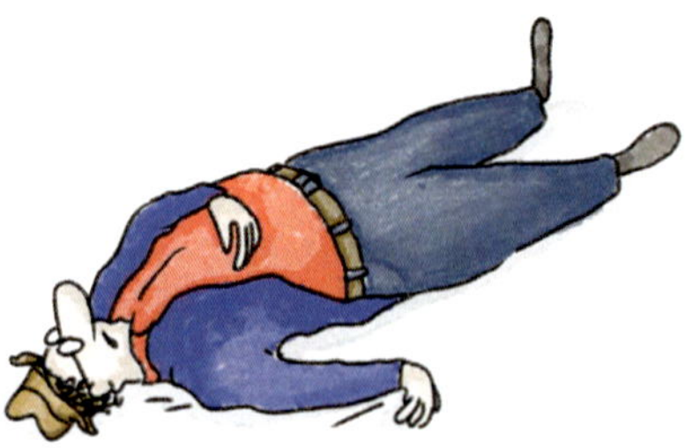

Cholesterol debates will continue, but the evidence is clear: cholesterol fuels heart disease, and lowering it saves lives. The science might be complex, yet the essentials are simple – lowering cholesterol is vital in secondary prevention, while imaging, risk scoring, and modern therapies guide primary prevention. Use this knowledge wisely and personally to turn complexity into confidence and better heart health.

chapter 24

CHOLESTEROL MYTHS AND MYSTERIES: ANSWERS, QUESTIONS, THE UNKNOWN

Cholesterol is often misunderstood and labelled as harmful, yet as we've seen throughout this book, its role in our health is complex and nuanced. Before concluding, it's important to revisit and dispel several persistent myths about cholesterol.

myths

From the idea that all cholesterol is harmful to overstating dietary cholesterol's impact, these widely held but misleading myths can strongly influence heart-health decisions. Often based on partial truths or mistaken beliefs, common examples include thinking only older adults should worry about cholesterol or that medications are the only solution.

So let's look at several myths that have no place in modern thinking:

- dietary cholesterol is the same as blood cholesterol
- only older adults need to worry
- no symptoms means no worries
- thin people don't have high cholesterol
- if the nutrition label says 'cholesterol free', then it must be healthy
- "I don't eat red meat, so my cholesterol must be fine"
- "I exercise so I will be okay".

dietary cholesterol is the same as blood cholesterol

The myth that dietary cholesterol directly translates into high blood cholesterol is a misunderstanding that simplifies the body's complex metabolic processes. While it's true that the cholesterol we eat can influence blood cholesterol levels, the impact is much less significant than once thought. The **body** produces cholesterol **daily** and, through **homeostasis**,

adjusts production in response to dietary intake, hormonal signals, genetics, and the body's broader metabolic needs.

For most people, dietary cholesterol has minimal effect on blood cholesterol levels. The more significant culprits are **saturated** and **trans fats** common in **processed** foods and some **animal** products. These fats stimulate the liver to produce more VLDL particles, ultimately increasing LDL particle numbers and LDL-C in the bloodstream. Understanding this distinction is key to managing cholesterol and targeting dietary changes only when they matter.

only older adults need to worry

The belief that cholesterol levels are only a concern for older adults is dangerous, as it overlooks the important understanding that atherosclerosis develops over many years, making early prevention and treatment critical.

Cholesterol build-up can begin in youth and progress silently, **setting the stage** for heart disease later in life. Studies show that the development of atherosclerotic plaques – which narrow and harden arteries – can start as early as adolescence. By maintaining healthy cholesterol levels from a younger age, individuals can significantly reduce their CVD risk.

It's crucial for **people of all ages**, including children and young adults, to be aware of their cholesterol levels and adopt heart-healthy habits **early**. This approach not only promotes better health outcomes in the long term but also emphasises the lifelong importance of cardiovascular health.

no symptoms means no worries

The assumption that the absence of symptoms means cholesterol levels are not a concern is misleading and can lead to neglect of cardiovascular health. High cholesterol levels do not cause any symptoms and neither does plaque build-up in the arteries. **People feel well until an event occurs.** Still, high cholesterol contributes significantly to the development of heart and vascular diseases, which can result in severe health issues such as heart attacks and strokes and the need for revascularisation.

The first 'symptom' of high cholesterol could be a catastrophic event such as a heart attack. This underscores why a person should not ignore cholesterol. This is why we advocate imaging the arteries of **well** people **before** they have an event.

Regular cholesterol screenings and appropriate artery scans are vital, enabling early detection and management of high cholesterol. This **proactive** approach allows timely medicinal and lifestyle interventions, promoting long-term heart health.

thin people don't have high cholesterol

The idea that only overweight or obese people have high cholesterol overlooks genetics, diet, and lifestyle factors affecting anyone. While weight can be a consideration, cholesterol levels depend more on genetics, types of fats consumed, and overall diet quality. Naturally thin individuals may have unhealthy eating habits, inadequate physical activity, or genetic predispositions like FH, causing elevated LDL-C. **Regular cholesterol screenings** and a **heart-healthy lifestyle** – balanced diet, regular exercise, and cholesterol monitoring – are important for **everyone**, regardless of body size or age.

if the nutrition label says 'cholesterol free', then it must be healthy

The label 'cholesterol-free' or 'low cholesterol' on food packaging can be **misleading**, as it may suggest the food is heart-healthy when that's not necessarily true. Such foods can still be high in **saturated** or **trans fats**, which influence the liver to produce more VLDL particles. As VLDL are broken down, this leads to higher LDL-C levels in the bloodstream. These fats may also lower HDL, the particles involved in reverse cholesterol transport. Additionally, many 'cholesterol-free' products are high in added sugars or salt, which can further contribute to cardiovascular risk. Therefore, it's essential to look beyond cholesterol content on nutrition labels and examine the **overall nutritional profile** of the food, including fats, sugars, and sodium, to determine its impact on heart health.

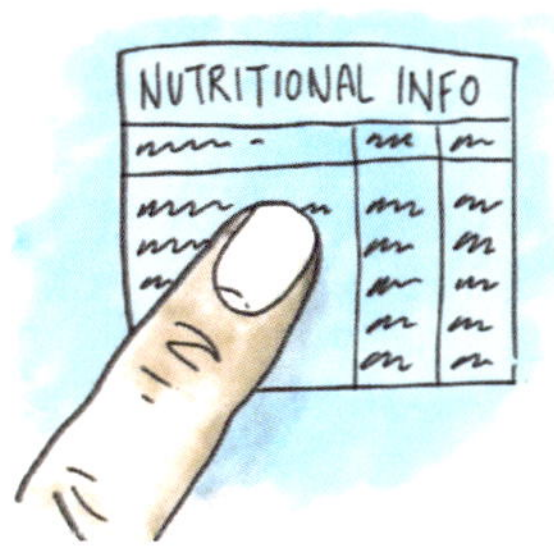

'Lite yoghurt' is a classic example of a low fat food that is high in sugar.

"I don't eat red meat, so my cholesterol must be fine"

Avoiding red meat alone doesn't guarantee healthy cholesterol levels, as other dietary factors also play a significant role. While reducing red meat, which is high in saturated fats, can help lower LDL-C, consuming other animal products, such as full-fat dairy, as well as certain oils, processed foods, and trans-fat-rich items like baked goods and fried foods, can still raise cholesterol levels. Effective cholesterol management requires a holistic view of your **entire diet**, not just one food group.

"I exercise, so I'll be okay"

This is a common but dangerous myth. Atherosclerosis doesn't care how many kilometres you run or laps you swim, and it isn't deterred by your training routine! Among athletes over 40, heart attacks remain a leading cause of sudden cardiac death.

Exercise is excellent for overall health (it provides some metabolic benefits, such as improving insulin sensitivity and mildly raises HDL-C), but typically it doesn't significantly lower LDL-C or remove plaque build-up.

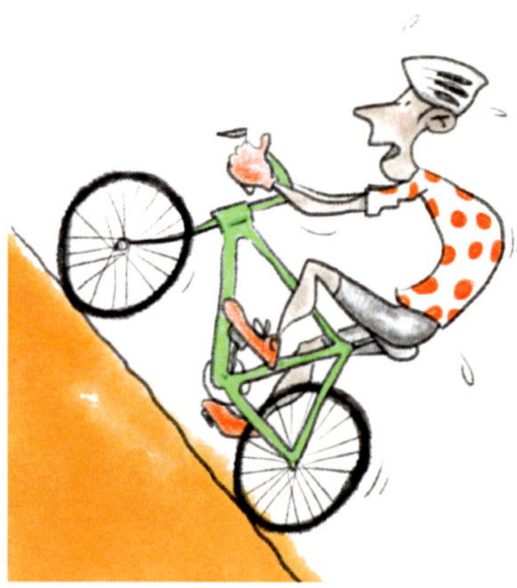

Fitness does not guarantee freedom from plaque; you can be fit yet still at serious cardiovascular risk.

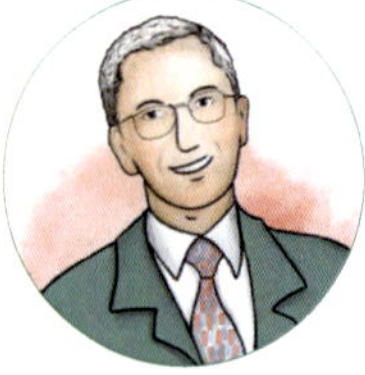

When confronted with a myth, especially one that could influence health decisions, it's crucial to be thoughtful and discerning. Base your judgments on facts and scientific research, not merely on popular opinion, catchy phrases, or trending fads on social media. Avoid being misled by complex terminology.

When discussing such topics, always approach conversations with sensitivity and respect for different viewpoints. Ask probing questions and critically analyse the information at hand. Being a critical thinker and fostering curiosity can help you, and encourage others, to seek genuine answers. Such an educational approach will improve your medical outcome.

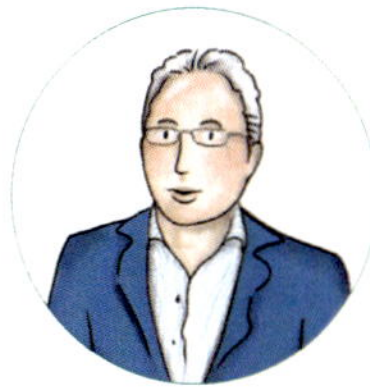

questions

Cholesterol raises many questions, and poorly answered ones only add to the confusion. The truth is, some questions we can answer confidently, while others remain unclear. The complexity of medical science and the uniqueness of each individual mean that definitive answers aren't always possible. Two important questions are:

- *How low can cholesterol be without it altering brain function?*
- *Do statins impact cognitive function?*

how low can cholesterol be without it altering brain function?

There are not many absolutes around this question. However, we can make strong inferences.

trials

Some trials have looked specifically at lowering LDL-C and assessing cognitive (mental) function using new PCSK9 inhibitor agents, which can reduce a person's cholesterol to very low levels.

For example, the EBBINGHAUS trial[1] looked at what happened to brain

1 *EBBINGHAUS (Evaluating PCSK9 Binding Antibody Influence on Cognitive Health in High Cardiovascular Risk Subjects) involved a subgroup of patients from the Further Cardiovascular Outcomes Research with PCSK9 Inhibition in Subjects with Elevated Risk (FOURIER) trial. Design and rationale of the EBBINGHAUS trial: A phase 3, double-blind, placebo-controlled, multicenter study to assess the effect of evolocumab on cognitive function in patients with clinically evident cardiovascular disease and receiving statin background lipid-lowering therapy – a cognitive study of patients enrolled in the FOURIER trial.*

function using the PCSK9 inhibitor, evolocumab. By blocking the protein PCSK9[2], evolocumab helps increase the number of LDLR on the surface of liver cells, leading to enhanced removal of LDL from the bloodstream and so lowering LDL-C levels. The EBBINGHAUS trial, conducted over several years, was unable to demonstrate any cognitive impairment by lowering cholesterol levels to very low levels for people who have very, very high risk of a heart attack. This is very reassuring.

babies

At birth, babies have very low cholesterol levels – LDL-C levels of 50 to 70 mg per decilitre, or around 1.3 to 1.8 millimoles per litre (mmol/L). These low levels are similar to the target levels when treating someone who has a high risk of heart disease. These baby levels are measured at the most metabolically active period of our lives, during the most rapid brain development we experience outside the womb. We can infer that the brain – at least the brain of an infant – works very well with those low levels. It's not proof, but it is reassurance.

PCSK9 – in families

We also know there are families who have **over-active** PCSK9 (see footnote 2). People with overactive PCSK9 have too much cholesterol in their bloodstream and run a high risk of coronary events. Others, however, have **non-functioning PCSK9** and very, very low levels of cholesterol. They appear to lead normal lives without any brain dysfunction or abnormality, tending to live long lives without incidence of coronary or vascular events.

Giugliano, R. P., Mach, F., Zavitz, K., Kurtz, C., Schneider, J., Wang, H., Keech, A., Pedersen, T. R., Sabatine, M. S., Sever, P. S., Honarpour, N., Wasserman, S. M., Ott, B. R., & Investigators, E. (2017). Design and rationale of the EBBINGHAUS trial: A phase 3, double-blind, placebo-controlled, multicenter study to assess the effect of evolocumab on cognitive function in patients with clinically evident cardiovascular disease and receiving statin background lipid-lowering therapy. A cognitive study of patients enrolled in the FOURIER trial. Clinical Cardiology, 40(2), 59-65. https://doi.org/10.1002/clc.22678

see also

Cognitive Function in a Randomized Trial of Evolocumab N Engl J Med 2017; 377:633-643 DOI: 10.1056/NEJMoa1701131

2 *Remember, PCSK9 made primarily in the liver, plays a key role in regulating cholesterol levels by binding to LDLR and promoting their breakdown. This reduces the number of receptors available to clear LDL-C from the blood.*

So, these data – the EBBINGHAUS trial, the cholesterol levels of newborns and families with very low cholesterol – while not absolute, **reassure** us when we are looking to lower cholesterol levels significantly.

some **short answers** to other important questions.

Does the use of a statin increase the risk of haemorrhagic stroke?

Earlier concerns suggested statins might raise this risk, but a 2025 systematic review and meta-analysis[3] found they were instead associated with a reduced recurrence of spontaneous intracerebral haemorrhage (a type of stroke caused by sudden bleeding into brain tissue, not related to trauma). Overall, evidence shows the benefits of statins, for the right individuals, outweigh any small historical concerns.

Should everyone follow the same cholesterol treatment strategy regardless of ethnic background or genetic differences?

No. Cholesterol management should be tailored to individual factors, including ethnic background and genetic differences.

Can infections contribute to the development of atherosclerosis?

Emerging research suggests that certain infections may contribute to atherosclerotic plaque development. For instance, *porphyromonas gingivalis*, a bacterium associated with periodontal disease, has been detected within atherosclerotic lesions, indicating a potential role in plaque formation. Similarly, *chlamydia pneumoniae,* known for causing respiratory infections, has been implicated in atherosclerosis, with studies suggesting it is a significant risk factor for plaque development. These findings highlight the complex interplay among many factors contributing to atherosclerosis risk – in **all** patients **regardless** of LDL-C levels.

Can I eat grapefruit and drink its juice while taking a statin?

Grapefruit can interact with some statins. Grapefruit and its juice block an enzyme in the gut (CYP3A4) that normally helps break down certain

---

3 *Statins reduce the recurrence of spontaneous intracerebral hemorrhage: A systematic review and meta-analysis. Li, Z., Xu, W.-q., Wang, J.-q., Yang, J.-h., Shi, X.-h., Wang, C.-b., Xu, Z.-x., & Jiang, J.-l. (2025). Clinical Neurology and Neurosurgery, 238, 108330. https://doi.org/10.1016/j.clineuro.2025.108330*

statins – including atorvastatin, simvastatin and lovastatin. If you take these, grapefruit can raise the level of medicine in your blood, which can increase the risk of side effects like muscle pain or liver irritation. Importantly, occasional consumption is rarely clinically significant. Other statins, such as rosuvastatin, pravastatin and fluvastatin, are not affected and can be taken safely with grapefruit. If you enjoy grapefruit, it is best to check with your doctor or pharmacist which statin you are taking. This also applies if you want to eat Seville oranges.

Should older adults maintain the same cholesterol targets as younger individuals?

Not necessarily. Cholesterol targets for older adults may be adjusted based on overall health, life expectancy, and individual risk factors.

How effective are alternative treatments like red yeast rice compared with traditional statins?

Red yeast rice can lower cholesterol as it naturally contains monacolin K, similar to statins. However, in contrast to quality-controlled and standardised statins, the **effectiveness and safety are less consistent** due to product variations. Furthermore, it can have side effects and drug interactions **similar to statins** – and is expensive and can be difficult to obtain. Consult a healthcare provider before use.

some **short comments** on questions **without** answers.

What are the precise biological mechanisms that cause statins to have varying effects on cholesterol levels among different individuals?

Essentially, we are all different: genetics, habits, age, sex, perhaps even microbiome. There are still plenty of mysteries for science to figure out.

Can we definitively determine the role of cholesterol in all forms of heart disease, considering the presence of heart disease in individuals with 'normal' cholesterol levels?

We have touched on cholesterol's amazing complexity – of particle size, composition, different proteins, electrical charge, shear stress, and even infection. Other factors are almost certainly at play but not yet identified. Cholesterol is wonderfully complex and will remain so.

What are the specific genetic factors that enable some individuals to maintain low cholesterol levels despite a high-cholesterol diet?

Basically, your parents.

Can a medication be developed that targets ApoB-100 only without any other effects?

Current therapies already focus on lowering LDL-C very effectively, while inclisiran, which blocks PCSK9 mRNA, can cut LDL-C by about 50 per cent for six months at a time. Gene therapies in development may offer lifelong cholesterol control with minimal side effects. Research is steadily moving towards even more precise and personalised treatments. *Watch this space!*

ongoing

Cholesterol research is robust and continuously evolving worldwide. Researchers continue to make exciting discoveries and develop more targeted treatments. Staying well-informed from reliable sources and taking a proactive approach ensures you base your health decisions on the most current and comprehensive information.

Regardless of your interest in cholesterol and the questions you may still have, it is important to **follow** the science, be **curious,** and always **consult** with your medical practitioner before taking any self-directed action.

To keep abreast of unfolding developments, join Dr Bishop's Healthy Heart Network, listen to his podcasts, and read his blogs.

Healthy Heart Network

podcasts

blogs

IMPORTANT POINTS

CHOLESTEROL MYTHS AND MYSTERIES

- A myth is a widely held but false belief. It may contain some truth, but without the full context, it can mislead. Myths can often stem from common misconceptions or mistaken ideas. They are accepted without solid evidence.
- Know the facts based on scientific data; be a critical thinker.
- The EBBINGHAUS trial indicated no cognitive impairment when cholesterol levels were lowered to very low levels using the PCSK9 inhibitor, evolocumab, in high-risk CVD patients.
- Babies are born with very low LDL-C levels, which suggests that such low levels do not impair brain function during significant developmental phases.
- Some families with overactive PCSK9 have high cholesterol levels and increased risk of coronary events, whereas those with non-functioning PCSK9 have very low cholesterol levels and lead normal, healthy lives.
- While many questions can be answered, there is still much about cholesterol that remains unknown and open to research.
- Cholesterol research is ongoing and robust.
- Always follow the science, be curious, and consult with your medical practitioner(s) before taking any self-directed action.

With the key messages now laid out, we bring our story of cholesterol to a close. We are privileged to have shared what we know, hopeful it has been of help, and mindful that the journey of discovery continues for all of us.

EPILOGUE

CHOLESTEROL AND CHOICE: INFORMED DECISIONS FOR THE FUTURE

Having made it this far, you've probably realised that cholesterol isn't just a number – it's a story. And like all good stories, it's full of perspectives: science, risk, prevention, uncertainty, and hope. In this unfolding narrative, the ending is yet to be written.

a final word from Dr Bishop

If I were speaking to a friend about cholesterol, I'd break it down into two parts: after and before.

After a coronary event, there is no question. All the evidence tells us that lowering cholesterol offers a clear benefit. Statins really do work and, contrary to popular belief, they are well tolerated by the vast majority of users.

An overwhelming body of data supports the principle that lower is better, and the newer cholesterol-lowering agents, acting as add-ons to statins, do a remarkable job of helping us achieve levels that may even lead to plaque regression. *That's pretty cool!*

Before an event, things are a little more complicated.

For those with a genetic mutation causing familial hypercholesterolaemia, there is little doubt. Cholesterol lowering is the way to go – and the sooner, the better.

For those with moderately high cholesterol, an intermediate risk profile, or a 'bad' family history, I believe there's an opportunity to apply precision medicine. By imaging the arteries, we can make better, more personalised decisions rather than relying solely on cholesterol levels in the blood.

The cholesterol story is fascinatingly complex. Despite decades of research, we are still uncovering its nuances. The idea that

- different cholesterol particles of different sizes and composition carry different risk profiles,
- coronary artery disease is patchy (pointing to local factors at play) and that even subtle differences in the amino acid sequences of particle proteins may alter the electrical charge of cholesterol particles, affecting how they pass through connective tissue,

is mind-blowing. Add to that the interplay between inflammation, plaque rupture, blood pressure, stress, and how they all interact, and you have a puzzle still being pieced together.

We've tried hard to share some of this wonder in *Cholesterol Explained.* I really do hope you've found it fascinating.

So, in summary, **please take action**:

- if you ***have*** had an event:
  - **lower your cholesterol** – as low as possible is best;
- if you ***haven't*** had an event:
  - have your **cholesterol checked**
  - have a coronary artery calcium **scan.**

That's it – simple, logical, and backed by the best science we have.

and a final word from Dr Kostner

As a cardiologist, I have witnessed the lives of many patients and their families be shattered by a diagnosis of cardiovascular disease, or in the worst cases, sudden cardiac death.

Cardiovascular disease can sneak up on you completely unannounced. The disease process occurs silently and painlessly over many years until, 'out of the blue', it takes a victim by surprise. Alarmingly, heart disease is known as the *silent killer*; it can cause immediate death without the victims ever knowing they were playing host to it.

I believe that **prevention is the best cure** – achieved through **education** and **informed decision-making**. Elevated cholesterol is common and lowering it is easy, safe and inexpensive. More importantly, it prevents heart attacks, strokes, and vascular dementia.

People with genetically elevated low-density lipoprotein and lipoprotein(a) genuinely benefit from early diagnosis and treatment.

We are now in the age of personalised risk assessment and can better predict who is at risk with better blood tests and imaging.

I hope that, after reading this book, you will be able to take advantage of these tools and reduce your chance of cardiovascular disease.

from us both

In the end, **cholesterol is not the enemy**. It is part of a larger conversation about risk, prevention, and personalised care. The more we understand, the better equipped we are to make informed, confident decisions.

Our ongoing aim is to offer clear, trustworthy information to help you take an active role in your health.

The choices are now yours to make –

guided by **knowledge**,

grounded in **evidence**, and

shaped by **your values**.

Wishing you good health and clarity on the journey ahead.

May you live as well as possible for as long as possible.

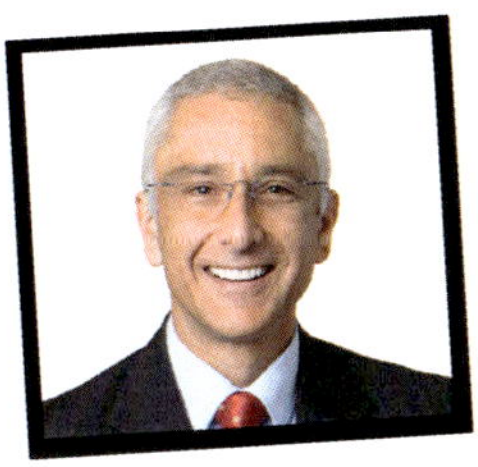

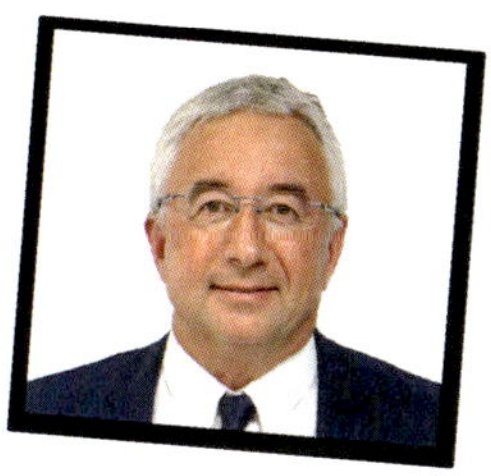

Warrick Bishop
Hobart, Tasmania
Australia

Karam Kostner
Brisbane, Queensland
Australia

CHOLESTEROL CHALLENGE

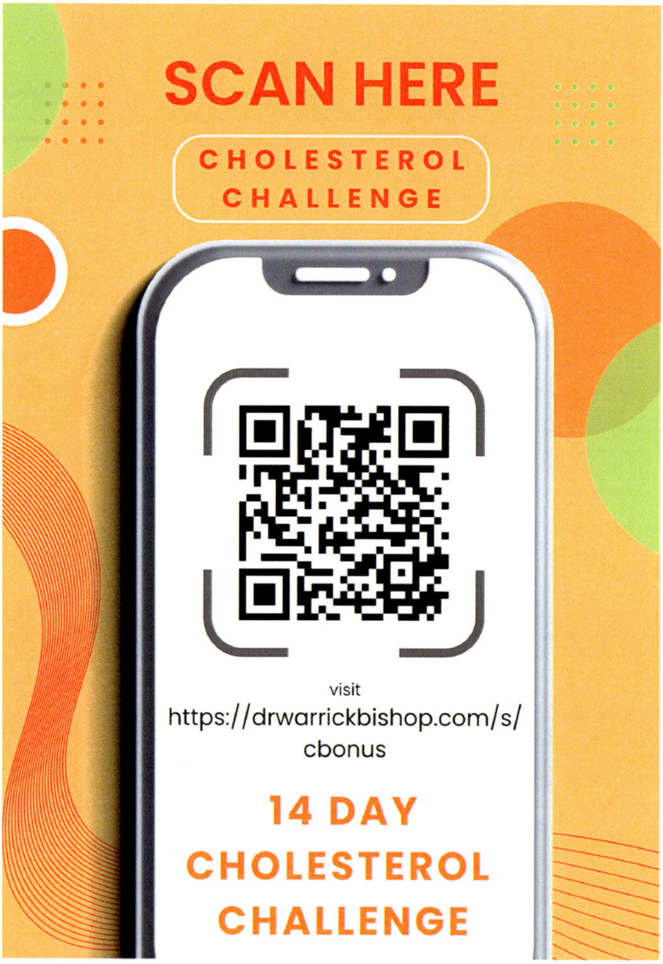

AFTERWORD

keep handy for reference!

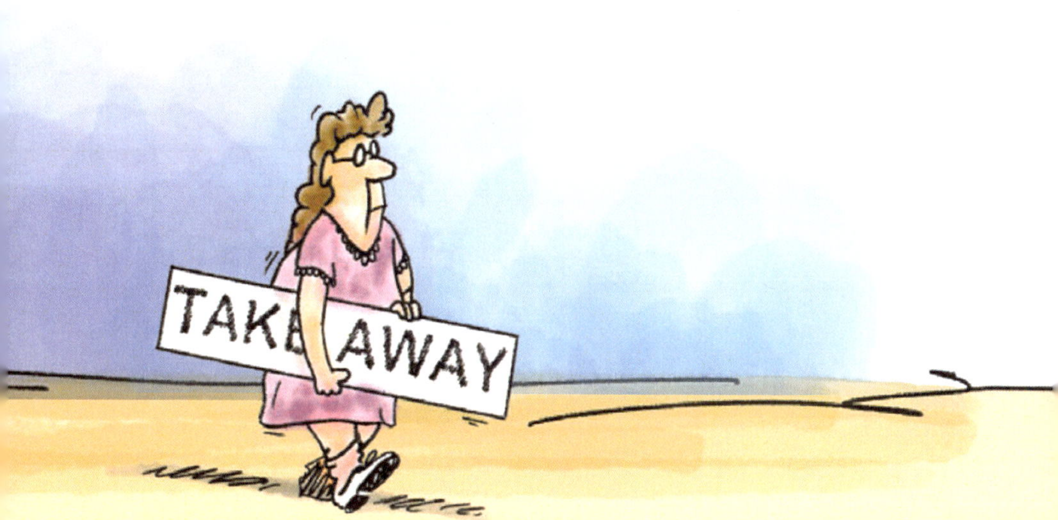

TOP 10 TAKEAWAYS

cholesterol at a glance

TOP 10 TAKEAWAYS
cholesterol at a glance

1. Cholesterol in cells is essential to the body. Cholesterol in particles in the blood, particularly LDL cholesterol, is our focus for cardiovascular risk.

2. Cholesterol metabolism and atherosclerosis are complex. Simplified 'sound bites' – often shared on social media – can distort the bigger picture, leading to confusion at best and harm at worst.

3. LDL-C is the most important treatable risk factor for cardiovascular disease.

4. LDL-C lowering is directly related to the reduction of cardiovascular risk.

5. High-risk patients – patients who have suffered events and those with high-risk plaque burden identified by imaging – need to achieve low LDL-C targets.

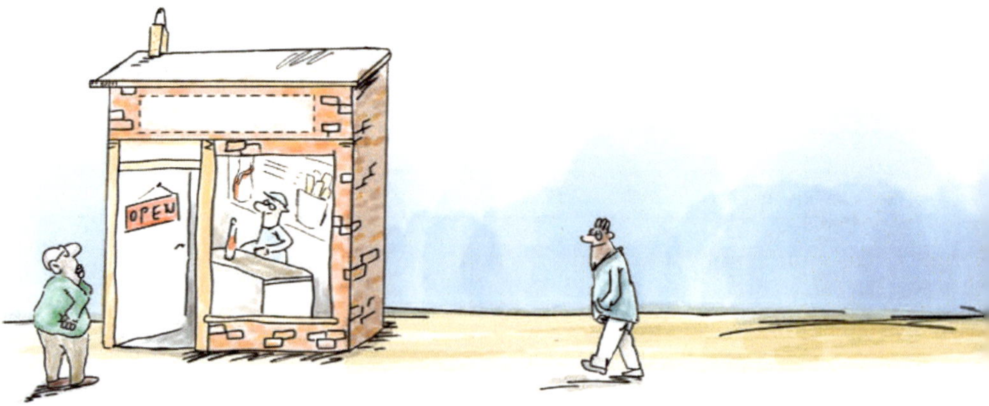

please copy, print & share!

6. Current therapies – statins, ezetimibe and PCSK9 inhibitors
   - achieve these low targets
   - are broadly well-tolerated, and
   - are cost-effective.

7. Primary and secondary prevention are part of the same continuum. Understanding this, and the cumulative damage caused by long-term LDL-C exposure, present an undeniable case for early detection (consider CAC) and sustained intervention. Such action could eradicate heart attacks.

8. Treating genetic dyslipidaemias and raised cholesterol, and recognising a family history of heart disease as early as possible, offer the best long-term outcome.

9. Beyond LDL-C levels, other risk stratifications, including lipoprotein(a) levels and imaging, will inform the best personalised care.

10. While diet and lifestyle changes are extremely important for heart health, on their own they are inadequate to achieve LDL-C targets in high-risk patients.

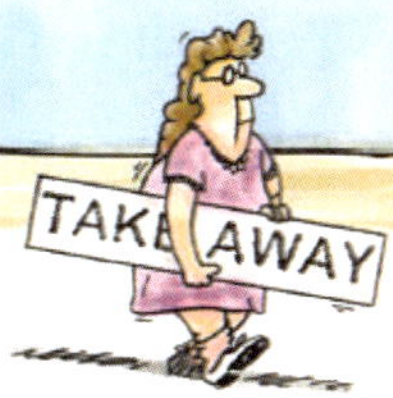

medications guide

statins *(atorvastatin and rosuvastatin are the most common)* ezetimibe
evolocumab (PCSK9 inhibitor; *alirocumab is not available in Australia)*
inclisiran (siRNA)
bempedoic acid (ATP citrate lyase inhibitor; *Austn approval pending, '25*)
omega-3 fatty acids
fibrates *(rarely used)*
bile acid sequestrants *(rarely used)*
lomitapide (MTP inhibitor, *compassionate use in Australia, '25*)
evinacumab (ANGPTL3 inhibitor, *compassionate use in Aust., '25*)

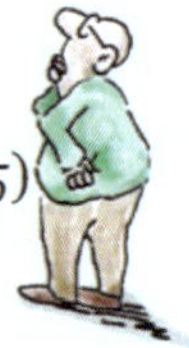

tests, markers and profiles

standard lipid profile

- total cholesterol (TC – *the overall amount of cholesterol in the blood*)
- LDL cholesterol (LDL-C)
- HDL cholesterol (HDL-C)
- triglycerides (TG)
- non-HDL cholesterol (TC minus HDL-C; *includes all atherogenic particles, LDL, VLDL, Lp(a)*)
- cholesterol/HDL ratio

lipoprotein(a)
omega-3 index omega ratio
apolipoproteins *(e.g. apoB – tests for all apolipoproteins are available)*
inflammation markers
genetics

- familial hypercholesterolaemia (FH) panel
- lipoprotein(a) [Lp(a)] genetic test
- polygenic risk score (PRS) for LDL-C
- ApoE genotyping

imaging

- coronary artery calcium (CAC) scan (to give a CAC score)
- coronary angiography
- carotid ultrasound
- intima-media thickness (IMT) measurement
- intravascular ultrasound (IVUS)
- intravascular ultrasound – virtual histology (VH-IVUS)
- optical coherence tomography (OCT)
- near-infrared spectroscopy (NIRS)

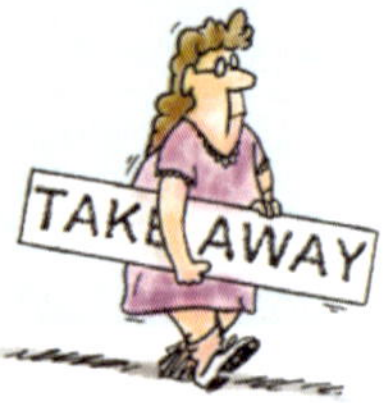

PATIENT, PROFESSIONAL RESOURCES

These Australian and international links offer valuable information about cholesterol for patients, health professionals, and anyone interested in learning more.

AUSTRALIAN RESOURCES

Australian Atherosclerosis Society (AAS) – https://www.athero.org.au
A leading organisation promoting research, education, and clinical guidelines on lipid management and CVD prevention in Australia.

FH Australia – https://fhaustralia.org.au/
Offering a voice and support for families and individuals with familial hypercholesterolaemia (FH).

Healthdirect Australia – https://www.healthdirect.gov.au/cholesterol
A government-funded service providing reliable, easy-to-understand information about cholesterol, heart disease, and healthy living, including links to local services and resources.

Healthy Heart Network – https://healthyheartnetwork.com
Dr Bishop's online platform offering tools and guidance to reduce CVD risk.

Heart Foundation – https://www.heartfoundation.org.au/
A leading Australian charity offering extensive resources for both health professionals and the public on every facet of CVD.

NSW Health Centre for Genetics Education –
https://www.genetics.edu.au
Provides education and resources on genetic conditions for individuals, families, and health professionals.

INTERNATIONAL

American Association of Clinical Endocrinology (AACE)
https://www.aace.co
Guidelines and patient information relating to lipids and metabolic health.

American Heart Association (AHA) – https://www.heart.org
Comprehensive resources on CVD prevention and cholesterol management.

British Heart Foundation – https://www.bhf.org.uk/
A prominent UK foundation offering high-quality resources for both patients and health professionals, including insightful videos, covering a broad range of conditions and risk factors.

Cleveland Clinic – cholesterol management (USA)
https://my.clevelandclinic.org/health/diseases/21656-hyperlipidemia
Detailed information on types of cholesterol, testing, treatment options, and lifestyle changes from a top-ranked US hospital.

European Atherosclerosis Society (EAS) – https://www.eas-society.org/
Professional organisation with guidelines, research updates, and resources on lipid disorders and atherosclerosis, suitable for clinicians and academics.

European Society of Cardiology (ESC) – www.escardio.org
A major European organisation providing clinical guidelines, research updates, and professional education on CVD, including cholesterol and lipid management.

International Lipid Expert Panel (ILEP) – https://www.ilep.eu
Evidence-based position statements and consensus documents from global lipid experts.

Learn Your Lipids – https://www.learnyourlipids.com/
A resource for patients living with dyslipidaemia, including familial hypercholesterolaemia (FH).

Mayo Clinic (USA) – https://www.mayoclinic.org
A world-renowned medical centre providing reliable, easy-to-understand information about cholesterol, diagnosis, treatment, and prevention.

National Lipid Association (NLA) – https://www.lipid.org
Professional education, patient resources, and lipid management guidance from the US-based lipid association.

US Centers for Disease Control and Prevention (CDC)
https://www.cdc.gov/cholesterol/
Trusted public health advice (stats, education, and prevention strategies).

World Heart Federation (WHF) – https://www.world-heart-federation.org
Global leadership in cardiovascular health, including reports on cholesterol and its global burden.

For a more exhaustive professional list of websites, please visit FH Australasia Network's **https://www.athero.org.au/fh/health-professionals/useful-links/**

Health professionals – FH and Lp(a) SPECIALISTS

The FH Australasia Network website at
https://www.athero.org.au/fh/health-professionals/fh-specialists/
lists FH and Lp(a) specialists in each **Australian State and Territory** as well as specialists/clinics in the **United Kingdom** and the **United States.**

REFERENCES

Cholesterol Explained has been informed by

Interpretation of the evidence for the efficacy and safety of statin therapy Rory Collins, Christina Reith, Jonathan Emberson et al; Lancet 2016; 388: 2531-61 Published online, September 8, 2016 http://dx.doi.org/10.1016/S0140-6736(16)31357-5

websites:

American Heart Association	https://www.heart.org
Australian Institute of Health and Welfare	https://www.aihw.gov.au
Diabetes Australia	https://www.diabetesaustralia.com.au
FH Australasia Network	https://www.athero.org.au
Food Standards Australia New Zealand	https://www.foodstandards.gov.au
Harvard Publishing, Harvard Medical School	https://www.health.harvard.edu
Healthy Heart Network	https://healthyheartnetwork.com
Heart Foundation (Australia)	https://www.heartfoundation.org
National Health and Medical Research Council (NHMRC Australia)	https://www.nhmrc.gov.au
National Heart, Lung and Blood Institute	https://www.nhlbi.nih.gov
National Library of Medicine (National Centre for Biotechnology Information)	https://www.ncbi.nlm.nih.gov
OpenAI ChatGPT-5 [Large Language Model]	https://chat.openai.com
ResearchGate	https://www.researchgate.net
The Lancet	https://www.thelancet.com
The New England Journal of Medicine	https://www.nejm.org
University of California San Francisco	https://www.ucsf.edu
World Economic Forum	https://www.weforum.org
World Health Organization	https://www.who.int
World Heart Federation	https://world-heart-federation.org

books:

Bishop, Warrick; *Have You Planned Your Heart Attack?* (2016)

Bishop, Warrick; *Know Your Real Risk of Heart Attack* (2018)

Bishop, Warrick, Begg, Alistair; *Cardiac Rehabilitation Explained* (2023)

Bishop, Warrick, Kostner, Karam; *10 Commandments of Heart Health Explained* (2024)

INDEX

*This index **highlights** the principal terms, themes, and examples discussed in* Cholesterol Explained, *and includes the footnotes. It is intended as **a guide** to key concepts rather than an exhaustive, encyclopaedic list.*

I

J

K

L

M

N

O

P

Q

R

S

T

studies/trials

ACKNOWLEDGEMENTS

Creating a book such as *Cholesterol Explained* is neither a result of mere chance nor a matter of fortuitous luck. It represents the culmination of the inspiration, expertise, and dedication of many remarkable individuals without whom this project would have remained an unfulfilled idea.

Our heartfelt thanks go to our distinguished colleague **Gerald Watts.** Gerald, who is based in Perth, Western Australia, is a globally recognised lipid expert with vast knowledge and depth of expertise. We are deeply honoured by his thoughtful foreword and are immensely grateful for his warmth, encouragement, and thoughtful reflections.

We extend our sincere appreciation to our esteemed colleagues, **David Colquhoun,** a clinical, research, and academic cardiologist from Brisbane, Queensland, and **Christian Hamilton-Craig**, a cardiologist, imaging specialist, and academic, based in Noosa, Queensland. Both are highly respected and experienced practitioners who generously contributed their time and expertise, providing invaluable feedback and encouragement. Their thoughtful reading and constructive comments helped refine this work. Our appreciation also extends to the **contributors** to the guideline papers that accompany this book. These documents represent the culmination of substantial efforts by dedicated professionals committed to advancing medical care.

A special debt of gratitude is owed to our **cardiac patients**. Their experiences have shaped our medical insights and life knowledge, enriching the pages of this book. We are particularly thankful to those whose case studies have added a practical, human perspective to the complex medical concepts explored within these pages.

Thanks are also due to our sharp-eyed practitioners of precision, **Michelle Kostner, Jacqueline Ryan, Fiona Scott, John Harbinson**, **David Thomas**, **Sandy Hancock, Carl Nilsson**, **Rachel Tope** and **Max Bishop,** whose candid real-world observations have enhanced the clarity and readability of the content.

This book would not exist without the talent and support of an exceptional technical team: creative powerhouses **Cathy McAuliffe** and **Beverly**

Waldie, marketing expert **John North** and his team, and our passionate and single-minded writing partner, **Penny Edman**. Each has played a vital role in bringing these pages to life; their expertise and commitment have been invaluable.

Finally, we extend our profound gratitude to our wives, **Chelle** and **Michelle**, and our families, for their unwavering support and patience during the long process of writing this book.

In the end, *Cholesterol Explained* is the result of a generous and respectful collaboration between two colleagues and friends united by a shared fascination with lipids and commitment to improving heart health. It has been a privilege to work together.

Warrick Bishop
Hobart, Australia
January 2026

Karam Kostner
Brisbane, Australia
January 2026

BEHIND THE SCENES

writer – **Penelope Edman** is a freelance writer, editor, high-performance coach, and photographer based in Hobart, Tasmania, Australia. She began her print journalism career in Bundaberg, Queensland, in the late 1970s and moved to Hobart in 1991. An award-winning journalist and editor, her articles and photographs have been featured extensively across Australia and internationally.

She authored four commissioned non-fiction books before assisting Dr Bishop with *Have You Planned Your Heart Attack?*, *Atrial Fibrillation Explained*, *Cardiac Failure Explained*, *Cardiac Rehabilitation Explained* (with Dr Alistair Begg), and, more recently in association with Dr Kostner, *10 Commandments of Heart Health Explained*, and now *Cholesterol Explained*.

Her in-depth engagement with the topics explored in each book has reinforced her commitment to managing her own heart health with regular checks and risk-factor control. She also encourages her family and friends to prioritise their cardiovascular well-being.

For readers who want to explore further …

other books by **Dr Warrick Bishop**

https://drwarrickbishop.com/s/books

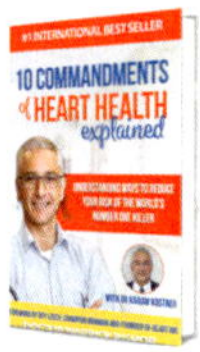

10 Commandments of Heart Health Explained is a practical guide to understanding and reducing your risk of heart attack. Drawing on up-to-date medical insights, it offers clear, actionable steps anyone can use to improve their heart health and prevent future problems. This book empowers you to take charge of your wellbeing and make confident, informed choices for a healthier life. (with Dr Karam Kostner)

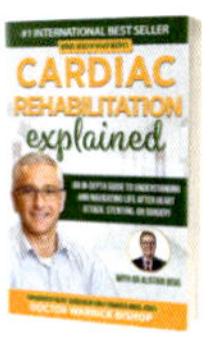

Cardiac Rehabilitation Explained outlines why cardiac rehabilitation matters, what brings a person to needing it, treatments involved, and the practical steps that support recovery and long-term heart health. It's also a helpful guide for people of any age who want to take a proactive approach to preventing future heart problems. (with Dr Alistair Begg)

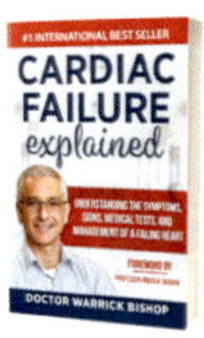

Cardiac Failure Explained is an accessible guide to understanding and managing heart failure. Written by an experienced cardiologist, it outlines diagnosis, key tests, medications and the practical steps that help you manage symptoms and improve daily life.

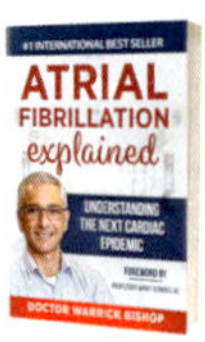

Atrial Fibrillation Explained is a comprehensive guide that provides an easy-to-understand overview of atrial fibrillation, covering its causes, symptoms, and treatment options.

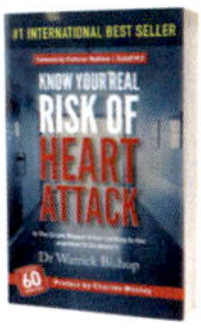

Know Your Real Risk of Heart Attack is an abridged version of *Have You Planned Your Heart Attack?*.

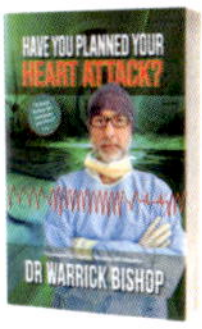

Have You Planned Your Heart Attack? offers a balanced and referenced discussion of coronary risk assessment using modern technology, specifically CT scans to evaluate the health of coronary arteries.

---

memberships and courses

Healthy Heart Network Membership https://healthyheartnetwork.com/page/join
Weight Loss Course https://healthyheartnetwork.com/page/weightloss
Atrial Fibrillation Kit
https://healthyheartnetwork.com/page/atrial-fibrillation-explained-premium-kit

other resources

Heart Attacks are Preventable Webinar
https://healthyheartnetwork.com/page/webinar
How Healthy is Your Heart Really? https://virtualheartcheck.com.au/index
download our free mobile app https://healthyheartnetwork.com/page/mobile
for podcasts, blogs, TV show, TEDx and more https://drwarrickbishop.com

the Healthy Heart Network will become the Healthy Life Network in 2026

---

other resources by **Dr Karam Kostner**

cholesterolcare.com.au

Cholesterol Care Australia
Dr Kostner's specialist cholesterol clinic,
private practice consulting, and
research facility
in the Taylor Medical Centre, Annerley Rd,
Woolloongabba (Brisbane), Australia.
0466 886 904
info@cholesterolcare.com.au
+61 7 37404777 (fax)

Among his other writing, Dr Kostner has published more than 150 peer-reviewed papers, as well as book chapters, review articles and editorials, and delivered numerous invitational lectures.

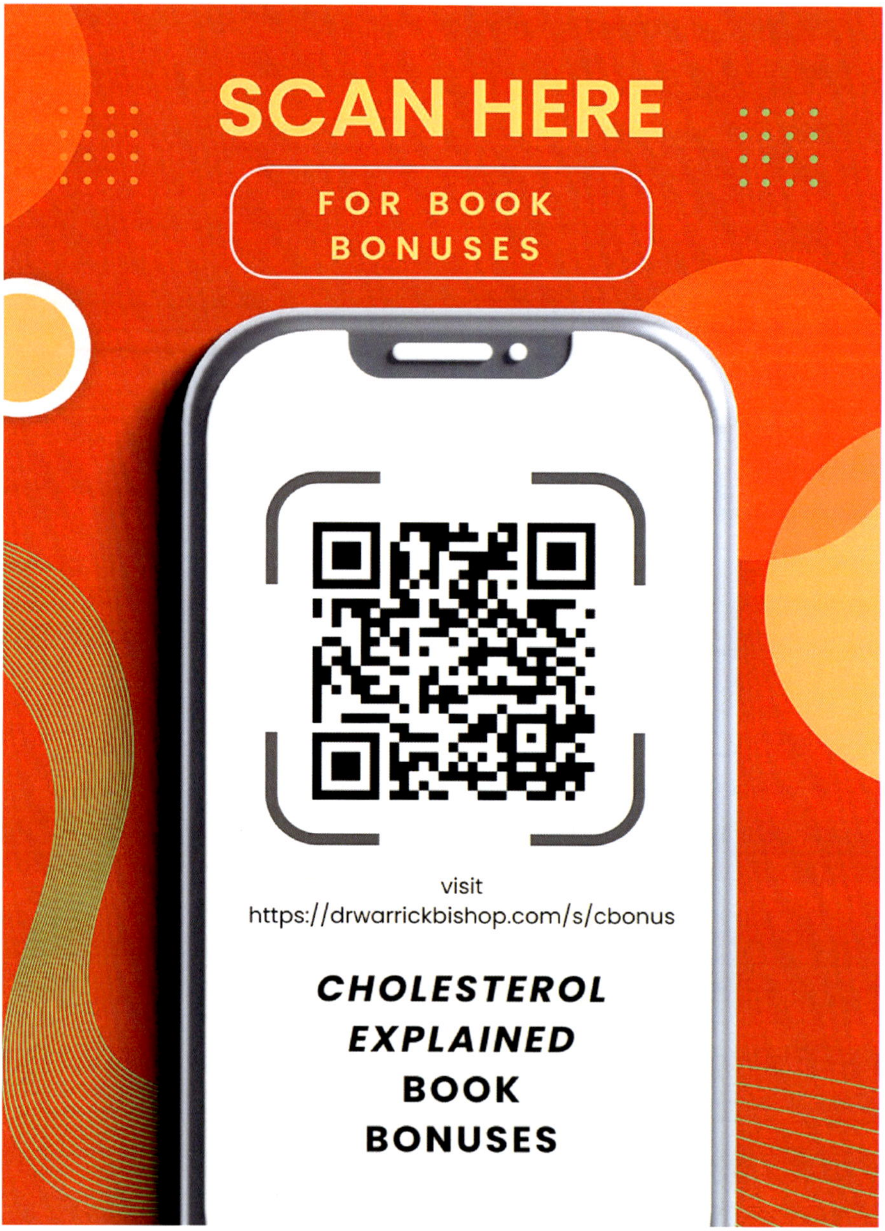
SCAN HERE
FOR BOOK BONUSES
visit
https://drwarrickbishop.com/s/cbonus
CHOLESTEROL EXPLAINED BOOK BONUSES

www.ingramcontent.com/pod-product-compliance
Lightning Source LLC
LaVergne TN
LVRC080205220926
848482LV00007B/337

* 9 7 8 0 9 7 5 6 3 1 0 9 6 *